Neurosurgical Critical Care

VOLUME 1: CONCEPTS IN NEUROSURGERY

Neurosurgical Critical Care

VOLUME 1: CONCEPTS IN NEUROSURGERY

EDITORS

FREMONT P. WIRTH, M.D.

Neurological Institute of Savannah
Director, Neurosurgical and Neurological
Intensive Care Unit
St. Joseph's Hospital
Savannah, Georgia

ROBERT A. RATCHESON, M.D.

Professor and Chief, Division of Neurological Surgery
Case Western Reserve University
University Hospitals of Cleveland
Cleveland, Ohio

ASSOCIATE EDITORS

Robert L. Grubb, Jr., M.D.
Julian T. Hoff, M.D.
Martin H. Weiss, M.D.

sponsored by the
Congress of Neurological Surgeons

WILLIAMS & WILKINS
Baltimore • London • Los Angeles • Sydney

Library of Congress cataloged this serial as follows:

Congress of Neurological Surgeons.
Neurosurgical critical care. (Concepts in neurosurgery: v. 1)

Includes index.
1. Nervous system--Surgery. 2. Critical care medicine. I. Ratcheson, Robert A. II. Wirth, Fremont P. III. Series. [DNLM: 1. Critical Care. 2. Nervous System--surgery. WL 368 N4953]
RD593.N4195 1987 617'.48028 86-13290
ISBN 0-683-07151-3

Accurate indications, adverse reactions, and dosage schedules for drugs are provided in this book, but it is possible that they may change. The reader is urged to review the package information data of the manufacturers of the medications mentioned.

Printed in the United States of America

Printed at the Waverly Press, Inc.

87 88 89 90 91
10 9 8 7 6 5 4 3 2 1

Dedicated to:

PENNY
PEGGY
JULIA
DEBBIE
DIANE

Foreword

The Congress of Neurological Surgeons was founded in 1951 with the prime purposes being to maintain high standards of neurosurgery and to promote continuing education. While the emphasis has been on the needs of the resident in training and the younger neurosurgeon, the programs of the Congress have benefited not only neurosurgery but also the neuroscience fields in general.

To help provide for the continuing education needs of its members, the Congress began publication in 1953 of an annual volume entitled, *Clinical Neurosurgery*, which presents in detail the invited presentations made at the annual meeting of the organization. This volume has become an important reference source for neurosurgeons. Then in 1977, after several years of planning, the Congress began publication of a monthly journal entitled, *Neurosurgery*, which proved to be an outstanding addition to the medical literature.

Now, under the direction of Doctors Fremont P. Wirth and Robert A. Ratcheson, the Congress is embarking on another publication series entitled, *Concepts in Neurosurgery*. The goals of this publication, as proposed by Dr. Ratcheson during his term as President of the Congress, are to provide a monograph that will cover a specific area in depth with basic scientific knowledge and theory applied to practical neurosurgical issues. For the resident in training this publication can supplement the educational program or provide knowledge in an area that might not be covered in depth in a training program. For the trained neurosurgeon, each monograph will provide the opportunity to review recent knowledge about a practical subject and supply up-to-date information in an important area of neurosurgery.

The Congress has selected Doctors Wirth and Ratcheson as editors, two individuals who have been members of the Executive Committee for several years and have recently been officers, who have also had considerable experience with educational programs. They will be aided by associate editors, Doctors Robert L. Grubb, Julian T. Hoff, and Martin H. Weiss, who also have had broad experience with publications and continuing education endeavors.

The Congress is again providing a leadership role in an important area that will benefit all of neurosurgery.

Robert G. Ojemann, M.D.

Preface

The neurosurgical patient often requires intensive management and monitoring. For the critically ill, this care is delivered in an intensive care setting and with increasing frequency it is in a dedicated neurosurgical unit. Many important advances in the practice of neurological surgery, as measured by decreased morbidity and mortality, parallel the development of specialized critical care. Concomitant with these advances is a body of new information of which the neurosurgeon managing these patients must have intimate knowledge in order to effectively carry out his or her responsibilities.

The first volume of this series, *Concepts in Neurosurgery*, addresses Neurosurgical Critical Care. This book is designed to provide neurosurgeons and neurosurgical residents with a compilation of modern concepts of intensive care management and an organized resource for basic information in this complex field. It is intended that this work, and those to follow in this series, will concentrate upon providing basic scientific knowledge and theory and relate this information to practical neurosurgical concerns. The book has not been designed to function as a "how to do it" manual or solely as a reference source. Hopefully, the material covered will enrich the reader's working background enabling the development of a sound basis for action.

The volume has been organized in a systems approach and emphasizes the effect of systems management and its importance for the neurosurgical patient. The sections on respiratory and cardiovascular physiology, fluid and electrolyte balance, metabolism, hematology, infection, and seizure disorders cover topics of which the neurosurgeon must have a sure working knowledge. Attention is also devoted to current concepts of cerebral homeostasis and protection and the evaluation and management of the patient with multiple trauma. In addition, suggestions are provided for the design and organization of the neurosurgical intensive care unit.

The most important aspect of neurosurgical intensive care has not received great attention in this volume. The feature that distinguishes neurosurgical intensive care from that of other highly technical specialties is the unequaled reliance upon clinical observation. In most instances, this observation is the responsibility of the neurosurgical intensive care nurse who represents the cornerstone upon which effective care is based. Although the sophisticated monitoring devices to which we have become accustomed are important, the efforts of the neurosurgical nurse are essential.

By initiating this series, the Congress of Neurological Surgeons is attempting to develop a vehicle to provide neurosurgeons with a foundation in topical pathophysiology and its application to contemporary clinical neurosurgery. The editors believe that in this manner, neurosurgeons will best be able to utilize the growing knowledge and technology available to them, and to effectively serve their patients.

Fremont P. Wirth, M.D.
Robert A. Ratcheson, M.D.

Contributors

EDITORS

Fremont P. Wirth, M.D.
Neurological Institute of Savannah
Director, Neurosurgical and Neurological Intensive Care Unit
St. Joseph's Hospital
Savannah, Georgia

Robert A. Ratcheson, M.D.
Professor and Chief, Division of Neurological Surgery
Case Western Reserve University
University Hospitals of Cleveland
Cleveland, Ohio

ASSOCIATE EDITORS

Robert L. Grubb, Jr., M.D.
Professor of Neurological Surgery
Washington University School of Medicine
St. Louis, Missouri

Julian T. Hoff, M.D.
Professor of Surgery
Head, Section of Neurosurgery
University of Michigan Hospital
Ann Arbor, Michigan

Martin H. Weiss, M.D.
Professor and Chairman
Department of Neurosurgery
LAC/USC Medical Center
Los Angeles, California

CONTRIBUTORS

Daniel L. Barrow, M.D.
Assistant Professor of Surgery
Department of Neurosurgery
Emory University School of Medicine
Atlanta, Georgia

W. Edwin Dodson, M.D.
Associate Professor
Departments of Pediatrics and Neurology
Washington University School of Medicine
St. Louis, Missouri

James A. Ferrendeli, M.D.
Professor of Neurology and Pharmacology
Washington University Medical Center
Barnes Hospital Plaza
St. Louis, Missouri

Fred H. Geisler, M.D., Ph.D.
Associate Professor of Neurological Surgery
University of Maryland
Medical Director of Neurotrauma
Maryland Institute for Emergency Medical Services/Systems (MIEMSS)
Baltimore, Maryland

Martin I. Griffel, M.D.
Assistant Professor
Department of Medicine
The Chicago Medical School
North Chicago, Illinois

Julian T. Hoff, M.D.
Professor of Surgery
Head, Section of Neurosurgery
University of Michigan Hospital
Ann Arbor, Michigan

Howard Kaufman, M.D.
Professor and Chairman
Department of Neurosurgery
West Virginia University Medical Center
Morgantown, West Virginia

Scott Litofsky, M.D.
Department of Neurosurgery
University of Southern California Medical Center
Los Angeles, California

Anthony Marmarou, Ph.D.
Division of Neurological Surgery
Department of Surgery
Medical College of Virginia
Virginia Commonwealth University
Richmond, Virginia

John McGilliguddy, M.D.
Associate Professor of Surgery
Section of Neurosurgery
University of Michigan Medical Center
Ann Arbor, Michigan

Carole A. Miller, M.D.
Associate Professor
Ohio State University Hospitals
410 West 10th Avenue
Columbus, Ohio

Richard J. Moulton, M.D.
Division of Neurological Surgery
Department of Surgery
Medical College of Virginia
Virginia Commonwealth University
Richmond, Virginia

J. Paul Muizelaar, M.D., Ph.D.
Division of Neurological Surgery
Department of Surgery
Medical College of Virginia
Virginia Commonwealth University
Richmond, Virginia

Paul B. Nelson, M.D.
Presbyterian University Hospital
230 Lothrop Street
Pittsburgh, Pennsylvania

Lawrence Pitts, M.D.
Associate Professor of Neurosurgery
Department of Neurological Surgery
University of California
San Francisco, California

Eric C. Rackow, M.D.
Professor and Vice Chairman
Department of Medicine
The Chicago Medical School
North Chicago, Illinois

Bryan J. Rowlands, M.D.
Professor and Head
Department of Surgery
Queens University of Belfast
Belfast, Northern Ireland

Michael Salcman, M.D.
Professor and Head Physician of Neurological Surgery
Director, Neurotrauma
University of Maryland School of Medicine
Baltimore, Maryland

Dennis Schaberg, M.D.
Associate Professor and Associate Chairman
Department of Internal Medicine
Division of Infectious Disease
University of Michigan Medical Center
Ann Arbor, Michigan

Warren Selman, M.D.
Assistant Professor of Neurosurgery
Case Western Reserve University
Cleveland, Ohio

Debra Tillman, R.N.
St. Joseph's Hospital
11705 Mercy Boulevard
Savannah, Georgia

George T. Tindall, M.D.
Professor of Surgery
Chief of Neurosurgery
Emory University Clinic
Atlanta, Georgia

Donald Trunkey, M.D.
Professor of Surgery
University of California
San Francisco, California

Patricia Valenzano, R.N.
St. Joseph's Hospital
11705 Mercy Boulevard
Savannah, Georgia

John Ward, M.D.
Associate Professor of Neurosurgery
Director of Neuroscience Intensive Care
Medical College of Virginia
Richmond, Virginia

Max H. Weil, M.D., Ph.D.
Professor and Chairman
Department of Medicine
Professor of Physiology and Bio-Physics
Chief, Division of Cardiology
University of Health Sciences
Chicago Medical School
North Chicago, Illinois

Fremont P. Wirth, M.D.
Neurological Institute of Savannah
Director, Neurosurgical and Neurological Intensive Care Unit
St. Josephs Hospital
Savannah, Georgia

Contents

CHAPTER 1

Respiratory System: Physiology, Pathophysiology, and Management

FRED H. GEISLER, M.D., PH.D., and
MICHAEL SALCMAN, M.D.

INTRODUCTION

Successful management of cerebral pathology and cerebral edema requires knowledge of the interaction of the central nervous system and the respiratory system. Studies suggest that 25% of all surgical mortalities are primarily related to pulmonary complications and that in another 25% pulmonary complications are a significant contributing factor (88, 160, 199, 278, 279, 291). The morbidity and mortality of pulmonary complications can be reduced by early recognition and subsequent modification of preoperative, intraoperative, and postoperative management (88, 262). The occurrence of preoperative abnormalities in pulmonary function is conditioned by genetic background, obesity, and smoking history (9, 114, 183). These factors are compounded by the normal aging process of lung function (160). Postoperative pulmonary complications occur in 3% of patients with pre-existing chronic obstructive pulmonary disease undergoing surgical operations (9, 157). After general anesthesia, hypoxemia is universally present due to incomplete reversal of muscle relaxants, central respiratory drive depression, increased oxygen consumption from shivering, increased pulmonary shunting, and a decrease in the functional residual capacity. Pulmonary complications are not always associated with respiratory insufficiency but the two are inter-related (108).

Overt respiratory failure occurs in 20% of isolated head-injured patients from hypoxemia, pulmonary edema, abnormalities of respiratory pattern, or aspiration (19, 94). Pulmonary abnormalities on post-mortem examination were present in 85% of isolated head injuries in the Vietnam study (251). Fifty-four percent of the deaths in severely brain-injured patients were associated with pulmonary failure (188). Elective brain tumor surgery in the elderly patient carries a 17.5% postoperative pulmonary complication rate and a 4% mortality from pulmonary complications (272). Pulmonary complications contribute to the morbidity and mortality of a wide variety of neurologic disorders (231). Thus, the respiratory system contributes more mortality and morbidity to neurologic disabled and postoperative patients than any other organ system (19, 88, 210, 249).

RESPIRATORY ANATOMY

The pulmonary system is functionally separated into the upper airway and the lower airway. The nose, nasopharynx, oral pharynx, oral cavity, laryngeal pharynx, and larynx comprise the upper airway. The tracheobronchial tree and the lung parenchyma comprise the lower airway.

The upper airway is the conduit for air passing to the lower airway. Foreign material is removed in the upper airway and thus provides protection for the lower airway. Half of the anatomic dead space in the entire pulmonary circuit is in the upper airway. Inspired air is warmed to body temperature and humidified by passage through the upper airway. The larynx connects the upper and lower airways. The epiglottis closes over the glottic opening in normal swallowing and prevents foreign substances from being aspirated into the lower airway. The tracheobronchial tree is a continually dividing conduit leading to the alveoli. The diameters of the conduit become progressively smaller with distal passage into the lung. The total number of airways of a particular size increases greatly as their size decreases; this results in a tremendous decrease in the effective total airway resistance of the smaller diameter conduits compared to the larger conduits.

The tracheobronchial wall contains three separate layers: an epithelial layer, the lamina propria, and a cartilaginous layer. Pseudostratified columnar ciliated epithelial cells are interposed with mucous and serous secreting glands to comprise the epithelial layer. The lamina propria contains the small blood vessels, lymph channels, nerves, and smooth muscle. The outer cartilaginous layer is a mechanical skeleton that is prominent in air conduits greater than 1 mm in diameter. Bronchioles are small airways that begin at the 9th to 11th branching of airways from the trachea; they are lined with cuboidal epithelial cells and the lamina propria is in direct continuity with the lung parenchyma. The bronchiolar blood supply is derived from the bronchial artery circulation. Bronchiolar diameters are less than 1 mm and airway patency is maintained by the elastic recoil of the surrounding tissues. The diameter of the bronchioles can be altered by spiral muscle bands in the lamina propria.

The lung parenchyma is composed of the respiratory bronchioles, alveolar ducts, alveolar sacs, alveolar epithelium, lung interstitium, and lung endothelium. The alveolar ducts are further subdivisions of the respiratory bronchioles. Fifty percent of the total lung alveoli arise directly from these ducts. The alveolar sacs are the last division of the airways and are blind passages. The alveolar epithelium is 95% covered by type I pneumocytes. These cells are very thin with a large surface area to enhance gas diffusion. The smaller but more numerous cuboidal secretory alveolar cells are the type II pneumocytes. These cells have a high metabolic activity and produce the pulmonary surfactant that is necessary to maintain the alveoli inflated. The lung interstitium contains the lymphatic system along with alveolar septa, smooth muscle, and nerves. The pulmonary capillary endothelium layer normally allows a portion of the serum electrolytes and colloid to enter the interstitium. This normal flow of fluid is greatly enhanced in some pathologic conditions.

The respiratory system has two protective airway mechanisms for removing foreign material: the mucous blanket and the ciliary escalator. A mucous blanket is formed in the tracheobronchial tree by secretion from surface goblet cells. The cilia from the epithelium extend into the mucous layer and provide the motion for moving the mucous blanket towards the larynx at a rate of about 2 cm per minute.

The muscles of ventilation are separated into three major groups: the diaphragm, the intercostal muscles, and the accessory muscles. The diaphragm is innervated predominately by the fourth cervical nerve root with some contributions from the third and fifth roots. The intercostal muscles are innervated by nerves leaving the spinal cord between T_1 and T_{11}. Although these muscles are capable of providing adequate ventilation when the diaphragm is not functional and aid in forced inspiration and expiration, they do not participate in normal resting inspiration. The accessory muscles comprise the scalene, sternocleidomastoid, and trapezius muscles. They are not used during normal resting respiration.

Inspiration is an active process dominated by the diaphragm in normal breathing. Although expiration during quiet breathing is a passive process of the chest, during active breathing—such as after exercise—the external oblique, rectus abdominus, internal oblique, and transversus abdominus muscles also participate in expiration. The nerves for the expiratory muscles leave the spinal cord between T_6 and L_1.

The autonomic nervous system also innervates the pulmonary tree. The sympathetic alpha response causes arteriolar smooth muscle constriction with a subsequent increase in pulmonary vascular resistance; beta-2 response results in bronchodilation (49, 119, 241, 288).

THE NORMAL CONTROL OF BREATHING

Arterial levels of oxygen and carbon dioxide are kept within tight tolerances despite variations in the metabolic rate through adjustment of alveolar ventilation (137). Control of the respiratory system, which enables it to perform this function, is dependent upon peripheral sensors, central controlling neurons, and effectors. The central controller for the automatic process of breathing resides in the lower brainstem but voluntary control directed by the cortex can modulate these centers. Voluntary hyperventilation can drop the Pa_{CO_2} to 20 torr and produce an arterial pH of 7.6. However, through voluntary hypoventilation it is not possible to effect such a broad range of physiologic values. Voluntary breath-holding not only increases arterial Pa_{CO_2} but also decreases arterial Pa_{O_2} such that the respiratory drive of hypoxia limits breath holding.

Three main groups of neurons participate in the respiratory cycle and are located in the medulla, lower pons, and upper pons (24, 288). The primary respiratory center is a diffuse collection of neurons in the reticular formation of the medulla. Inspiration is associated with a group of dorsal neurons whereas expiration is associated with a group of ventral neurons. The inspiratory area contains intrinsic periodic neurons believed to be the origin for the basic rhythm of ventilation. The firing rate of the inspiratory area is inhibited by impulses from the pneumotaxic center in the upper pons. Dysfunction of this pneumotaxic center decreases inhibition of the inspiratory area of the medulla and increases the breathing rate. The inspiratory cells in the reticular formation of the medulla lie close to the tractus solitarius and are modulated by inputs from the vagal and glossopharyngeal nerves. The expiratory area in the medulla is inactive during the breathing cycle, since normal expiration is a passive relaxation of the chest wall. During exercise when forceful breathing is needed for the greater movement of air, the expiratory cells assume activity during the expiratory phase.

In the lower pons an apneustic center has been identified in animals and lesions there produce prolonged inspiratory gasps. This area apparently sends excitatory information to the inspiratory area in the medulla. The pneumotaxic center in the upper pons helps determine the respiratory rate by making fine adjustments to the normal rhythm.

The effectors concerned with the regulation of respiration include the diaphragm, intercostal muscles, abdominal muscles, and accessory muscles. These muscles act in a co-ordinated fashion during the normal respiratory cycle.

Chemical sensors sensitive to changes in the arterial concentrations of oxygen and carbon dioxide are located within the central nervous system and peripherally. The central control of ventilation is determined by chemoreceptors near the ventral surface of the medulla; these are bathed in extracellular fluid in direct contact with the cerebrospinal fluid (CSF). Although the blood-brain barrier is impermeable to hydrogen and bicarbonate ions, molecular CO_2 readily diffuses across the barrier. When the CO_2 concentration in the blood rises and diffuses into the CSF, hydrogen ions are liberated, the pH is depressed, and the chemoreceptors are stimulated.

The peripheral chemoreceptors are located in the common carotid arteries and in the aortic bodies above and below the aortic arch. They respond to a decrease in arterial Pa_{O_2} and pH or an increase in arterial Pa_{CO_2}. Responsiveness to Pa_{O_2} is nonlinear with a rapid rise in firing rate below 100 torr and a peak intensity of discharge near 50 torr. The peripheral receptor response to changes in arterial concentrations of gases and pH is rapid.

Pulmonary receptors also participate in the regulation of ventilation. Lung distention is assessed by pulmonary stretch receptors in the smooth muscles of the airways that are maximally active during inflation. The neural impulses are transmitted centrally in the vagus nerve by large myelinated fibers. The Hering-Breuer inflation reflex is operated via these stretch receptors and involves the slowing of the respiratory rate together with an increase in the expiratory duration. These receptors also contribute to a negative feedback mechanism in which inflation of the lungs inhibits further inspiratory muscle activity and in which deflation excites inspiratory activity.

A second group of receptors is located between the airway epithelial cells and responds to irritants. The impulses travel up the vagus nerve and have reflexive actions that include bronchoconstriction and hyperpnea. A third type of receptor is called the juxtacapillary receptor and is located in the alveolar wall close to capillaries. Its impulses also pass up the vagus nerve and reflex action produces rapid shallow breathing that can progress to apnea. Evidence suggests that increased interstitial fluid volume in the alveolar walls may activate these receptors and play a role in dyspnea.

The overall purpose of the multiple components that control normal ventilation is to regulate arterial Pa_{CO_2}, Pa_{O_2}, and pH in response to changes in metabolic demand. These interactions are nonlinear, interrelated, and augmented by various acute and chronic pulmonary diseases. The normal control of respiration is dominated by sensitivity to Pa_{CO_2} except in advanced chronic obstructive pulmonary disease where it can be dominated by sensitivity to oxygen (24, 93, 137, 140, 288).

ABNORMAL BREATHING PATTERNS FOLLOWING NEUROLOGIC INJURY

Dysfunction of central nervous system structures can result in abnormal respiratory patterns (144). Plum and Posner (209) have categorized these abnormalities and correlated them with the anatomical locations of particular lesions. Other workers have reported abnormalities in respiratory changes secondary to unilateral brainstem infarctions (92, 161).

Cheyne-Stokes respiration, although commonly seen in chronic pulmonary disease, is also associated with bilateral dysfunction of the cerebral hemisphere or of the basal ganglia projections to the brainstem. It is categorized by a periodic breathing pattern of several minutes duration in which hyperpnea alternates with apnea in a decrescendo/crescendo cycle. This pattern is often an early indication of an expanding supratentorial mass and increased intracranial pressure. The cyclic pattern of Cheyne-Stokes respirations results from an increased ventilatory response to carbon dioxide. This results in overbreathing with a decrease in Pa_{CO_2} to a level that produces apnea. Once apnea occurs, carbon dioxide reaccumulates until it exceeds the respiratory threshold and the cycle repeats. When clear periods of apnea are present, patients are usually in coma and the mortality rate exceeds 50%. When a cyclic variation occurs without an apnea phase, the cerebral lesions are usually unilateral, the patient is arousable, and the prognosis for survival is good.

Central neurogenic hyperventilation results from dysfunction within the pons. It is categorized by a pattern of rapid, deep, sustained hyperventilation and severe respiratory alkalosis. Tissue hypoxia results from the leftward shift of the hemoglobin dissociation curve due to alkalosis and the increase in oxygen demand resulting from the tremendous increase in the work of breathing. This respiratory pattern is seen with midbrain compression secondary to transtentorial herniation. The associated mortality rate is high and patients are usually unresponsive and posturing (164, 200).

Irregular cluster breathing and apneustic periods may accompany extensor posturing. Chaotic or ataxic breathing consists of inspiratory and expiratory phases that are irregular in both timing and volume. Variable periods of apnea may be interposed and the outcome for these patients is usually fatal. Ataxic breathing is a sign of medullary failure (19, 92, 137, 209).

PULMONARY SYSTEM EVALUATION

Pulmonary pathology is investigated with four types of tests: roentgenographic, pulmonary function, arterial blood gas, and biopsy/culture. The chest x-ray most commonly obtained in critically ill patients in the intensive care unit is a portable anteroposterior (AP) film. This study along with lateral or decubitus chest x-rays, pulmonary fluoroscopy, and pulmonary ultrasonography can be performed with portable equipment. Other studies for investigation of pulmonary pathology, such as ventilation perfusion lung scans, pulmonary angiograms, and standard posteroanterior (PA) chest x-rays, require transportation of the patient to a radiologic suite. Portable AP films of the chest are obtained on a daily basis in all intubated patients (106, 304). Forty-three percent of daily chest films in intensive care patients demonstrate an abnormality important to clinical management (111). Since portable AP films are often taken in the supine position, they overestimate the size of the heart and mediastinal structures. Futhermore, the vessels of the upper lobe routinely distend in the supine position so that they cannot be used to indicate passive congestion within the lungs. When a lateral chest film is taken in addition to the AP chest film, the diagnosis of pleural effusion, lobar atelectasis, pericardial effusion, and sternal fracture is enhanced. The lateral chest film also localizes the position of various tubes and lines in the thorax. Portable fluoroscopy is useful during the insertion of pulmonary arterial lines and pacemaker electrodes. When phrenic nerve dysfunction is suspected, the motion of the diaphragm can also be assessed. Portable ultrasonography is useful in detecting the difference between pleural and subphrenic fluid. When thoracentesis is required in a patient on positive pressure ventilation, the needle is guided with ultrasound as the safest method to prevent an iatrogenic pneumothorax. Ventilation/perfusion lung scans evaluate pulmonary blood flow and ventilation in patients suspected of pulmonary embolism (179). Selective pulmonary arteriography follows the ventilation/perfusion scan to investigate regions of abnormality (40). In post-traumatic patients, mediastinal widening on the chest x-ray is investigated by an aortogram to look for an aortic dissection.

Endotracheal tubes are easily visualized on the chest x-ray and their location is assessed immediately after insertion and on a daily basis (106, 304). The ideal location for the tip of the endotracheal tube is 5 to 7 cm from the primary carina or midway between the carina and the vocal cords. In patients with a tracheostomy the chest x-ray verifies the position of the tube to be half the distance from the stoma to the carina. The tracheostomy tube should be approximately two thirds the width of the trachea and positioned parallel to its long axis. The appearance of air in the subcutaneous tissues of the neck or mediastinum indicates a problem at the tracheostomy site. Central lines are checked to verify correct position and absence of pneumothorax. The central venous catheter should be above the right atrium. The correct position for the tip of the Swan-Ganz pulmonary artery catheter is below the level of the left atrium for accurate measurements (242). Nasogastric tubes should be in the stomach and not coiled in the esophagus or inadvertently placed in the trachea. In patients with a chest tube, position of the tube combined with the amount of drainage and the purpose of insertion determines whether a second chest tube is to be placed and when chest tubes are to be removed.

Positive pressure mechanical ventilation can produce dramatic changes in the appearance of the pulmonary fields (304). When positive pressure ventilation is instituted, especially with positive end-expiratory pressure (PEEP), infiltrates appear to vanish in many areas of the pulmonary parenchyma secondary to the increased aeration. The reverse can occur during the weaning process or the removal of PEEP. Complications of mechanical ventilation occur in 5 to 10% of critically ill patients and include: pneumomediastinum, subcutaneous emphysema, and pneumothorax. Pleural effusions can be detected on an erect AP film or on a lateral film as a ground-glass hazy density. The presence of a pleural effusion can limit lung expansion and removal of the fluid can increase respiratory function. A pneumothorax is diagnosed when the lung parenchyma does not fill the chest cavity. Pneumomediastinum or subcutaneous air in the neck can arise from a ruptured esophagus or traumatic rupture of the bronchus, but most commonly arises from spontaneous barotrauma in a ventilated patient. A clinically significant pneumothorax is searched for in any patient with pneumomediastinum or subcutaneous air. Pulmonary embolism does not cause any characteristic sign on routine chest roentgenograph, although a majority of studies contain some abnormality such as an elevated hemidiaphragm, plate-like atelectasis, pleural effusion, or consolidation. When any of these signs appear in conjunction with clinical signs suggesting a deep venous thrombophlebitis or pulmonary embolism, a nuclear ventilation/perfusion scan is indicated. Parenchymal infiltrates are seen in aspiration pneumonia, bacterial pneumonia, and traumatic pulmonary contusions. They can exist as patchy or diffuse infiltrates or involve a segment or lobe in consolidation. Parenchymal infiltrates due to congestive heart failure are gravity dependent and change position with a change in the patient's position; the location of an inflammatory infiltrate remains stationary (162).

Ventilatory mechanics are assessed in awake and co-operative patients by measurement of the lung volumes and gas flow rate on forced expiration with spirometry (10, 87). Figure 1.1 diagrammatically presents the subdivisions of the lung volume along with a representative tracing from a spirometer. The total lung capacity (TLC) is the gas volume in the lungs and conducting airways at maximum inspiration. The vital capacity (VC) is the maximum volume of gas that can then be exhaled. When maximal exhalation force is used to empty the lungs, the amount of air exhaled is the forced vital capacity (FVC) and the volume expired in the first second is termed FEV_1. The volume of gas remaining after maximal expiration is the

Subdivisions of Total Lung Capacity

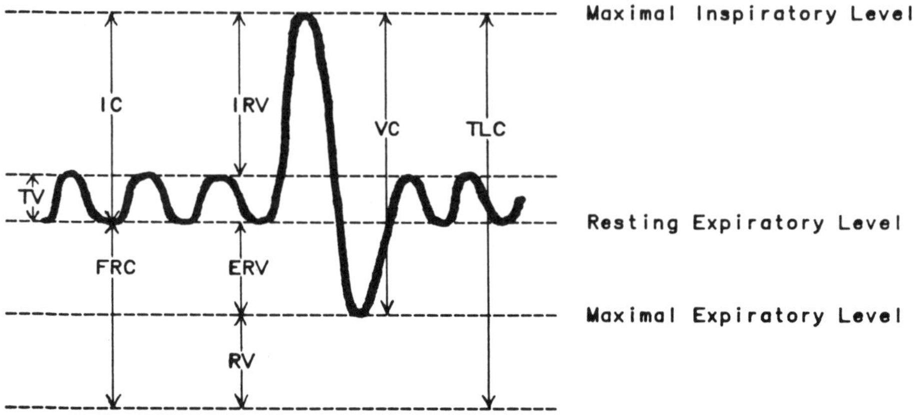

Figure 1.1. Diagram representation of the subdivision of lung volume with a typical spirometry tracing superimposed. See text for definitions of abbreviations.

residual volume (RV). The tidal volume (TV) is the volume of gas inhaled during a normal breath at rest. The functional residual capacity (FRC) is the lung volume remaining at the end of normal tidal volume expiration. The inspiratory capacity (IC), inspiratory reserve volume (IRV), and the expiratory reserve volume (ERV) are geographically defined in Figure 1.1 The ratio of FEV_1 and FVC is a sensitive indicator of pulmonary obstructive pathology in the large airways as it decreases early in disease. In contrast, restrictive disease reduces both FEV_1 and FVC proportionally without affecting the ratio.

The lung volumes in restrictive disease typically have a normal RV with a mild reduction in FRC and TLC. Etiology of restrictive disease includes: chest wall abnormalities from kyphoscoliosis or obesity; neuromuscular disorders such as myasthenia gravis, Guillain-Barré syndrome, muscular dystrophy, cervical cord injury, or phrenic nerve injury; pleural diseases including pneumothorax and pleural effusion; abdominal masses; pulmonary parenchymal lesions including sarcoidosis, interstitial fibrosis, pulmonary edema, and local fibrosis; and pain during the forced expiration.

Obstructive disease in the large airways is caused by asthma, chronic bronchitis, emphysema, and bronchiectasis. RV and FRC are typically elevated with a normal TLC. The FVC is near normal but the FEV_1 is markedly decreased so that the FEV_1/FCV ratio is lowered. When the obstructive disease becomes severe the RV is greatly elevated and the expiratory flow rate can be so slow that the patient cannot complete the expiration from maximum inspiration and must stop exhaling to take a new breath. The FEV_1/FVC ratio in these patients is extremely low.

Combined obstructive and restrictive pulmonary disease is seen with sarcoidosis, chronic bronchitis, emphysema, and pneumonectomy. A low FEV_1/FVC ratio with FEV_1 reduced more than the reduction of FVC is typical (2, 10, 87).

Normal values for pulmonary function tests along with limits that have been associated with poor surgical risk are presented in Table 1.1. The comparison of pulmonary tests with control values requires taking into account the gender, height, and age correction factors (10, 87, 147, 167, 287).

TABLE 1.1.
Pulmonary Function Tests

	Normals		Poor Surgical Risk
	Females	Males	
FVC (liters)	4.28	5.80	
FEV_1 (liters)	3.68	4.54	< 1
FEV_1/FVC (%)	> 75	> 75	< 50

Spirometry requires an awake co-operative patient. To obtain an assessment of pulmonary function in comatose or paralyzed individuals, a computer-based evaluation of cardiopulmonary function based on flow and pressure signals at the endotracheal tube is useful (26). The volume of gas inspired or expired is obtained by integrating the gas flow electronically or with computer software. The Siemens-Elema 900B and 900C servoventilators (Siemens Corp., Union, N.J.) electronically measure the airway pressure and flow so that no extra respiratory monitoring equipment is needed in the airway tubing circuit. An example of flow-volume-pressure waveform generated with this analysis and the measurement of pulmonary compliance with this procedure is presented in Figure 1.2 (250). Special pulmonary function tests include measuring the FRC by using a helium tracer in a washout curve and tests for the uniformity of ventilation by using multiple inert gases or an analysis of the N_2 washout curve (99, 100, 101). The production of carbon dioxide and the consumption of oxygen are calculated by the Fick principle and are used to estimate the metabolic rate and respiratory coefficient (137, 287, 288).

The minute ventilation is the total amount of air inspired in a 1-minute period. This parameter is important in the evaluation of a patient during weaning from ventilatory support. Normal minute ventilation in adults is 5 to 8 liters per minute. A large increase over this normal value indicates an inability of the patient to successfully wean and the presence of pulmonary dysfunction such as: increased dead space, increased CO_2 production, or a large pulmonary work load.

The dead-space fraction (DSF) is the fraction of tidal volume that ventilates non-air-exchange areas in the lung. The non-air-exchange areas include the large airways and the pharynx. Carbon dioxide is not normally present in the inspired air and is not exchanged in the anatomic dead space. Thus, the DSF can be approximated by the Bohr equation:

$$\frac{V_D}{V_T} = \frac{Pa_{CO_2} - PE_{CO_2}}{Pa_{CO_2}} \qquad \text{(eq. 1)}$$

where V_D is the physiologic dead space volume, V_T is the tidal volume, Pa_{CO_2} is the arterial CO_2 partial pressure, and PE_{CO_2} is the average mixed expired CO_2 partial pressure (288). This ratio is typically less than 0.4. In patients with a ratio greater than 0.6 mechanical ventilation is almost universally required. Negative inspiratory pressure (NIP) is measured by occluding the airway with a pressure sensor. Spontaneous breathing requires a pressure more negative than 20 cm of water to inspire a vital capacity large enough to sustain normal respiration, coughing, and sighing.

The arterial blood gas evaluates both respiratory and metabolic disorders. Respiratory failure is usually defined on arterial blood gas analysis by an oxygen pressure of less than 50 torr or a carbon dioxide pressure of greater than 50 torr. The transport of carbon dioxide is the major buffer in the blood and determines the acid-base status of the body.

The arterial blood sample is obtained from an artery by direct puncture or through an arterial pressure monitoring line. The radial artery is easily palpated in the wrist and is the site most commonly used for direct puncture. The sample is collected in a glass or a specifically designed plastic syringe that allows the arterial blood to pump itself into the syringe when the needle enters the artery. The needle and syringe are first coated with sodium heparin solution to prevent clotting of the blood sample. Any air bubbles in the syringe are expelled and the blood sample is rolled between the sampler's hands for 20 seconds to mix the blood and heparin. The capped sample is placed on ice and sent to the laboratory for prompt analysis. Errors in values of arterial blood gas samples can occur when suction is applied to the syringe allowing air bubbles or venous blood to enter the sample; an excess amount of heparin is left in the syringe reducing the measured carbon dioxide level; a delay exists in analyzing the uncooled sample resulting in a fall in the pH and Po_2 and rise in the Pco_2 from metabolism of the red cells of the sample; and sampling a vein instead of an artery. When an arterial blood gas value does not correlate with the clinical situation it should be immediately repeated (240).

The oxygen in the arterial blood is carried both dissolved in plasma and bound to hemoglobin. The bound oxygen accounts for 98.5% of the content in the blood. The hemoglobin dissociation curve describes the content of oxygen at different levels of oxygen partial pres-

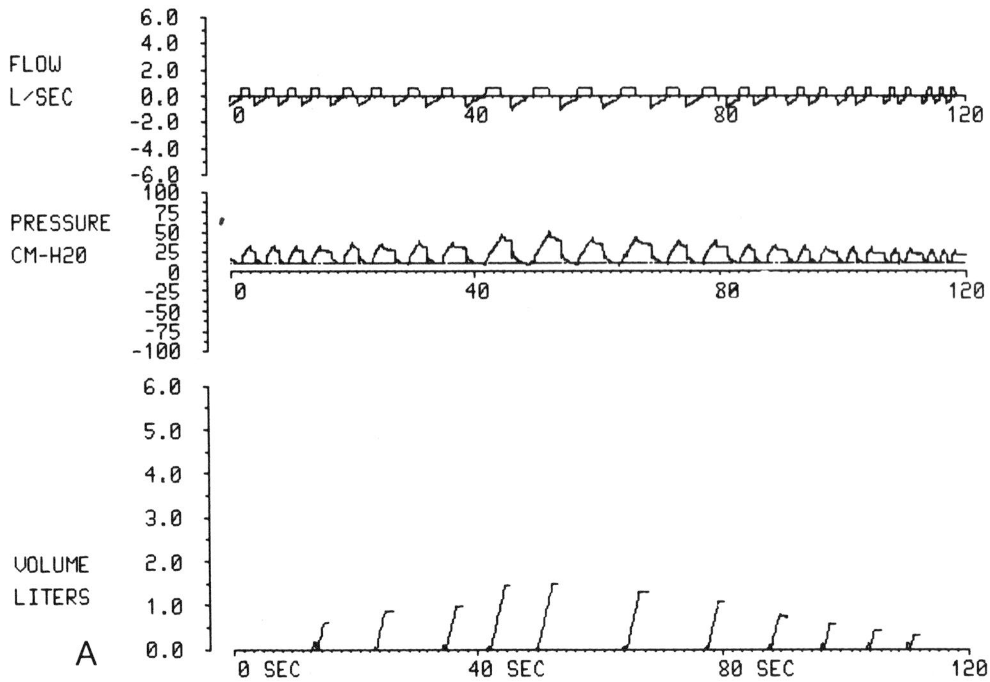

Figure 1.2. Respirator flow-pressure calculation of pulmonary compliance. *A)* The airway flow and pressure are measured at the endotracheal tube. The volume is estimated by numerical integration of the flow on a breath by breath basis with interactive computer analysis. The inspired volume is varied after each breath while maintaining a constant maximum flow rate by altering the effective breathing rate on the Siemens-Elema 900C Servo ventilator. *B)* A single breath of the current tidal volume is selected for flow-pressure-volume two- and three-dimensional analysis. *C)* A dynamic compliance curve derived from the different inspired volumes and plateau pressures of *A* with a calculated effective PEEP of 13.6 cm H_2O and a dynamic compliance of 0.0536 liter/cm H_2O. Representative compliance curves of early ARDS and chronic fibrous ARDS are also presented for comparison.

sure. The curve rises rapidly between O_2 partial pressure of 15 to 50 torr and is relatively constant at high partial pressures of oxygen (80 to 600 torr). The shape of the dissociation curve has several physiologic consequences: if the alveolar oxygen partial pressure is reduced, the blood continues to be saturated; the peripheral tissues can withdraw a large amount of oxygen with only a small drop in oxygen partial pressure thereby enhancing tissue oxygenation; and the plateau in the dissociation curve at high oxygen partial pressures prevents correcting right-to-left pulmonary shunts with increases in the inspired oxygen fraction and resultant higher alveolar oxygen partial pressure. The oxygen dissociation curve is shifted to the right by decreased pH, rise in partial pressure of carbon dioxide, rise in temperature, and increase in 2,3-diphosphoglycerate. The shift in the dissociation curve is assessed by measuring the pressure of oxygen required to reach 50% saturation (P_{50}). The normal P_{50} is 27 torr (33, 49, 57, 119, 137, 225, 287, 288).

Carbon dioxide is carried in the blood dissolved in plasma, as bicarbonate, and combined with protein in carbamino compounds. They account for 10%, 60%, and 30%, respectively, of the transport of carbon dioxide expired by the lungs. The dissociation curve for carbon dioxide is more linear than that for oxygen. The concentrations of oxygen and carbon dioxide modulate the dissociation curve of each other. The transport system for carbon dioxide is the main controller of the acid-base status in the body. The lung excretes the equivalent of 10,000 mEq of carbonic acid per day and the kidneys excrete 100 mEq of fixed acids per day. The acid-base status can be altered acutely by variations in the elimination of carbon dioxide through changes in the alveolar ventilation and chronically by differences in renal function. The acid-base status is described

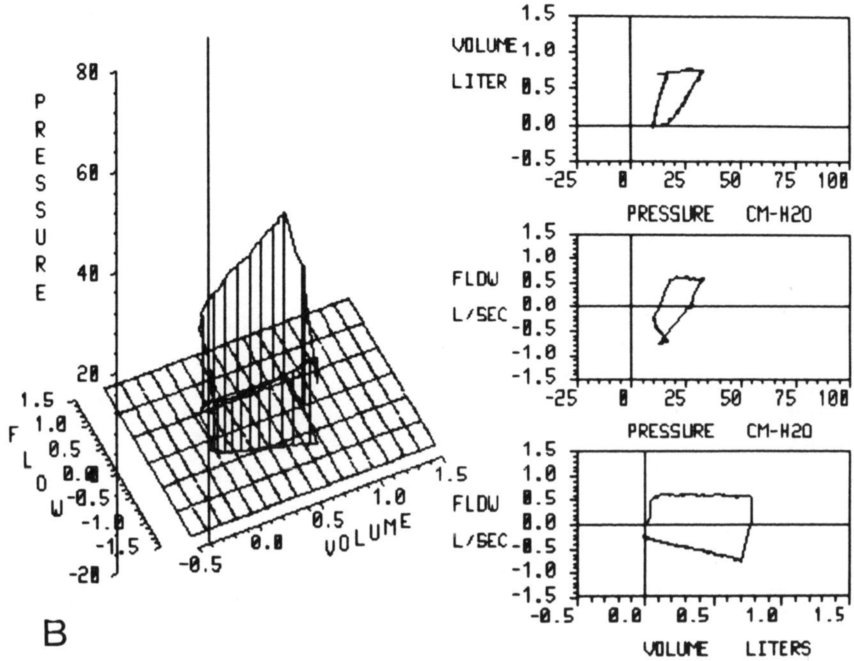

B

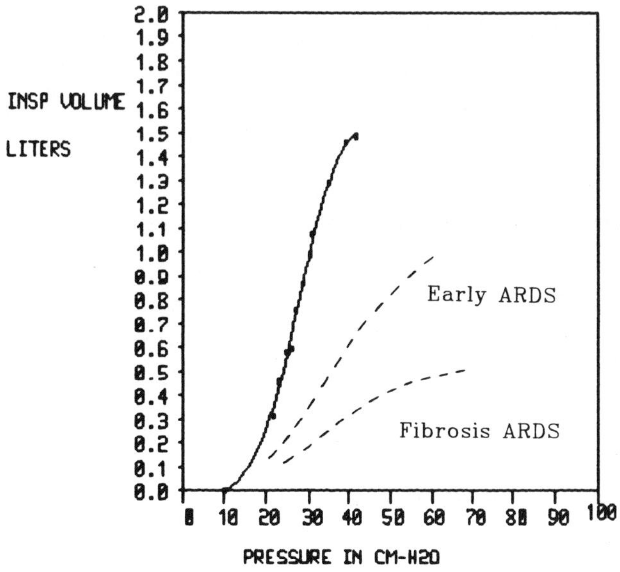

C

Figure 1.2 *B* and 1.2 *C*.

by three parameters: the largest component of the abnormality as respiratory or metabolic, the acid-base status relative to normal, and the degree of compensation which usually is to normalize the pH. It is clinically useful to plot and follow the acid-base status on a graphical inter-relationship of pH, Pco_2 and HCO_3^-. Figure 1.3 is such an inter-relationship and Table 1.2 defines the definitions of the acid-base regions in the figure. Detailed acid-base management of clinical problems and the corresponding pathophysiology is beyond the scope of this chapter and is covered in the references. Normal blood gas values are pH 7.35 to 7.45, Pco_2 36 to 44 torr, and Po_2 70 to 100 torr with the patient breathing room air (49, 57, 119, 137, 148, 226, 240, 247, 276, 287, 288).

The exact diagnosis of pulmonary dysfunction may require the collection of specimens or obtaining biopsies of tissues. Sputum examination is necessary for the diagnosis of pulmonary infections and is obtained by nasotracheal suction. The fiberoptic bronchoscope is useful in clearing the large airway of major aspirations and for obtaining cultures when nasotracheal cultures do not yield a specific organism. In some patients with large pleural effusions, thoracentesis is necessary for both diagnosis and improving mechanical pulmonary function (241).

AIRWAY MAINTENANCE IN PATIENTS WITH DEPRESSED LEVEL OF CONSCIOUSNESS

Obtunded or comatose patients require special airway and respiratory management (134). Regardless of the cause of a depressed level of consciousness, patients without airway protective mechanisms are subject to large airway obstruction, decreased lung inflation, hypoxia, and hypercarbia. The assessment and mainte-

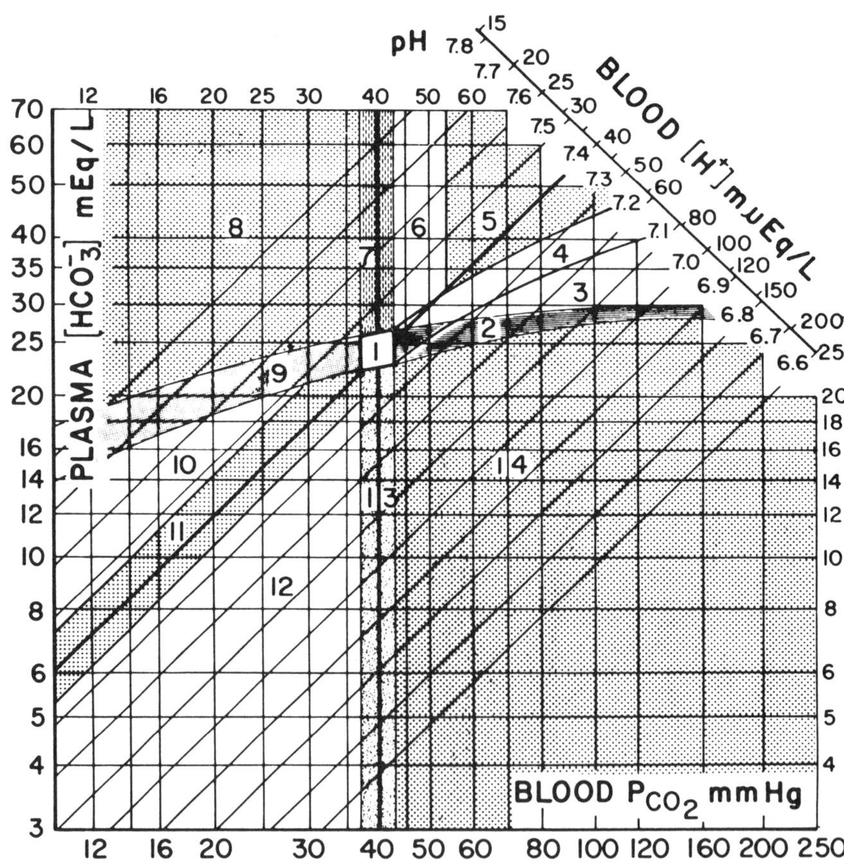

Figure 1.3. Graphical inter-relationship of pH, Pco_2 and HCO_3^- used to determine acid-base status.

TABLE 1.2.
Acid-Base Regions of Arterial Blood Gases

1) Normal
2) Respiratory acidosis
3) Respiratory acidosis—partially compensated
4) Respiratory acidosis—compensated
5) Respiratory acidosis and metabolic alkalosis (mixed)
6) Metabolic alkalosis—compensated
7) Metabolic alkalosis
8) Respiratory alkalosis and metabolic alkalosis (mixed)
9) Respiratory alkalosis
10) Respiratory alkalosis—compensated
11) Metabolic acidosis and respiratory alkalosis (mixed)
12) Metabolic acidosis—compensated
13) Metabolic acidosis
14) Metabolic acidosis and respiratory acidosis (mixed)

nance of the airway is the first and most important step in patient resuscitation and management.

Upper airway obstruction results from pharyngeal soft tissue displacement or damage or from laryngeal obstruction. The most common site of upper airway obstruction with decreased level of consciousness is in the pharynx. Functional patency of the upper airway is lost secondary to decreased motor tone and posterior displacement of pharyngeal soft tissues. This posterior displacement results from the combined effect of gravity in the supine position and the intrinsic elastic forces of the tissues. Trauma patients may additionally have local edema or hemorrhage in the region of the pharynx contributing to airway compromise. The upper airway can also be obstructed by vomitus, false teeth, or foreign bodies. Functional patency between the base of the tongue and the posterior wall of the pharynx is absent in all of these types of upper airway obstruction. In partial upper airway obstruction, the inspiration is noisy and has a snoring quality. When obstruction is complete there may be markedly ineffective inspiratory efforts with clinical signs of sternal retraction, intercostal spasm, and epigastric retraction. In conscious patients, the obstructed respiratory distress of upper airway obstruction produces an extreme anxious state. In unconscious patients, spasmodic efforts at ventilation can be misinterpreted as posturing or seizures.

The proper ventilation of an obtunded or comatose patient can be the single most important lifesaving manuever in his management. Pharyngeal soft tissue obstruction can be relieved with extension of the neck and elevation of the chin. Placing the patient in the lateral position with the neck extended permits gravity to aid in moving the base of the tongue forward. Visual inspection and palpation of the mouth are performed to search for foreign body obstruction. Since head-injured patients have a 5% incidence of cervical spine fracture, the head is maintained in neutral position while using the jaw thrust manuever until the cervical spine has been evaluated by a lateral x-ray (48).

Oropharyngal and nasopharyngal airways are useful in deeply lethargic patients who do not require artificial ventilation. The oropharyngeal airway is inserted so the distal end lies between the posterior pharynx and the base of the tongue. Lateral grooves maintain a patent airway past the potential occlusion of the tongue base and the posterior pharyngeal wall. Catheter suction of the pharynx can be easily accomplished with an oropharyngeal airway in place. This airway is frequently not tolerated by conscious patients because it activates the gag reflex, which produces gagging, vomiting, and even laryngospasm. The oral pharyngeal airway can also help prevent airway occlusion in unconscious patients with an endotracheal tube due to chewing or biting motions (241).

A nasal pharyngeal airway is adequate in many lethargic or obtunded patients. It is constructed from a flanged soft rubber tube with a gentle curve. This design allows insertion through one of the nares with the airway following the curvature of the posterior wall in the nasal and oral pharynx. The tip of the nasal pharyngeal airway is between the base of the tongue and the posterior wall of the pharynx and hence prevents posterior displacement of the pharyngeal structures. This airway is usually well tolerated in both lethargic and awake patients. Suctioning of the pharynx is possible through a nasal pharyngeal airway (241).

All posturing neurosurgical patients and head-injured patients with an initial Glasgow Coma Score of 7 or less usually require endotracheal intubation. Transtracheal intubation corrects any airway obstruction, provides protection of the airway from aspiration, aids in tracheal suctioning, and is required for positive pressure artificial respiration. A nasal or an oral endotracheal tube can almost always be safely passed, and only rarely is an emergency tracheostomy necessary to secure an airway. Tracheostomy may be required in head trauma patients in the presence of massive facial trauma or a fractured larynx. The choice between nasal and oral endotracheal intubation is determined by the experience of the person placing the tube and the speed required for tube placement. Although it is faster to insert an oral tube, some extension of the neck is usually required. In trauma patients with a potentially unstable cervical fracture, the insertion of a nasal tube without neck movement is a safer alternative. Nasal tracheal tubes need to be removed within a few days or sinusitis is a predictable complication (67).

A transtracheal airway relieves all types of upper airway obstruction by bypassing them. The cuff on the transtracheal tube seals the lower airway from the pharynx and decreases the incidence of aspiration of gastric contents, oral secretion, and foreign bodies. This protective role is normally provided by the pharynx, vocal cords, and epiglottis, but this reflexive action is impaired in patients who are obtunded or comatose.

The protective airway reflexes can be separated into four types: the pharyngeal, the laryngeal, the tracheal, and the carinal. The pharyngeal reflex is composed of the gag and swallowing reflexes. The afferent limb of the reflex is in the glossopharyngeal nerve and the efferent limb in the vagus nerve. The laryngeal reflex is vagovagal and produces opposition of the vocal cords and closure of the glottis with laryngeal stimulation. The tracheal reflex is also vagovagal and produces coughing on irritation of the tracheal mucosa. The carinal reflex is another vagovagal response that initiates coughing upon irritation in the region of the carina. The tracheal and carinal reflexes are responsible for the coughing observed in intubated comatose patients during suction.

The protective airway reflexes are lost in a predictable manner with depression of the level of consciousness. First the pharyngeal reflex is lost, then the laryngeal, and finally the tracheal reflex. It is unusual for even posturing patients in coma to have lost the carinal reflex. A patient with a clinical diagnoses of brain death has lost all brainstem reflexes, including all protective airway reflexes. Patients recovering from coma regain their protective airway reflexes in the reverse order in which they were lost. Thus, the first to be lost, the pharyngeal is the last to return. During recovery, patients often have strong carinal, tracheal, and laryngeal reflexes; however, extubation or feeding may not be safe because the pharyngeal reflex has not returned and pulmonary aspiration can still occur (137, 241, 287, 288).

Most severely head-injured patients and many of the moderately injured with traumatic pulmonary complications require endotracheal intubation for longer than 2 weeks. The oral tracheal tube in these patients should be changed electively to a tracheostomy tube since it is more comfortable for the patient and eliminates laryngeal damage secondary to relative tube motion. Patients who wake up in a combative or agitated state are especially prone to such damage. At our Institute, no difference in laryngeal damage was found in rigid or posturing head-injured patients who receive an early tracheostomy at 3 to 4 days or a delayed tracheostomy at 2 weeks (78). Early tracheostomy in head-injured patients carries the potential risks of transporting a critically ill patient and being unable to elevate the head for treatment of intracranial pressure during the procedure. Similarly, a rise in arterial carbon dioxide is associated with the insertion of the tracheostomy tube and subsequent suctioning may cause an increase in the intracranial pressure when brain compliance is low. For these reasons, it is preferable to delay tracheostomy for 2 weeks until the patient is past the initial stage of critical swelling. In stroke, aneurysm, and brain tumor patients requiring ventilatory support beyond 2 weeks a tracheostomy is advised.

When endotracheal intubation is unsuccessful or impossible and an emergency surgical entrance to the trachea is required, the procedure of choice is a cricothyroidotomy. Cricothyroidotomy is safer to perform under emergency circumstances than a tracheostomy since the surgical landmarks are easier to locate and no major vessels cross directly beneath the incision. The latter is located directly below the thyroid cartilage and by using a transverse incision for the cricothyroidotomy, a clean surgical site for a subsequent tracheostomy has been protected. Emergency cricothyroidotomy has two major limitations as a long-term airway: the entrance for the transtracheal tube is located close to the vocal cords and the procedure is usually carried out under less than optimal conditions of sterility. Thus, an emergency cricothyroidotomy should be followed by placement of an endotracheal tube or by a formal tracheostomy within 12 to 48 hours (32, 48, 154).

Oral tracheal intubation is accomplished with the aid of a laryngoscope. The techniques of intubation have been described (197). The average adult trachea is 11 to 13 cm in length and can be completely traversed by the endotracheal tube. It is essential to verify that the cuff of the tube is inserted past the vocal cords to prevent vocal cord damage and to seal the airway. If the first attempt to intubate is not successful, then it should be discontinued, the airway cleared with suction, and the patient ventilated with jaw thrust and manual bag-mask ventilation. An assessment as to why the intubation failed should be made during this brief period and a second attempt made to intubate the patient (197).

The nasotracheal tube can be inserted either blindly or under direct laryngoscope vision. The technique of nasotracheal intubation requires special training and successful blind nasotracheal intubation requires an alert patient capable of spontaneous ventilation. This form of transtracheal intubation is thus seldom appropriate in comatose patients. In elective nasotracheal intubations, the nose and pharynx are premedicated with topical anesthesia and vasoconstrictors. Then, with a laryngoscope in the oral cavity, the tip of the nasotracheal tube can be grasped in forceps and steered into the glottis under direct vision (241).

Advocates of the nasotracheal tube emphasize the ease of stabilizing the tubing and improved patient comfort. The superior stability allows fewer accidental extubations and results in less movement than the endotracheal tube. However, significant pressure necrosis can occur near the ala nasi from the pressure of the tube on the skin. The nasotracheal tube can also cause acute sinusitis by obstructing nasal sinus drainage (67). Although sinusitis is easy to diagnose in conscious patients, the only sign of acute sinusitis in comatose patients may be high fever (261). The nasotracheal tube also may cause functional obstruction of the eustachian tube in the nasopharynx and subsequent middle ear infections. Although the curvature of the nasotracheal tube is less angular than that of the oral tracheal tube and should allow passage of a suction catheter more easily, difficulties are sometimes encountered during suctioning because of its small diameter (241).

A tracheostomy tube is the best artificial airway. It completely bypasses all upper airway obstructions and pathology. A tracheal tie around the neck effectively stabilizes the tube and prevents its motion in the trachea. Suctioning of the bronchi is more complete, the tube is comfortable, and patients can swallow normally when their mental status and pharyngeal reflexes are intact. The mortality of tracheostomy performed under elective conditions is from 0.9% to 5.1% and significantly related to the critical nature of the patient (182, 192, 235). Immediate complications of tracheostomy include bleeding, pneumothorax, air embolism, subcutaneous emphysema, and the potential of tension pneumothorax. Delayed complications include infection, hemorrhage, airway obstruction, swallowing difficulties, and tracheal esophageal fistulas. The overall late morbidity approaches 40% in high risk groups (124, 183, 192). When the air inspired by the tracheostomy is humidified, the tracheostomy tube does not need to be routinely changed. The surgical tract is not well established for the first 4 to 5 days and changing the tracheostomy tube within this period carries a significant risk of being unable to rapidly re-establish the airway at the bedside. The addition of stay sutures in the inferior tracheal ring of the tracheostomy can aid in re-insertion of the tracheostomy tube during the postoperative phase by elevating the trachea to the skin edge (93, 241).

HYPERVENTILATION THERAPY AND INTRACRANIAL PRESSURE

The cerebral blood flow (CBF) in normal brain is regulated to match local blood flow to local metabolic demand by varying the resistance of the cerebral vessels. The control is mediated by metabolically determined local extracellular pH. This chemical control for modulating CBF is therapeutically manipulated by changing the Pa_{CO_2} which changes the cerebral extracellular fluid pH. Hypocapnia causes the cerebral vessels to vasoconstrict with a 4% decrease in CBF for every torr change in Pa_{CO_2} down to 25 torr. Below this level, the vasoconstrictive effect of hypocapnia is diminished or absent (31, 125, 159, 187, 238, 239, 302).

Hyperventilation results in an acute reduction of Pa_{CO_2}. Since carbon dioxide rapidly equilibrates across the blood-brain barrier and the bicarbonate ion requires 12 to 72 hours to equilibrate, an abrupt rise in the extracellular fluid pH results and is hypothesized to mediate the prompt vasoconstrictive effect on the cerebral vessels (13, 19, 45, 81, 86, 115, 122, 149, 236, 237).

The cerebral blood volume (CBV) decreases as a result of vasoconstriction concomitant with decreases in CBF. The change in CBV from variation of carbon dioxide is 0.05 ml/100 gm torr Pa_{CO_2} in normal volunteers. For example, a reduction in the Pa_{CO_2} from 40 to 25 torr produces a decrease of 10.5 ml in the intracranial blood volume. This reduction in CBV persists for approximately 15 minutes after the arterial carbon dioxide tension returns to its original value (112). The magnitude of the acute drop in intracranial pressure (ICP) following hyperventilation is similar to that produced by the ventricular drainage of a few milliliters of CSF (158).

Hypoxemia causes an increase in the CBF when the Pa_{O_2} is below 40 torr. The brain undergoes anaerobic metabolism with production of lactate that decreases local cerebral pH. The increase in CBF of hypoxemia is thus regulated by the same chemical mechanism as alters cerebral blood flow to changes in Pa_{CO_2} (69, 125, 153).

Pure metabolic acidosis or alkalosis has no effect on the cerebral blood flow unless accompanied by compensatory Pa_{CO_2} changes since the bicarbonate ions cannot readily enter the cerebral extracellular fluid.

Hyperventilation therapy can alter cardiopulmonary physiology secondary to the increase of intrathoracic pressure required for the rapid respiratory rate. These changes include a decrease in venous return, a depression of cardiac output, and an elevation of central venous pressure. These effects are monitored with the use of a Swan-Ganz cardiac output catheter and compensated for with fluid and inotropic drug therapy (92).

Severe hypocapnia to levels of 20 torr or less can cause tissue hypoxia and may be contraindicated in head injury or subarachnoid hemorrhage with cerebral vasospasm contributing to brain ischemia (149, 187, 302). Hyperventilation therapy is begun in neurosurgical patients with elevated ICP secondary to expanding mass lesions and severe head injuries with the Pa_{CO_2} adjusted in the range of 25 to 30 torr; diagnostic tests and surgery are then performed. After approximately 8 to 16 hours, the Pa_{CO_2} is gradually elevated to 30 or 32 torr with careful monitoring of the intracranial pressure. When control of the ICP below 15 torr is maintained at this mild degree of hypocapnia, the nursing staff can acutely hyperventilate the patient to abort further rises in ICP from spontaneous pressure wave or suctioning pressure elevations. When hyperventilation is abruptly discontinued, cerebral vasodilation can result from the decrease of extracellular cerebral pH; this is the reverse phenomenon from the vasoconstriction produced by acute hyperventilation and can precipitate increases in ICP. This elevation can be blunted or eliminated by tapering the hyperventilation over 24 to 48 hours (19, 52, 123, 138, 191, 244).

Vessels in damaged regions of the brain lose chemical control of vessel caliber and remain in a maximally dilated state. Thus, hypocapnia therapy causes a decrease of blood flow to normal cerebral tissues and effectively diverts a larger percentage of the cerebral blood flow to the damaged tissues supplying their high nutrient and oxygen demands. The alkalosis of hyperventilation therapy may aid in reversing local tissue acidosis and subsequent damage. Hyperoxia is another benefit of hyperventilation therapy that may aid in the protection of borderline ischemic regions of the brain. Hyperventilation also reduces the rate of CSF production and hence may augment the control of the intracranial pressure (19, 125, 302).

DIAGNOSIS OF RESPIRATORY FAILURE

Respiratory insufficiency can be diagnosed by several criteria summarized in Table 1.3 (30, 35, 92, 137). A patient with a respiratory rate in excess of 40 breaths per minute soon is exhausted because the effort of breathing is too high to be sustained. Rapid breathing also causes severe respiratory alkalosis with shift of the oxygen dissociation curve to the left so that oxygen is tightly bound to the hemoglobin. The net effect is to decrease the amount of oxygen available to the tissues. A respira-

TABLE 1.3.
Criteria for Diagnosis of Respiratory Insufficiency

Respiratory rate	>40	br/min
	< 8	br/min
Tidal volume	< 3.5	ml/kg-br
Vital capacity	<15	ml/kg
Negative inspiratory force	<20	cm-H_2O
Arterial oxygen	<50	torr
Arterial carbon dioxide	>50	torr
Pulmonary shunt	>10	%

tory rate below eight breaths per minute leads to an increase in the arterial carbon dioxide tension and respiratory acidosis. The hypercapnia causes cerebral vasodilation, increased CBV, and ultimately a rise in the ICP. A low rate of shallow respirations is extremely dangerous in neurosurgical patients with expanding mass lesions or head-injured patients with significant cerebral contusion. Hypercapnia can lead to brain swelling and death (77, 173).

TV is defined as the amount of air inspired at rest during a single breath. It is approximately 375 ml in a 70-kg man. When the TV falls below 250 ml (3.5 ml/kg-br) respiratory insufficiency follows. The VC is a measurement of the maximum amount of air that can be moved between inspiration and expiration. Young healthy males have a VC approaching 5 liters. Respiratory insufficiency occurs with a reduction of VC to below 1 liter (15 ml/kg). The VC is a measure of the patient's ability to expand the lungs and prevent miliary atelectasis.

The maximum negative inspiratory force (NIF) is measured with the patient inspiring against an occluded airway. A maximum inspiratory force less negative than 20 cm of water indicates respiratory insufficiency. Measurements of NIF, TV, and VC are easily obtained in awake patients and accurately predict the need for respiratory assistance. They are also useful for assistance in weaning from a respirator.

Arterial blood gas analysis is the laboratory test most useful for evaluating respiratory insufficiency (196, 288). Respiratory insufficiency can be defined as an arterial blood gas sample with an oxygen tension of less than 50 torr or a carbon dioxide tension of greater than 50 torr. The pulmonary shunt fraction is calculated by

$$\frac{\dot{Q}_s}{\dot{Q}_T} = \frac{Cc_{O_2} - Ca_{O_2}}{Cc_{O_2} - Cv_{O_2}} \quad \text{(eq. 2)}$$

where $\dot{Q}_s$ = pulmonary shunt blood flow, $\dot{Q}_T$ = cardiac output, Ca_{O_2} = O_2 concentration in arterial blood, Cv_{O_2} = O_2 concentration in mixed venous blood, Cc_{O_2} = O_2 concentration in end pulmonary capillary blood. The Cc_{O_2} is estimated from the calculated alveolar $P_{A_{O_2}}$ (see eq. 3) and the hemoglobin dissociation curve (288). A pulmonary shunt can result from true anatomic right-left communication or ventilation-perfusion mismatch. Pulmonary insufficiency is diagnosed with an effective shunt of greater than 10%.

Abnormal pulmonary gas exchange is separated into two major classes with different pathophysiology and treatment: hypoxemia and hypercapnia. This separation is based on an analysis of the arterial oxygen and carbon dioxide partial pressure and the alveolar-arterial oxygen gradient [(A-a)O_2 gradient]. The normal oxygen partial pressure of the arterial blood is between 90 and 100 mm Hg. The alveolar-arterial oxygen gradient is calculated by using the alveolar oxygen pressure obtained from the alveolar gas equation. The alveolar oxygen concentration is estimated by:

$$P_{A_{O_2}} = F_{I_{O_2}}(P_b - P_{H_2O}) - P_{A_{CO_2}}\left[F_{I_{O_2}} + \frac{1 - F_{I_{O_2}}}{R}\right] \quad \text{(eq. 3)}$$

where $P_{A_{O_2}}$ = alveolar oxygen partial pressure, $F_{I_{O_2}}$ = inspired oxygen fraction, P_b = barometric pressure, P_{H_2O} = water vapor pressure (47 torr at 37°C), $P_{A_{CO_2}}$ = alveolar carbon dioxide partial pressure (estimated as Pa_{CO_2} the arterial partial pressure), and R = respiratory coefficient estimated as 0.8 or calculated as the ratio of the production of carbon dioxide to the consumption of oxygen as calculated by the Fick principle (49). When the patient is breathing 21% oxygen at sea level and has a normal Pa_{CO_2} of 40 torr, then the alveolar gas equation predicts an alveolar oxygen concentration of 100 torr. A normal (A-a)O_2 gradient is thus 5 to 10 torr. The (A-a)O_2 gradient is a sensitive indicator of all respiratory diseases in which ventilation-perfusion mismatch or anatomic pulmonary shunts are present. An $(A\text{-}a)O_2$ gradient of greater than 20 torr represents pulmonary gas exchange insufficiency. The level of the arterial concentration of CO_2 varies directly with the CO_2 production and inversely with the alveolar ventilation. Hypocapnia in a ventilated patient results from an increase in the alveolar gas exchange from a high minute ventilation.

There are five major conditions causing hypoxemic respiratory failure as listed in Table 1.4. A low Pa_{O_2} corresponds to a ventilatory malfunction delivering a suboptimal level of oxygen or an occluded airway. Diffusion impairment as a cause of hypoxemia is rarely clinically important in neurologic patients. In alveolar hypoventilation, the $(A\text{-}a)O_2$ gradient is normal, with both Pa_{CO_2} elevated and Pa_{O_2} decreased. Patients with a ventilation/perfusion mismatch or a right to left pulmonary shunt have an increased $(A\text{-}a)O_2$ gradient; the Pa_{CO_2} is initially in the normal range and the Pa_{O_2} is decreased corresponding to the size of the shunt. In patients with a ventilation/perfusion mismatch there is generally a dramatic rise in the Pa_{O_2} in response to breathing 100% oxygen, whereas in patients with a large right to left shunt only a small increase in the Pa_{O_2} is obtained (163, 224, 285, 286). Ventilation/perfusion mismatch has been described as causing hypoxemia in isolated head trauma and is attributed to neural or humoral derangements from the central nervous system injury (234).

Arterial hypercapnia results from three clinical conditions. Ventilating patients with a gas mixture containing CO_2 is rarely used clinically and is an obvious cause of arterial hypercapnia to diagnose. Alveolar hypoventilation as a cause of hypercapnia is diagnosed by a normal $(A\text{-}a)O_2$ gradient. A severe ventilation/perfusion mismatch is clinically the most common cause of arterial hypercapnia in patients with severe intrinsic lung disease. The degree of ventilation/perfusion mismatch required to cause arterial hypercapnia is larger than that needed to cause arterial hypoxemia and an $(A\text{-}a)O_2$ gradient of 30 to 40 torr is typical (62, 214, 271, 284).

TABLE 1.4.
Hypoxemic Respiratory Failure

Low inspired oxygen pressure
Alveolar hypoventilation
Ventilation/perfusion mismatch
Right-to-left pulmonary shunt
Gas diffusion impairment in alveolar membrane

INSTITUTING VENTILATORY THERAPY

Ventilatory therapy is instituted in neurosurgical patients for hyperventilation, protection of the airway, or as necessitated by respiratory failure. Mechanical ventilatory support with sedation or muscle paralysis may be required to ensure delivery of hyperventilation therapy. In neurologic patients with mass lesions, dangerous rises in carbon dioxide can occur in sedated or obtunded patients as the tongue falls against the posterior pharynx and partially occludes the upper airway. This can occur during the 15 to 20 minutes of computed tomography (CT) scan while observation of the patient is compromised. The carbon dioxide pressure in apnea rises at the rate of 4 torr/min. It is safer to electively intubate lethargic patients before sedation and all obtunded patients to ensure an adequate airway and ventilation (241).

The first step is the establishment of an airway and manual support of the ventilation. Manual ventilation is immediately available and offers the clinician direct control of the air flow for aeration of both lung fields and as well as manual assessment of the pulmonary compliance.

The second step in establishing ventilatory control is to assess cardiovascular instability usually manifest as hypotension or arrhythmia. Hypotension may occur immediately after placement of an airway due to the physiologic stress of intubation, from delays in obtaining an airway with subsequent blood gas abnormalities, from untoward responses to pharmacologic agents used during intubation, and secondary to unrecognized hypoventilation during intubation. The instability is enhanced when positive end-expiratory pressure (PEEP) is utilized. Autonomic nervous system responses are triggered by hypoxemia, hypocarbia, acidemia, mechanical tracheal stimulation, and, in conscious patients, anxiety and fear. The autonomic nervous system stimulated in this manner produces both arterial and venous vasoconstriction and myocardial stimulation. Mechanical ventilation comfortably ventilates many patients when the increased work of breathing is eliminated and the blood gases and pH are returned to normal. The abrupt physiologic improvement can cause a large decrease in the autonomic system outflow with elimination of vasoconstriction resulting in hypotension. Pharmacologic sedation or unconsciousness can also reduce sympathetic outflow in ventilated patients and cause hypotension. The relaxation of sympathetic tone results in a relative hypovolemia as the arterial and venous vessels are no longer constricted. Fluids and colloids are used to correct the hypovolemia acutely as the body cannot mobilize extravascular fluids rapidly enough to correct the acute hypotensive response.

The third step in initiating ventilatory support is to establish base line measurements and to start a continuous record of ventilatory and cardiorespiratory parameters along with arterial blood gas and pulmonary function values. Trends in the peak airway pressure and pulmonary compliance reflect changes in ventilatory mechanics. Arterial blood gases, pulmonary artery wedge pressures, and cardiac output trends are useful in cardiopulmonary management. Trends in parameters are often more important than the individual values themselves.

The fourth step is to ventilate the patient at the desired rate and approximate tidal volume manually before connecting the patient to the ventilator. Patients unable to tolerate this manual ventilation require sedative or paralyzing agents for successful ventilatory support. The fifth and final step is to connect the patient to the ventilator. The ventilator is used to deliver hyperventilation therapy or for temporary pulmonary support while respiratory pathology is treated.

Arterial blood pressure variations are monitored during the inspiratory phase of ventilation. In some mildly hypervolemic patients, a rise in the arterial blood pressure occurs with the inspiratory phase of ventilation and ranges as high as 30 mm Hg. This elevation in blood pressure can be detrimental in the management of patients with impaired cerebral autoregulation. A state of mild dehydration appears to eliminate or blunt this rise in systemic arterial pressure.

Neurosurgical patients are managed on positive pressure ventilators. These ventilators provide a cyclic pressure gradient in the upper airways which pushes gas into the lower airways. In normal physiologic respiration, the diaphragms create a cyclic negative pressure within the thorax and suck air into the lower airways. Positive pressure ventilators are separated into two separate classes of mechanical ventilators: pressure preset ventilators and volume preset ventilators (180). The pressure preset ventilators deliver inspired flow until a specific preset pressure is reached at which time the inflow of gas is turned off and the expiratory phase is started. These ventilators are not recommended in neurosurgical patients because the minute ventilation is not directly controlled, and hence the arterial pressure of carbon dioxide is not tightly controlled. If a bronchus is occluded with a mucous plug, for example, the tidal volume may be substantially reduced and lead to an elevation in Pa_{CO_2}.

Volume control ventilators deliver breaths at measured volumes and set intervals. These ventilators control the amount of inspiratory time and expiratory time and in some cases the length of inspiratory pause before the start of expiration. The modes of operating a volume cycle ventilator are listed in Table 1.5. In assisted ventilation, the patient triggers the ventilator with an NIF and the ventilator delivers a positive pressure breath at the preset tidal volume. The patient determines only the rate of breathing, and multiple NIF in an agitated patient can result in severe hyperventilation. Hence, this mode is rarely useful in neurosurgical patients. In controlled ventilation, the ventilator delivers breaths at the tidal volume and inspiratory rate set on the machine irrespective of the patient's breathing efforts. Paralyzation or heavy sedation is required to prevent bucking the ventilator and producing high intrathoracic pressures as no extra breaths are allowed by the mode. In assist-controlled ventilation, the ventilator responds to the patient's NIF as in assisted ventilation with the additional guarantee that the delivery of a preset automatic

TABLE 1.5.
Respiratory Modes for Volume Cycled Ventilators

Assisted ventilation
Controlled ventilation
Assist control ventilation
Intermittent mandatory ventilation (IMV)
Synchronized IMV (SIMV)
Pressure support ventilation

number of breaths is assured even in the absence of any patient inspiratory efforts. The intermittent mandatory ventilation (IMV) mode has a preset tidal volume and breathing rate but allows the patient to breath spontaneously between the controlled breaths. During these spontaneous breaths, the patient breathes the quantity of gas he wishes as opposed to receiving a full tidal volume as is the case in assisted or assist-controlled ventilation. Synchronized IMV (SIMV) is a combination of spontaneous and assisted ventilation. In this mode, the respirator waits for an NIF and then delivers the preset volume in synchrony with the patient's inspiratory effort. If the required minimum number of breaths per minute are not triggered, then the machine originates ventilatory cycles to guarantee that the preset minute ventilation is delivered. The patient is free to breathe at his own desired volume in between these triggered breaths. This mode is thought to be more comfortable for the patient than IMV (68, 71, 72, 181, 184, 219, 241, 243). Pressure support ventilation is a new form of respiratory support available on the Siemens-Elema 900C servo-ventilators (Siemens Corp., Union, N.J.). This mode requires a conscious patient and is most useful in respiratory insufficiency from an inability to perform the required work of breathing. The respirator is set to assume a large or small fraction of the work of breathing with the patient triggering the onset of breaths and determining the amount of minute ventilation. It can be combined with intermittent mandatory ventilation during weaning from the respirator. This mode has been most useful at our institution in weaning patients with preoperative/injury pulmonary disease who are unsuccessful in traditional weaning protocols (144).

In neurosurgical patients, controlled ventilation is the initial ventilation pattern of choice. This mode allows precise delivery of minute ventilation. When the need for hyperventilation in the control of ICP is no longer necessary, the patient is weaned from respiratory support by either an IMV or SIMV. Sedating drugs useful in ventilated patients include morphine, fentanyl, pentobarbital, lorazepam, and diazepam. Neuromuscular blocking drugs are used for control of neurologic patients only when all sedating drugs are contraindicated as the neurologic examination is totally lost and the patient is exposed to the risk of delayed diagnosis of neurologic deterioration (19).

High frequency ventilation is a new technique of ventilatory support that has been investigated for a variety of applications in recent years. The technique of high frequency ventilation includes a spectrum of frequency and ventilatory delivery modes. The common thrust of all the methods of high frequency ventilation is to provide breathing rates between 100 and 3,000 breaths per minute to enhance the diffusion process of gas exchange within the lower airways of the lung. High frequency ventilation eliminates the normal cyclic variations of the intracranial pressure present in positive pressure breathing. Most head-injured patients and general neurosurgical patients with low intracerebral compliance do not permit optimal utilization of this technique because of a concurrent pulmonary pathology. When the high frequency ventilator settings are adjusted to achieve the desired arterial oxygen and carbon dioxide levels, an effectively high PEEP in the pulmonary circuit results and raises the intracranial pressure. At the current time, high frequency jet ventilation is experimental and has no place in the routine management of head-injured patients (16, 37, 89, 90, 110, 152, 201, 202, 253).

When lung disease is extremely asymmetric, independent lung ventilation can be useful for optimum management of the patient's respiratory status. This technique may be particularly useful in unilateral adult respiratory distress syndrome or atelectasis of one lung when there is a major ventilation/perfusion mismatch between the two sides. This technique requires two synchronized ventilators and a critical care staff to support the ongoing effort of this experimental form of pulmonary therapy (18, 98, 213).

POSITIVE END-EXPIRATORY PRESSURE

Positive end-expiratory pressure (PEEP) is often a necessary adjuvant therapy for treatment of respiratory failure in ventilated patients. PEEP is active during the exhalation phase of the ventilator cycle by restricting expiration of pulmonary air to periods where the airway pressure is greater than the present PEEP pressure. PEEP is added to the ventilatory circuit by placing the expired outlet port under water or by inserting a calibrated springball pressure pop-off regulator in the exhalation circuit. The major effect of PEEP on lung pathophysiology is to increase the FRC and thereby normalize ventilation/perfusion maldistribution. In atelectatic regions of the lungs the increased FRC is reflected as an opening of airways and recruitment of previously collapsed alveoli. The change in FRC with the institution of PEEP can be directly measured by assessing ventilatory gas flows. Figure 1.4*A* shows the endotracheal gas flow and pressure along with a breath by breath integration of inspiration and expiration volumes from a ventilated patient before and after PEEP. The derived flow-volume loop of an initial and post-PEEP breath in Figure 1.4*B* demonstrates an increase in FRC of 0.82 liters when 25 cm-H_2O PEEP is acutely applied. The increase in FRC can also be measured by washout of inert gases.

PEEP is clinically indicated for hypoxic respiratory failure of acute respiratory distress syndrome (ARDS) and cardiogenic pulmonary edema (CPE) requiring supplemental oxygen greater than 50%. The pathologic increase in interstitial fluid is not removed from the lungs by PEEP but is redistributed. PEEP improves the arterial blood gases in pulmonary disorders with ventilation/perfusion maldistribution and pulmonary right-left shunting by expansion of previously collapsed alveoli along with redistributing the alveolar ventilation and pulmonary blood flow to provide a better match (14, 275).

PEEP is a potentially dangerous form of respiratory therapy resulting from effects on and complex interaction of the cardiovascular, pulmonary, and intracranial physiology. PEEP has a variable effect on the cardiac output. In patients with highly compliant lungs, PEEP reduces cardiac output by impairing the venous return. This reduction is accentuated by hypotension or hypovolemia (216). Severely ill patients with poorly compliant lungs, however, often demonstrate stable hemodynamics or an increase in cardiac output related to better oxygenation of the arterial blood with PEEP. When patients are in a high cardiac output state, PEEP may cause a mild reduction in it. Successful management of the cardiovascular system with PEEP requires careful fluid balance; the use of a pulmonary artery catheter is recommended. Inotropic agents are often necessary to augment the cardiac output when PEEP is used (84, 155, 168).

The pulmonary complications of PEEP are dominated by barotrauma. The incidence of pneumothorax from positive pressure ventilation with PEEP in intensive care patients has been reported from 7% to 39%. The incidence of pneumothorax in similar patients on only positive pressure ventilation without PEEP has been reported from 7% to 14%. The incidence of pneumothorax increases with high airway pressures resulting from low compliance lungs and high PEEP (53, 65, 150, 156). PEEP has also been associated with pneumomediastinum and subcutaneous emphysema. PEEP greatly increases the work of breathing and the successful weaning of patients while on PEEP is difficult or impossible (83, 128).

The effect of PEEP on the intracranial pressure is variable with increases in ICP more common in the presence of low cerebral compliance (11). During PEEP, the intrathoracic pressure is raised as is the pressure in the large veins and right atrium of the heart. The increase in central venous pressure may impair cerebral venous return and cause an elevation in ICP. The intracranial effects of PEEP can be blunted or eliminated by positioning head-injured patients at a 30- to 45-degree head-up position and limiting PEEP to 12 cm-H_2O (91). In this position the cerebral venous system is physically higher than the level of PEEP and hence the dural sinuses are not directly elevated in pressure by PEEP and easy run-off of cortical venous blood is assured. Transmission of PEEP pressure to the intrathoracic and hence the intracranial compartments is less with a low pulmonary compliance as seen in ARDS, and in these patients PEEP of 25 cm-H_2O can often be tolerated without dangerous ICP elevations (131, 135, 245).

Patients with an expanding intracranial mass lesion or low cerebral compliance with concomitant pulmonary pathology require hemodynamic and intracranial pressure monitoring. The cerebral perfusion pressure (CPP) is calculated from the arterial and intracranial pressure measurements:

$$CPP = MAP - MICP \quad \text{(eq. 4)}$$

where MAP is the mean arterial pressure and MICP is the mean intracranial pressure. Inotropic administration, positioning of the pa-

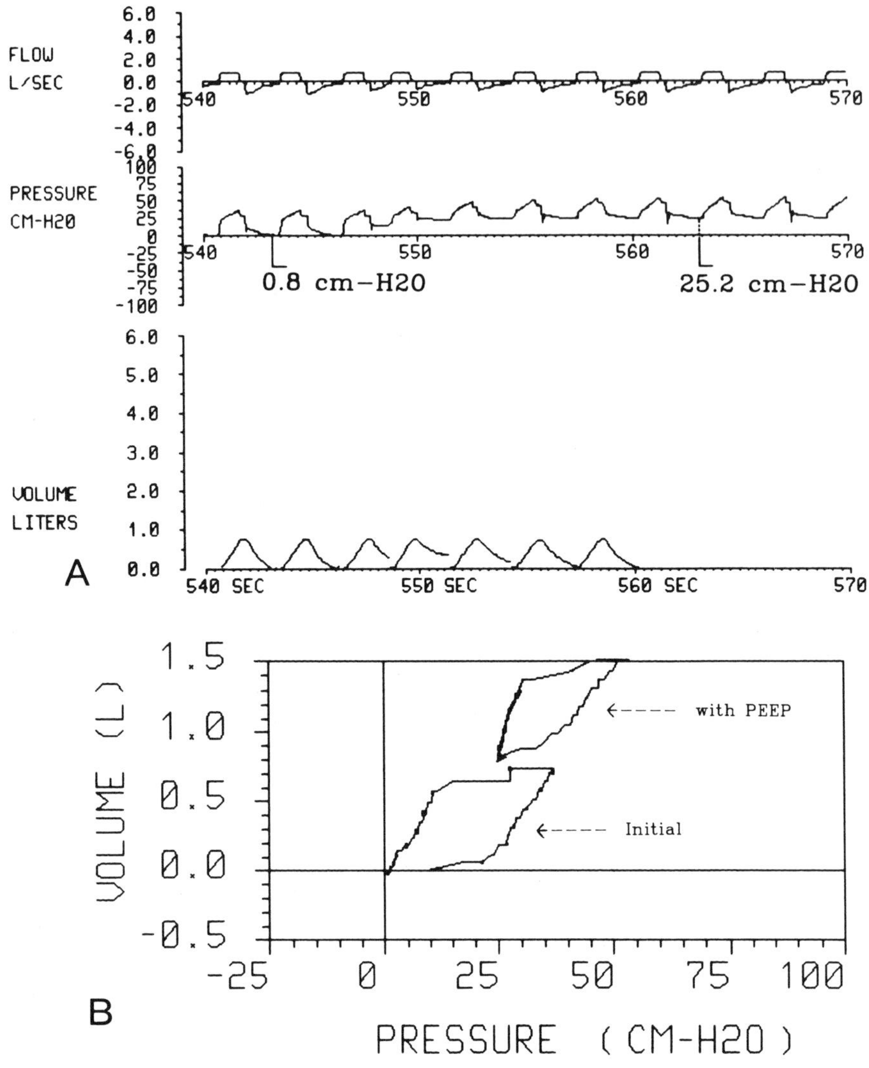

Figure 1.4. Increased FRC with PEEP measured by integrating flows. *A)* Airway flow and pressure measured at the endotracheal tube. After the end expiration of the second breath 25 cm H_2O PEEP was added. Note the measured end-expired pressure is changed from 0.8 to 25.2 cm H_2O as measured and recorded on the graph. The volumes of the two base line breaths along with the first five breaths following institution of PEEP are separately integrated. Note that the inspired and expired volumes are equal for the first two base line breaths by the return of the integrated flow to zero at end expiration. However, the inspired volume is greater than the expired volume for the first four breaths following institution of PEEP as evidenced by the integrated flow over each breath remaining with a positive valve at end expiration. This quantity of gas remains in the lung and is the increase of FRC. *B)* Two breaths are presented on the pressure-volume graph; the lower loop is a base line breath with an end expiration retained volume normalized to zero when no PEEP was used. The upper loop is the fifth breath after PEEP is instituted. The end expiration retained volume is 0.82 liters greater with PEEP of 25 cm H_2O airway pressure. This directly measures the increase in FRC by 0.82 liters when a PEEP of 25 cm H_2O is applied in this patient.

tient, and PEEP are adjusted to continuously obtain a CPP greater than 50 torr and adequate oxygenation. The measurement of cardiac output (CO) and pulmonary artery wedge pressure (PAWP) with a thermal dilution Swan-Ganz catheter aids in fluid and inotropic management (4, 245).

Optimal PEEP to the respiratory system has been defined by a variety of methods: maximum oxygen transport; minimum dead-space fraction; static compliance; or intra-esophageal balloon manometry. The optimum level of PEEP cannot, however, be defined solely with arterial blood gas samples. Delivering PEEP at the maximum pulmonary compliance is a clinically useful method for optimum PEEP therapy (36, 60, 63, 267).

Termination of PEEP is performed in a stepwise fashion with careful monitoring of hemodynamic parameters and the arterial blood gas over 1 to 2 days. This lessens the chance that unstable alveoli opened by PEEP will recollapse. Abrupt discontinuation of PEEP can lead to a reflexive hypertension with subsequent elevation of ICP through engorgement of cerebral tissues with defective autoregulation (4, 19).

WEANING FROM VENTILATORY SUPPORT

Neurologically impaired patients require special consideration during weaning from ventilator support. The time of weaning may be determined by cessation of hyperventilation therapy or return of protective airway reflexes and not solely on resolution of pulmonary failure. Traditional tests for predicting successful weaning and extubation are: NIF more negative than 20 cm-H_2O; VC in excess of 10 ml/kg; and minute ventilation (MV) less than 10 liters/min. In unco-operative neurologic patients these measurements are not reliably made except for the MV measured directly on the ventilator. Co-operative patients are asked to maximally ventilate for 1 minute and the MV typically at least doubles compared to resting minute ventilation in patients ready for extubation; this test assesses respiratory reserve.

Two basic methods are available for weaning patients from mechanical ventilatory support: the traditional T-tube and intermittent mandatory ventilation (IMV) weaning protocols. The T-tube weaning procedure involves disconnecting the patient from the ventilator abruptly and placing him on a T-tube with an inspired oxygen concentration enriched by an additional 10% from that used with the ventilator. Arterial blood gas samples are followed at 5-, 15-, and 30-minute intervals to verify that the patient's blood is adequately oxygenated. The vital signs are watched along with continuous assessment for any respiratory distress signs. If the patient fails the initial weaning step, he is placed back on the ventilator and weaning is tried at a later time. During the first 24 hours off the ventilator, the patient is monitored carefully for respiratory distress, change in vital signs, or cardiac arrhythmias (85, 230).

The IMV protocol utilizes the IMV mode of the ventilator. The IMV rate is slowly decreased and hence the patient gradually assumes a greater burden of the work of breathing. Initial weaning rates are 10 to 12 breaths per minute and when stable blood gases are obtained at this setting, the rate is gradually decreased at a 1-hour to 4-hour interval by two breaths per minute. After each change, the arterial blood gases are checked. Conventionally, the rate is gradually decreased to four breaths per minute, to two breaths per minute, and when the IMV setting is zero breaths per minute, the ventilator is functioning as a T-piece. Since the inspired and expired resistance of the IMV ventilatory circuit is significant when compared to a T-piece, some patients can be weaned on T-tubes when they cannot be weaned on a zero IMV setting. It is thus useful to blend the IMV and T-piece protocols so that when a low IMV rate of four or six breaths per minute is reached, the patient is switched to the T-piece weaning protocol. Patients intubated more than 4 days generally require a period on low IMV settings or T-pieces for 6- to 24-hours before extubation to lessen the incidence of reintubation (166). The combined use of pressure support ventilation with IMV aids in the weaning of patients requiring respiratory muscle strengthening (144).

Any time extubation is done on an elective basis, all the equipment for a reintubation must be present at the bedside in the intensive care unit (ICU). Reintubation can be necessary due to intrinsic pulmonary failure, glottic edema, or cerebral decompensation. Most patients requiring reintubation have respiratory failure in the first few hours after extubation. Serial arterial blood gases are diagnostic and essential (102).

If a patient fails to wean successfully, then underlying causes must be sought. The principal reason for failing to wean is fatigue of the inspiratory muscles. The effects of fatigue can be overcome by increasing respiratory muscle strength or decreasing the respiratory muscle demand. Respiratory muscle strength is increased by correcting malnutrition in the post-trauma or postoperative period. Sedative drugs are discontinued since they depress respiratory muscle drive. Theophylline both stimulates respiration and increases diaphragm contractability (15). Progesterone is useful in selected patients difficult to wean as a respiratory stimulant (105, 254). Drug-induced neuromuscular dysfunction can decrease ventilatory strength and is most frequently caused by aminoglycoside antibiotics (12).

The respiratory muscle demand can be decreased by minimizing the metabolic requirements of the body. Infections cause large metabolic requirements and can surpass the ability of the pulmonary system to provide respiration. Diuretics may be helpful in increasing the compliance of the lung and thereby decreasing the work of breathing. Airway resistance may be modified with theophylline or beta-adrenergic agonists when bronchoconstriction is a significant component of residual respiratory dysfunction. The work of breathing is increased by endotracheal tubes with an internal diameter of less than 7 mm and can even be a significant factor in patients with endotracheal tubes of 8 mm internal diameter. These patients often ventilate adequately with the decreased airway resistance of their own natural airway (61, 266). In patients with a component of obstructive disease, beta-adrenergic blocking drugs are discontinued and other drugs substituted to eliminate any bronchoconstrictive effects delaying weaning.

In patients on PEEP, the weaning process requires weaning of PEEP along with the oxygen and ventilatory support. Generally, the oxygen therapy is weaned first and the PEEP is not weaned until the inspired oxygen concentration is less than or equal to 40%. The PEEP is decreased in steps of 2 cm of water until it is in the range of 3 to 5 cm of water. PEEP can then be safely discontinued. The T-tube or IMV weaning protocol is then started as outlined previously. The entire process is guided by arterial blood gas samples. When difficulties are encountered in the weaning process, ventilatory support is reinstituted and weaning is attempted later (4, 19, 185).

PULMONARY TOILET MANAGEMENT DURING VENTILATORY SUPPORT

Pulmonary toilet is an essential component of the clinical management of all intubated and mechanically ventilated patients (133, 171). The two main modalities used to maintain pulmonary toilet are endotracheal suctioning and chest physiotherapy. Both of these modalities affect intracranial pressure and require tailoring to prevent detrimental effects on the central nervous system. Endotracheal suctioning is required to clear secretions since physiologic methods of clearing secretions are eliminated in intubated patients. Suctioning removes pulmonary mucous plugs and secretions and reduces subsequent atelectasis. The irritation of the trachea during suctioning stimulates the cough reflex and elevates the mean arterial blood pressure and heart rate. There is a rise in the mean intracranial pressure with the cerebral perfusion pressure remaining relatively constant since both the mean arterial and intracranial pressures are elevated by similar amounts. The cough reflex has the potential to produce pressures as high as 300 torr within the chest cavity; when particularly severe or prolonged, the reflex can interfere with venous return and lead to an increase in intracranial pressure by impairing cerebral venous return (59, 64, 273). If the intracranial pressure rise associated with coughing falls to base line values in 15 to 30 seconds, then normal intracranial compliance is inferred. However, if the intracranial pressure remains significantly elevated for many minutes, then the presence of a low intracerebral compliance is inferred. The small increase in intracranial blood volume resulting from venous impairment due to coughing is comparable to a fluid challenge test for the direct measurement of intracranial compliance (19, 170). The effect of raising the intracranial pressure from the stimulation of the cough mechanism can be blunted or eliminated with morphine, fentanyl, sodium pentothal, succinyl choline, or lidocaine. The choice of drugs is determined by the patient's individual response to previous therapy and concurrent medication (19, 70, 203, 211).

Suctioning acutely alters the Pa_{CO_2} and Pa_{O_2}. The Pa_{CO_2} can rise at a rate of up to 10 torr per minute during the apnea period of suctioning (244). This rise in CO_2 can produces a rise in the intracranial pressure that may precipitate a cerebral pressure wave or cerebral herniation. Limiting suctioning intervals to 10 or 15 seconds at a time minimizes this effect. Pretreatment before each suctioning with 100% oxygen manual hyperventilation alleviates the hypoxemia associated with endotracheal suctioning (19).

Patients receiving PEEP therapy as part of ventilatory support cannot be disconnected from the ventilator to be suctioned. An abrupt loss of PEEP may produce an abrupt hemodynamic change affecting intracranial pressure and perfusion. Typically, both the systemic arterial pressure and venous pressure are elevated enhancing cerebral edema and increasing ICP. Patients on PEEP are best suctioned through a porthole on the end of the endotracheal tube designed for bronchoscopy. PEEP can thus be maintained during the suctioning with the ventilator connected during therapy and hence changes in arterial oxygen and carbon dioxide are minimized (4, 19).

Chest physiotherapy involves postural drainage with percussion and vibration. In the compromised patient, the mucociliary escalator is greatly aided by the use of gravity. To effectively drain mucous from various segments of the lung, several positions are used. Basal segments of the lung most commonly become atelectatic and require the head-down position to obtain gravity drainage. Standard physical therapy positioning is used for all neurosurgery patients except when cerebral compliance is extremely low. In patients with a low cerebral compliance a 15-minute time limit for the head-dependent position is mandatory. In patients with an ICP monitor a record is kept of the ICP response to physical therapy both for the elevation in ICP and the time necessary for the ICP to return to base line. A return of the ICP to base line values 10 to 15 minutes following chest physiotherapy after the patient is returned to the 30° head-up position indicates relative safety of repeating physical therapy (170).

Chest percussion is used in combination with postural drainage to loosen thickened bronchial secretions and aid in the gravity drainage. The clapping of the chest wall starts a wave at the surface that transmits energy into the lung parenchyma. Percussion elevates the ICP only when associated with elevations in the systemic arterial pressure while intracranial autoregulation is defective. The chest physiotherapist watches the intensive care monitors during the clapping procedure and minimizes changes. Care is taken during positioning the patient to avoid rotations of the head that may occlude veins in the neck and cause increases in the ICP by increasing cerebral venous pressure. A loose fitting Philadelphia collar can maintain the head in neutral position and prevent venous occlusion in the neck (170).

COMPLICATIONS OF TRANSTRACHEAL AIRWAY MANAGEMENT

Many neurosurgical patients require artificial airways for hyperventilation, depressed protective reflexes, or concurrent pulmonary disease. Management of these patients can be accomplished either with an endotracheal tube or a tracheostomy. There is no unequivocal answer as to whether an endotracheal tube or a tracheostomy is superior in many patients. There is universal agreement that short-term airway management for up to 3 to 5 days is best accomplished by nasal or oral trachael intubation and that airway management more than 3 weeks requires a tracheostomy. We have found the conversion point from an oral tracheal intubation to a tracheostomy optimum at about 10 to 14 days. However, neurologically impaired patients who wake up in a combative and agitated state have a tracheostomy performed as an urgent procedure when concurrent pulmonary dysfunction requires respiratory support for several more days. The motion of any combative patient causes repeated laryngeal trauma that may lead to long-term complications. Conversion from an endotracheal tube to a tracheostomy is performed electively by a surgeon experienced in the technique. The major complication of tracheostomy is infection. A morbidity rate of under 2% is expected (241).

Insertion of an endotracheal tube results in a high incidence of contamination of the lower airways due to its passage through the contaminated oral pharynx. Nosocomial infections are easily transmitted via hand contact from patient to patient in the densely populated intensive care unit. Hand washing significantly reduces the possibility of cross-contaminating infections. In addition to contamination of the lower airway with bacteria the placement of an artificial airway compromises the normal defense mechanism of the lower airways by blockage of normal ciliary motion in the trachea causing dysfunction of the mucociliary escalator and blockage of the cough mechanism for effectively removing retained secretions (127, 139).

Suctioning of the airway is required in almost all patients with an artificial airway and those with copious secretions require frequent suctioning. Complications can occur during suctioning and include hypoxemia and hypercarbia, cardiac arrhythmias, systemic hypotension, and partial collapse of lung parenchyma. Hypoxemia and hypercarbia are serious complications of suctioning in neurosurgical patients since both tend to increase cerebral blood flow and cerebral blood volume and thus increase intracranial pressure. Suction causes the oxygen enriched mixture within the large airways supplied by the ventilator to be removed and replaced by room air with 21% oxygen; this effect can be blunted by pre-oxygenating the patient with 100% oxygen shortly before suctioning or providing oxygen to the air that would enter around the catheter. The first effect of hypoxemia during suctioning would be an initial bradycardia that occurs without arrhythmia. This abnormal cardiac rhythm reverts as soon as oxygen is resupplied to the patient. Cardiac arrhythmias can occur following either arterial hypoxemia or vagal stimulation from tracheal irritation. Premature ventricular contractions can occur during the suctioning process for either reason. Profound bradycardia can occur in individuals with a strong vasovagal reflex (6, 59, 273).

Hypotension can result during suctioning as a direct result of the bradycardia or from prolonged coughing. The severe coughing caused by stimulation of the tracheal or carinal reflexes results in hypotension by interfering with venous return and cardiac output. Pre- and intermittent oxygenation with 100% oxygen and limiting the suctioning process to 10 or 15 seconds with close cardiac monitoring provide the best protection against hypotension.

Lung collapse is a potential complication of suction catheter technique when a large catheter is used in a small diameter airway. If the suction catheter completely blocks the surrounding airspace, then the vacuum in the catheter is applied directly to the lung and may cause a portion of that parenchyma to collapse. This complication is avoided by using a suction catheter no larger than one-half the internal diameter of the pulmonary tube requiring suction (241).

A high incidence of mucosal damage is found in autopsy series in patients who have received only a few days of tracheal suctioning. Fiberoptic bronchoscopy of the mucosa has further demonstrated the mucosal damage. This damage occurs even when meticulous technique is used. The suction catheter appears to invaginate the mucosa in the side ports when vacuum is applied; these areas then immediately become hemorrhagic and eventually will show erosion. The use of suction levels in the minus 80 to minus 120 torr range are recommended but even they do not fully exclude this process (229). Mucosal damage is thought to further compromise the host defense mechanism and encourage infection. All gas delivered to the patient must be 100% humidified and warmed to body temperature to prevent secretions from drying and obstructing the airways (241).

Emergencies requiring immediate attention can exist in any patient with an artificial airway. Cuff-leaks can occur causing a large fraction of the tidal volume to escape from the oral cavity and thus not contribute to pulmonary ventilation. The fastest emergency measure for this situation is to increase the tidal volume on the ventilator to compensate for the leak until a new tube can be placed on an elective basis. This technique is successful except in patients who are on high levels of PEEP. In these patients the loss of the cuff results in a loss of PEEP and an emergent changing of the airway may be necessary as the only means of re-establishing full respiratory support. Since cuff failure is relatively common, all patients requiring an intact cuff for respiratory therapy should have a spare at their bedside.

Obstruction of the artificial airway will result in the suffocation of the patient unless the condition is quickly corrected. Tubes can be kinked and slight movement of the head may correct this. An endotracheal tube can be occluded if the patient bites down on it and the suffocation that results can cause the patient to panic and perpetuate the process. Sedative or paralyzing medications followed by insertion of a bite block are useful in these situations. Occlusion of the distal end of the airway is possible by herniation of the cuff over the open end. Deflation of the cuff relieves this obstruction. Tracheal secretions can plug the lumen of the airway. The tube may migrate down in the trachea and the open end bevel contact the carina causing an airway obstruction, which can be relieved by simply withdrawing the tube.

When an airway obstruction occurs, investigation as to the cause should proceed rapidly through manipulating the tube and head, deflating the cuff, and then suctioning the airway. If these steps are unsuccessful, then the artificial airway must be immediately removed and ventilation provided by mouth-to-mouth or mask-bag technique until a new airway can be inserted. When all these techniques are unsuccessful, the presence of a pneumothorax or other primary lung pathology should be considered responsible for the inability to ventilate the patient. The insertion of a chest tube can be lifesaving and should not be delayed pending chest x-ray in patients who cannot be ventilated.

A laryngeal occlusion can happen immediately after extubation as a result of vocal cord spasm. This causes total airway obstruction with inability of the patient to inspire. Such spasms are usually of short duration, lasting less than 30 seconds. However, if laryngeal spasm persists it is necessary to relieve it with a muscle relaxant and ventilation of the patient (241).

The most common complication of endotracheal intubation is edema in the glottic area. It is seldom severe and reintubation can be prevented in many cases by early recognition and appropriate treatment. Glottic edema can result from trauma during intubation, management of an agitated patient, insertion of an oversized endotracheal tube, poor endotracheal hygiene, or allergic responses.

Inspiratory stridor is the most common clinical presentation of glottic edema and develops when the glottic opening is reduced by 50%. A high-pitched musical sound caused by the narrowed glottic opening is commonly heard on inspiration. Edema occurs in the connective tissue directly below the epithelium in the glottic area. Submucosal swelling begins upon removal of the artificial airway and increases over several hours to its maximum extent at 24 hours. Patients with inspiratory stridor on extubation must be considered at high risk of developing significant edema (142). The topical application of the adrenergic drug racemic epinephrine provides vasoconstrictor activity and decreases the edema (66). The anti-inflammatory effects of steroids also decrease the severity of glottic edema. Subglottic edema commonly requires reintubation and is assumed to be present when measures to prevent glottic edema have been unsuccessful.

Vocal cord ulceration, granuloma, and polyp are investigated when hoarseness persists for more than 7 days after extubation. The diagnosis is made by indirect visualization of the glottis. These problems are believed caused by intubation trauma or by patient movement during agitation or coughing (241).

Tracheal stenosis may occur from a few weeks to years following endotracheal intubation. The stricture in the airway is produced by the healing process of the trachea in response to injury by the artificial airway. A reduction in the tracheal cross sectional area of less than 50% does not result in clinical symptoms. Tracheal malacia is a destruction of the tracheal cartilage by intubation with resulting collapse of the trachea during inspiration. Elements of both stenosis and malacia can exist together. The incidence of tracheal stenosis is between 1% and 20% for patients receiving mechanical ventilation with cuffed tubes. However, only 0.5% to 2% require surgical correction of the stenosis for symptomatic relief (121, 241).

The cuff pressure of the artificial airway forming the air seal to the tracheal wall can cause pressure-induced ischemic damage to underlying mucosa. The arterial pressure in the adult tracheal wall is approximately 30 torr and the capillary bed pressure at the venous end is approximately 18 torr. The pressure in the cuff must be below 12 torr to allow adequate tracheal mucosal blood flow. However, cuff pressure must exceed peak airway pressure to eliminate leaking of the delivered tidal volume around the cuff. In some patients on positive pressure ventilation these two pressure restrictions are almost identical. Mucosal damage that results from overinflation of the cuff is entirely reversible unless it is circumferential (241). A variety of special cuffs have been designed to provide high residual volumes and low pressure to reduce mucosal damage (42, 79, 113). High pressure cuffs have no place in the modern ICU care of patients requiring prolonged intubation.

ACUTE HYPOXEMIA ON VENTILATORY SUPPORT

Acute respiratory failure on ventilatory support with development of hypoxia requires prompt recognition and treatment to avoid morbidity and mortality (93). Conscious patients are in distress with the onset of acute respiratory failure whereas stuporous patients manifest a decrease in their level of consciousness. The earliest physiologic sign is bradycardia, occasionally coupled with ventricular arrhythmia. Hypotension may occur as may hypercarbia. The arterial blood is cyanotic. When the Hering-Breuer reflex is not abolished by the sedation or paralyzation, then some patients have gasping respiration or hiccoughing. A rapid diagnosis of hypoxia on respiratory support must be made and immediately corrected to prevent anoxic brain damage. The causes of hypoxemia are listed in Table 1.6 and are separated into three categories: mechanical, pulmonary, and central nervous system. Disconnection of the respiratory circuit is continually anticipated and all ventilator alarms are immediately assessed. Secure taping of the endotracheal tube prevents migration downward to occlude a main stem bronchus or unplanned extubation.

Hypoxia can gradually develop when the patient is placed prone or in other positions compromising the mechanical motion of the chest cavity. If the peak inspiratory pressure is greater than 50 cm H_2O, the patient's position is adjusted to allow free movement of the chest cavity. The use of lower ventilator pressures decreases the incidence of barotrauma and the possibility of intraoperative spontaneous pneumothorax.

Arterial hypoxemia can result from an increase in pulmonary shunting as a result of sedation or paralyzation required for ventilatory support. This increases pulmonary shunting by decreasing the FRC of the lung and results in an effective shunt of less than 9%. Inspired oxygen concentration of 40% corrects this hypoxemia. Serial blood gas determinations with adjustment of inspired oxygen are usually all that is required but occasionally 5 to 8 cm H_2O of PEEP is necessary to prevent this hypoxemia. Venous air embolism can cause respiratory insufficiency and originates from either an open wound with venous sinuses, diploic veins exposure, or an opening or disconnection in a central venous line. A decrease in arterial oxygen concentration is not present until several minutes after the initial embolism. Treatment consists of blocking the site of entry to prevent further air embolism and full cardiovascular collapse while 100% oxygen is administered (3, 103, 135, 141, 258).

TABLE 1.6.
Causes of Hypoxemia on Ventilatory Support

Mechanical
Ventilator dysfunction
Oxygen not added to ventilation mixture
Disconnection or kinking of the respiratory tubing
Dislodgement of endotracheal tube inserted to occlude mainstem bronchus or extubation
Occlusion of endotracheal tube with mucous plug
Herniation of endotracheal cuff to occlude distal lumen
Pulmonary
Increased severity of pulmonary pathology
Ventilation/perfusion mismatch induced by sedation drugs
Pneumothorax or hemothorax
Venous air embolism
New onset of pulmonary pathology
CNS
Neurogenic pulmonary edema secondary to brain damage

Massive intracranial damage from trauma may produce a sudden large sympathetic discharge yielding an intense vasoconstrictive response shifting peripheral blood to the pulmonary system and producing severe pulmonary hypertension, pulmonary edema, and hypoxia. This problem is related to central neurogenic pulmonary edema and is covered in a subsequent section on pulmonary edema.

Pulmonary causes of hypoxia include pneumothorax, emphysematous blebs, or small air leaks. A chest film is necessary after placement of all central venous lines to investigate for pneumothorax (see Fig. 1.5). A normal chest film does not, however, exclude the later development of a pneumothorax during positive pressure ventilation.

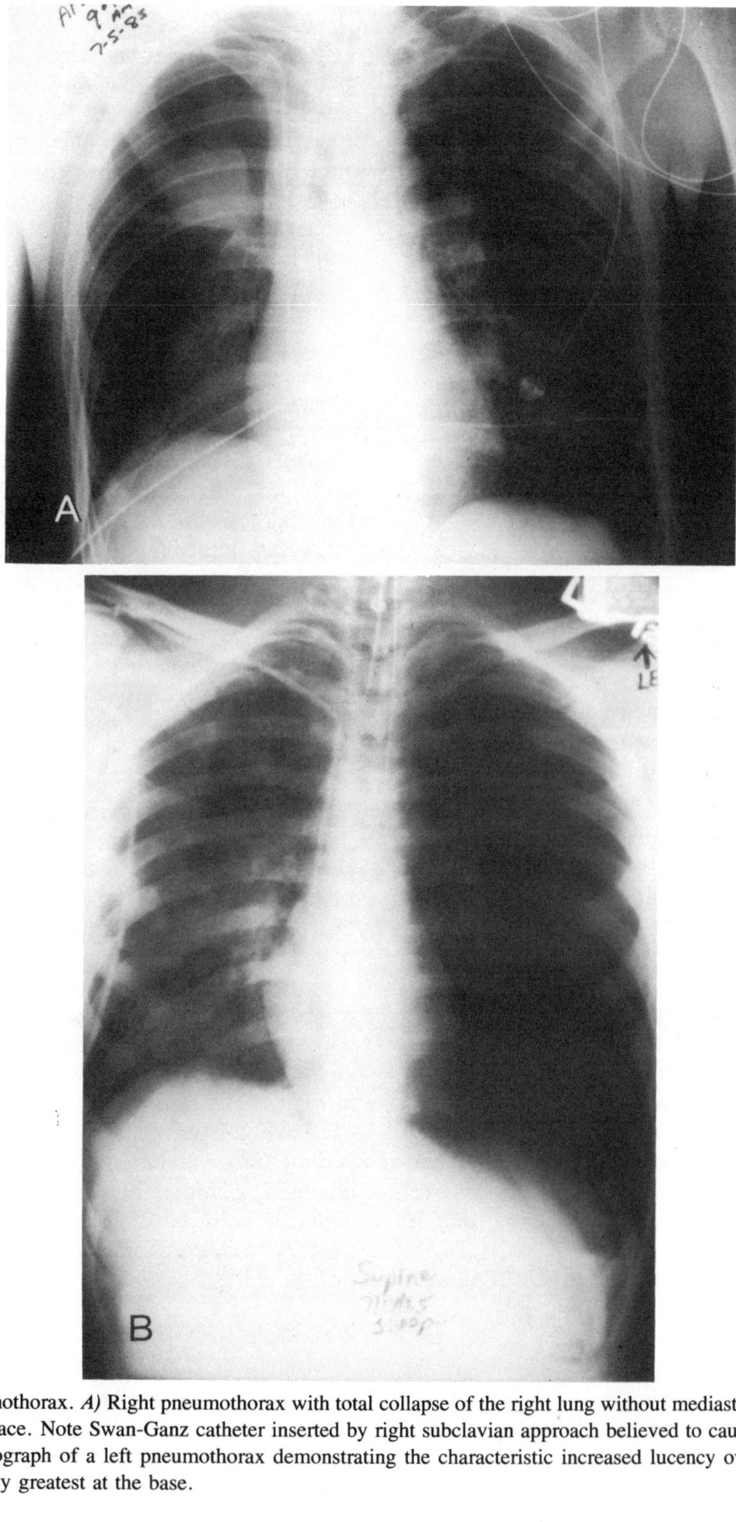

Figure 1.5. Pneumothorax. *A)* Right pneumothorax with total collapse of the right lung without mediastinal shift. Bilateral chest tubes are in place. Note Swan-Ganz catheter inserted by right subclavian approach believed to cause the pneumothorax. *B)* Supine radiograph of a left pneumothorax demonstrating the characteristic increased lucency over the entire lung field with the lucency greatest at the base.

ATELECTASIS

Atelectasis is defined as lung tissue in which the alveolar air space has collapsed. A diffuse pattern of atelectasis is termed miliary atelectasis and is not imaged by routine chest films. Blood gas analysis, however, reveals an increased (A-a)O_2 gradient from the right-to-left pulmonary shunting of blood past collapsed segments of the lung.

Atelectasis in many clinical situations involves discrete areas of the lung and is termed segmental or lobar atelectasis. Several examples are shown in Figure 1.6. An increased density is visualized on chest films in the area of collapsed segments or lobes when a portion of a lung is collapsed secondary to external pressure from pleural fluid or pneumothorax and is termed compression atelectasis. The treatment of compression atelectasis involves removal of the compressive mass and general supportive respiratory therapy.

The most common type of lung collapse seen in an intensive care unit setting is absorption atelectasis. It results when retained secretions block airways and prevent distal ventilation. Pulmonary blood flow then absorbs the remaining trapped alveolar air and the alveoli collapse. Suctioning by nasotracheal or bronchoscopy methods only removes secretions in the large airways. The secretions in bronchioles and small bronchi must be mobilized to the large airways by chest physiotherapy before they can be removed. Routine bronchial hygiene remains the cornerstone of the prevention and treatment of absorption atelectasis. When a segment or lobe of the lung collapses, the TLC is markedly decreased. Although pulmonary blood flow through the collapsed region is decreased, it represents a true physiologic shunt since an unventilated segment of lung is perfused with blood. Oxygen therapy can only reverse part of the arterial hypoxemia due to pulmonary shunting.

Absorption atelectasis is common in all critically ill patients and especially prevalent in patients with ineffective cough and gag reflexes. The atelectatic secretions that fill the alveoli are rich in nutrients that promote bacterial growth. The body's defense mechanisms are compromised in atelectasis because of compromised blood and lymph flow in the affected area. Pneumonia is a common sequel and is a serious complication in an already compromised patient.

Retained secretions occur in almost all patients with transtracheal airways or a depressed level of consciousness. The normal bronchial hygiene mechanisms in these patients are interrupted by foreign bodies, the lack of defensive reflexes, CNS depression, or chest trauma. Retained secretions cause an inflammatory response in the pulmonary mucosa which reduces the diameter of the smaller airways by mucosal swelling and results in an increased resistance to air flow. Bronchial lumens are further narrowed by the presence of retained secretions. The secretions and resultant inflammatory response cause an uneven distribution of increased resistance to air flow. Ventilation perfusion mismatches result in these regions of the lung. As the amount of retained secretions increases, total plugging of the bronchioli with distal absorption atelectasis occurs. The entire atelectatic process is reversible with proper mobilization of the retained secretions and re-aeration of the lung.

Miliary atelectasis occurs secondary to failure of the lungs to fully expand at normal intervals. The dependent sections of the lung are most affected and are usually situated along the lung base in normal nursing positions. The activity of the surfactant that normally reduces surface tension within the alveoli and aids in maintaining open alveoli is decreased by inactivity. In poorly ventilated areas, the available oxygen molecules diffuse into the blood from the alveoli at a greater rate than they can be replaced and this promotes collapse. High inspired oxygen concentrations accelerate the absorption process by reduction in alveolar nitrogen. The nitrogen molecules hold the alveoli open longer because they are poorly absorbed into the blood. When the gas in the alveoli is completely absorbed, the air spaces collapse and contribute to the right-to-left pulmonary shunt enhancing hypoxic inspiratory failure (116, 241, 248).

PULMONARY EDEMA

Pulmonary edema is an abnormal accumulation of fluid in either the lung interstitium or alveolar spaces. It is produced by a wide variety of diseases as a final common pathophysiologic response (29, 223, 239, 259, 260). The normal blood free lung weighs about 500 gm in an adult human and is composed of 80% water. Normal lung fluid is a filtrate crossing the capillary endothelium into the lung interstitium. The fluid then flows from the alveolar interstitial spaces into the perivascular interstitium and lymph channels. This forms a continuous irrigation of the lung parenchyma with a flow rate of approximately 20 ml/hr. Endothelial damage enhances the outward hydrostatic flow of fluid. Oncotic forces oppose the hydrostatic forces and thus encourage a fluid balance favoring the intravascular space and a relatively dry pulmonary parenchyma (259, 287).

The etiology of pulmonary edema can be divided into two major pathologic processes: increased capillary hydrostatic pressure and increased capillary permeability (104, 257). Increased capillary hydrostatic pressure is the most common cause of lung edema (7, 186). It occurs as a consequence of left ventricular failure with myocardial infarction the most common cause. Mitral stenosis, functional obstruction of the pulmonary venous system, systemic hypertension, or cardiac contusion can also produce left ventricular failure with increased capillary hydrostatic pressure and edema. The capillary permeability is preserved and the protein content of the edema fluid is low with the ratio of the protein in the edema fluid to the protein in the serum being less than 0.46. The hydrostatic mechanism for production of lung edema is documented by right-heart catherization with the Swan-Ganz pulmonary artery catheter. The pulmonary artery wedge pressure (PAWP) in hydrostatic-produced edema is elevated with 20 to 25 torr range typically measured (257). An elevation in PAWP, however, does not always produce pulmonary edema (8).

Two stages of parenchymal edema can be separated roentgenographically. In the interstitial stage, there are ring shadows in the hilar regions and Kerley A, B, and C lines (143). As pulmonary edema advances to the alveolar stage, coalescence of shadows and air bronchograms becomes evident. It is thought that the progression from interstitial to alveolar edema results from excess fluid in the interstitial space flooding the alveolar air sacs and causing local collapse.

Pulmonary edema caused by increased capillary permeability occurs due to several different insults to the lung parenchyma. Once the capillary endothelial lining is damaged, edema fluid with a protein content approaching that of serum leaks out of the capillaries and into the lung interstitium. This is the predominant type of edema in acute respiratory distress syndrome (ARDS). The capillary endothelial damage is typically caused by a pathologic process and at first no lung damage is perceived by the patient or measured by chest x-ray. This asymptomatic clinical course is followed 6 to 36 hours later by acute respiratory failure, with interstitial and alveolar edema prominent on chest films. The protein content of the edema fluid compared to the protein content of the serum is greater than 0.72. The pathophysiology and treatment of ARDS is discussed in the next section (17, 222).

Other causes of pulmonary edema include a decreased colloid oncotic pressure as occurs in hypoproteinemia following liver failure, the nephrotic syndrome, or overhydration with intravenous fluids (55). Pulmonary edema is likely when the systemic colloid oncotic pressure is less than 4 torr greater than the PAWP (217). An extremely negative interstitial pressure can cause lung edema. Clinically this occurs during acute bronchial asthma or periods of total airway obstruction, such as hanging or occlusion of the upper airway. In these settings, an extremely negative pleural pressure is generated by the patient attempting to breathe through the physiologically occluded upper airway. Lymphatic obstruction can cause lung edema in cases of carcinoma or silicosis. Pulmonary edema can also be produced by high altitude exposure.

Pathophysiologic changes secondary to head injury and brain damage can result in formation of pulmonary edema by a process termed neurogenic pulmonary edema (NPE) (73–76, 92, 97, 129, 143, 215, 227, 232, 269, 277, 298). NPE is thought to be caused by either a massive sympathetic discharge to the entire vascular bed of the body or a release of catecholamines that results in generalized vasoconstriction with systemic hypertension. An acute elevation in systemic arterial pressure results in initial left ventricular overload, followed by engorgement of the pulmonary veins, and finally pulmonary artery hypertension. The pulmonary capillary bed is subjected to increased capillary pressure by hypertension in both the pulmonary venous and pulmonary ar-

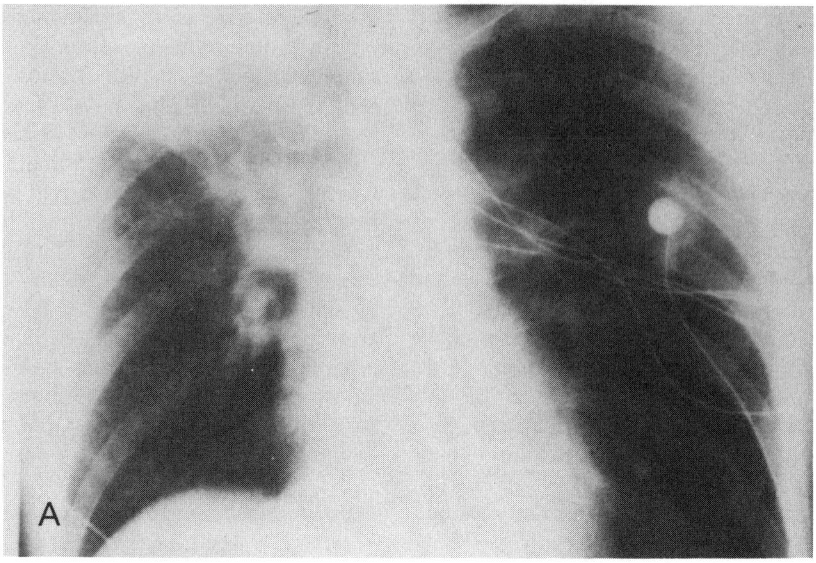

Figure 1.6. Regional pulmonary atelectasis. *A)* Partial right upper lobe atelectasis with elevation of the minor fissure. *B)* Partial right lower lobe atelectasis marginated by the major fissure. The right middle lobe remains aerated because the right cardiac border is evident. *C)* Partial left lower lobe atelectasis projecting in the cardiac shadow from the retrocardiac region.

terial systems. Direct endothelial damage results with extravasation of serum and blood into the interstitial spaces and eventually into the alveoli (28, 232, 298). Once the capillary endothelial damage has occurred, a further progression of pulmonary dysfunction can produce ARDS. The incidence of NPE is reported from a low of two cases per 2,100 serious head injuries to a high of 17 in 20 victims with fatal gunshot wound to the head (109, 251).

In experimental studies, cervical cord transection is protective against the subsequent development of NPE (277). Hypothalamic dysfunction is hypothesized as the origin of the massive sympathetic response initiating NPE (218). The initiation of the sympathetic response and systemic hypertension often occurs at the scene of an accident and may precede any medical observation. Thus, endothelial damage to the lung may occur before medical therapy can be begun. NPE with hypoxic respiratory failure develops on a delayed basis 6 to 36 hours following the endothelial damage.

The diagnosis of NPE is made following CNS damage by the presence of hypoxic respiratory failure relatively refractory to oxygen therapy. The treatment of NPE involves general cardiopulmonary support as indicated by monitoring with arterial and Swan-Ganz catheters. Cardiac output and PAWP measurements along with hemodynamic assessment guide the fluid and inotropic therapy. Alpha-receptor blocking agents have been investigated in animals as a means to prevent NPE by blocking the systemic hypertensive response to circulating catecholamines (28, 169, 277). Direct myocardial function is often affected by the hemodynamic changes that precipitated the neurogenic pulmonary edema and inotropic support is often required to elevate the cardiac output and enhance left ventricular function.

ACUTE RESPIRATORY DISTRESS SYNDROME

Acute respiratory distress syndrome (ARDS) is the common pathologic response of the lung parenchyma to a variety of pulmonary insults (193, 221). More than 150,000 cases of ARDS occur annually in the United States. The causes of ARDS share in common damage to the pulmonary endothelium with a subsequent plasma leak into the alveoli. Common conditions associated with ARDS in neurologic patients are listed in Table 1.7 (241). ARDS can be caused by processes directly damaging the lung parenchyma or by remote disease processes that cause indirect damage to the lung. Direct dam-

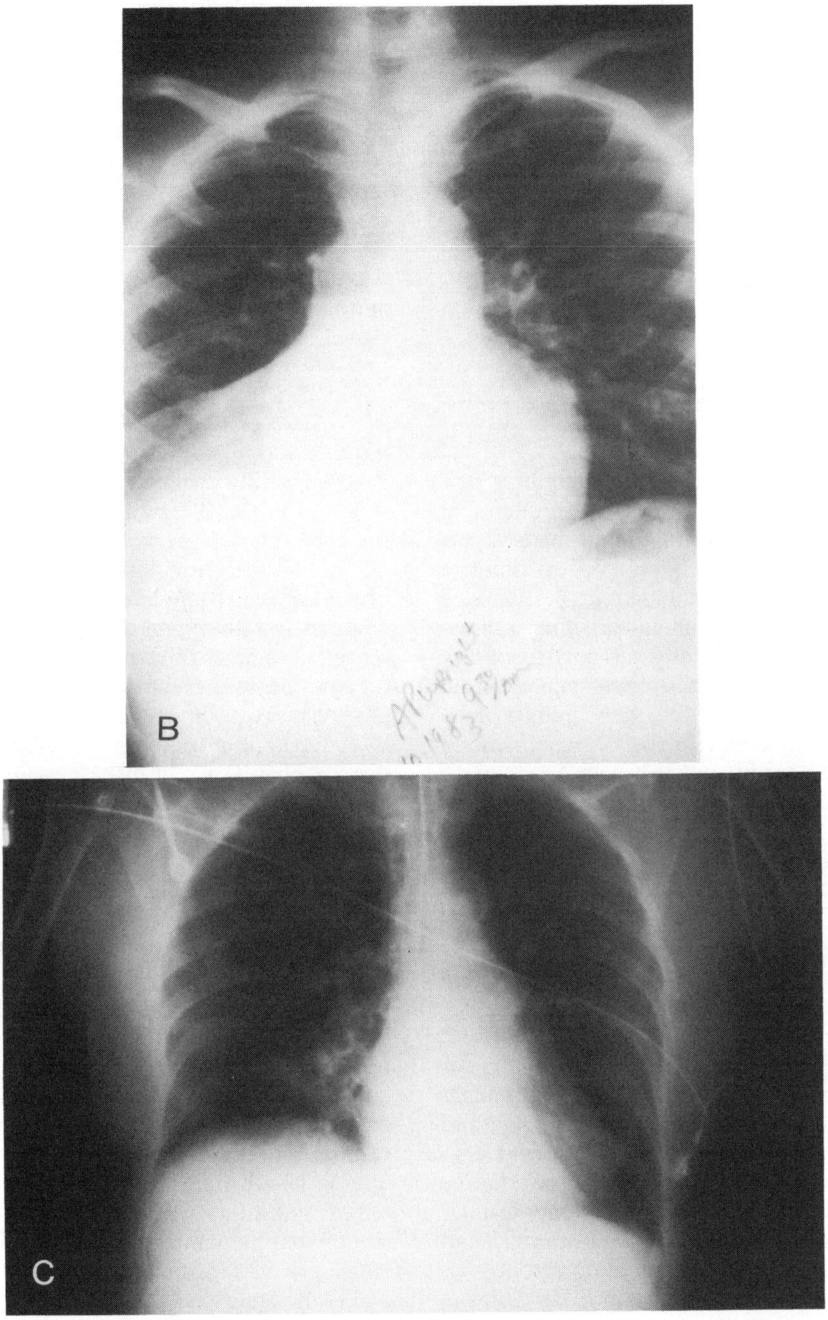

Figure 1.6 *B* and 1.6 *C*.

TABLE 1.7.
Common Causes in Neurologic Patients for Acute Respiratory Distress Syndrome (ARDS)

Pulmonary contusion
Aspiration
Fat emboli syndrome
Smoke inhalation
Anaphylactic reaction
Neurogenic pulmonary edema
Pneumonia
Bacteremia
Radiation toxicity
Drowning
Complement system activation
Gram-negative sepsis
Massive trauma
Pancreatitis
Transfusions

age to the alveolar capillary membrane is caused by contusion, infection, or chemical agents. In aspiration, the acidity of the contents or the enzymes present is believed to produce the damage. In smoke inhalation, the damage is thought to be direct chemical injury. In radiation and oxygen toxicity, alveolar capillary damage is associated with free oxygen radicals. In near drowning, the alveolar capillary cells are damaged by either hypo- or hyperosmolar forces during fresh- and salt-water drowning, respectively. Pulmonary infections cause inflammation and local accumulation of toxins from the micro-organism; the host immune responses include activation of the complement system that further enhances damage to the alveolar lining (17, 130, 136, 205, 301).

ARDS is also associated with several disorders that do not directly affect the pulmonary parenchyma. Alveolar capillary injury is produced through blood-borne mediators or massive hemodynamic changes. Complement activation causes neutrophils to aggregate and these clumps are filtered in the pulmonary capillary bed where they release toxic substances that locally injure the capillary membrane. Gram-negative sepsis, massive trauma, and pancreatitis all activate the complement system. In the fat emboli syndrome, fat globules are filtered by the pulmonary capillaries where lipases digest the emboli and produce local endothelial damage. Massive transfusions have been implicated in forming platelet-leukocyte aggregates that are filtered by the pulmonary capillaries, obstructing the microcirculation, and damaging the endothelium. The massive hemodynamic changes associated with the production of neurogenic pulmonary edema can also lead to endothelial damage and the ARDS picture (17, 301).

The mortality rate for ARDS and ARDS combined with multiple organ failure was investigated in an 18-month study in nine medical centers covering 686 patients. The respiratory failure entrance criteria of the study required patients with transtracheal airway, PEEP for greater than 24 hours, and inspired oxygen concentration greater than or equal to 50%. The overall mortality of the patients was 68%. Patients over 65 years of age had a poorer prognosis with a mortality of 81% overall and 68% in the absence of multiple organ failure. The entire group had a 41% mortality when only respiratory failure was present, 50% when respiratory failure plus one other organ was involved, 72% mortality when respiratory failure and two other organs were involved, an 84% mortality when respiratory failure and three other organs were involved, and a 100% mortality when respiratory failure was combined with four other organ systems (198, 294).

The pathophysiology of ARDS has four distinct phases: latent disease, acute interstitial edema, acute intra-alveolar edema, and subacute chronic fibrosis. The latent period can last from a few hours to 48 hours. During this phase there is little evidence of pulmonary failure clinically or on blood-gas analysis. Ultrastructural evidence, however, indicates the presence of damage to the pulmonary capillary endothelial cells (17). The clinical picture of the patient is dominated by the primary disorder in this phase of the disease. In the acute interstitial edema phase, arterial blood-gas analysis demonstrates a respiratory alkalosis with hypoxic respiratory failure. The chest film remains normal or demonstrates minimally increased interstitial markings. The pulmonary capillary membranes are damaged and high protein interstitial edema accumulates. Lung compliance is markedly decreased (see Fig. 1.2*C*) and a ventilation-perfusion mismatch is present causing hypoxemic respiratory failure. The decrease in compliance increases the work of breathing and intubation with mechanical ventilation is necessary.

In the intra-alveolar phase of ARDS, arterial blood-gas analysis reveals severe arterial hypoxemia with an elevated $(A\text{-}a)O_2$ gradient that is unresponsive to supplemental oxygen. During this phase many alveoli are completely filled with high protein content edema fluid. The functional residual capacity (FRC) is decreased along with the lung compliance. When the alveoli in a section of lung completely fill with high protein fluid the ventilation-perfusion mismatch converts to a right-to-left physiologic shunt (56). Type I alveolar cells undergo cytoplasmic changes in responses to hypoxemia that open cellular junctions and permit interstitial fluid to enter the air spaces. When type II cells are damaged, surfactant production is compromised. Damage to the alveolar cells is compounded by a decrease in the blood and oxygen supply available to them. Chest films in this stage demonstrate a diffuse fluffy pattern of pulmonary edema (241).

The subacute chronic fibrosis stage of ARDS develops when recovery from the pulmonary failure cannot be achieved within the first few days. In such patients, hyaline membranes appear in the interalveolar spaces. If the primary disease process can be aborted and the respiratory failure reversed, a complete resolution of ARDS lung pathology is possible. However, if ARDS continues, fibrogenesis begins and progresses to pulmonary fibrosis over the next few weeks. This process begins with destruction of the normal alveolar capillary structures and replacement with interstitial fibrosis. The ventilation/perfusion mismatch becomes severe and lung compliance is further decreased. Peak ventilator pressures necessary to ventilate the patient require progressive increases to provide adequate gas exchange. The arterial blood gases show a progressive widening of the $(A\text{-}a)O_2$ gradient. With increasing respiratory failure, carbon dioxide accumulation becomes a predominant feature. The chest film demonstrates increasing fibrosis and edema and CT of the lung demonstrates parenchymal opacification and cystic changes. During this stage, high frequency ventilation or high frequency ventilation combined with pressure cycle ventilation may be clinically useful in providing enhanced gas exchange. Pneumothorax secondary to high ventilation pressures are common in these patients. Mortality in this group is high and results from either complications of the primary disease, multiple organ failure, or massive pulmonary failure.

ARDS is distinguished from CPE by analysis of PAWP. In ARDS the PAWP is typically normal, less than 12 torr, and the pulmonary artery diastolic minus pulmonary capillary wedge pressure gradient will be increased due to the increase in pulmonary vascular resistance. The caliber of the pulmonary vessels in ARDS is reduced in areas of consolidation and accounts for the increased pulmonary resistance. In CPE the PAWP is usually increased over 15 torr with a pulmonary artery diastolic minus PAWP gradient of less than 5 torr indicating no increase in the pulmonary vascular resistance (257, 274).

The treatment of ARDS involves both reversal of the initiating disorder responsible for the alveolar capillary injury and support for the pathophysiologic consequence of ARDS. Treatment of the initiating disorder varies with the etiology: antibiotics for bacterial infections, volume replacement for hypovolemic shock, and hemodynamic management of increased sympathetic outflow following neurologic injury. There is no treatment to block the alveolar capillary injury. There is some evidence to suggest that high dose corticosteroids augment the C5A induced neutrophil aggregation component of the capillary damage (120).

The pathophysiologic consequences of ARDS can be minimized by controlling the amount of pulmonary edema and correcting the respiratory failure. The pulmonary edema is managed by a relative state of intravascular hypovolemia produced by diuretics. Inotropic support may be necessary if left ventricular function is compromised due to initial trauma or the stress of the precipitating disease. Colloids have not been shown to be of great benefit in this form of pulmonary edema because the alveolar capillary injury does not confine the colloid to the vascular compartment.

The pathophysiologic consequences of ARDS gas exchange can be treated with a combined use of oxygen, mechanical ventilation, and PEEP. An increase in the inspired oxygen fraction improves the alveolar oxygen partial pressure and reverses a majority of the hypoxemia caused by ventilation/perfusion mismatch. As ARDS pathology progresses to alveolar collapse and significant right-to-left pulmonary shunting occurs, increasing the inspiratory oxygen fraction alone is ineffective in correcting the respiratory hypoxemia. Mechanical ventilatory support is necessary in these patients because the work of breathing with the low pulmonary compliance of ARDS and increased expiratory effort of PEEP therapy is too high for sustained spontaneous breathing.

PEEP increases the FRC in patients with ARDS by opening alveoli collapsed by edema fluid and low surfactant. As alveoli are opened with PEEP, this component of hypoxemia is reversed. The inspired concentration of oxygen can often be dramatically reduced after PEEP therapy is begun and this decreases pulmonary damage from oxygen toxicity. PEEP is a supportive measure and there is no evidence that PEEP affects the underlying alveolar capillary injury or decreases the amount of pulmonary edema present (257).

ASPIRATION

Aspiration is common in patients with a depressed level of consciousness (132). The incidence is high in the perioperative period and during intubation. Head-injured patients may aspirate at the scene of the accident. Aspiration is common in unconscious patients because they lack protective airway reflexes including an effective cough. Aspiration often begins a sequence of pneumonia, respiratory failure, ARDS, and death (301). The diagnosis of aspiration is made by combining the clinical signs of tachypnea, fever, localized rales; arterial blood gas evidence of hypoxemia; and chest films demonstrating localized or diffuse infiltrates that develop over a 24- to 36-hour period. Particulate matter must be removed by bronchoscopy whereas aspirated liquids can be adequately removed by nasotracheal suction techniques (1, 21, 241).

The acidity of the gastric contents causes a chemical pneumonitis with a pulmonary inflammatory reaction that reaches maximum severity between 12 and 36 hours following aspiration. If bacterial infection does not occur during this period, the inflammatory reaction decreases and is clinically insignificant by 72 hours postaspiration. Re-aspiration restarts the physiologic response cycle. The primary irritant in gastric aspiration appears to be the pH. Aspiration of gastric contents above a pH of 2.5 results in an inflammatory reaction similar to water aspiration, whereas an aspiration of gastric content below a pH below 2.5 produces a severe inflammatory reaction. The duration of the reaction is not affected by the pH of the solution. The aspiration of fluid with a pH of below 1.5 in humans results in a pneumonitis throughout both lung fields (38, 264, 299).

The diagnosis of massive aspiration in conscious patients is usually obvious; however, diagnosis in patients with a depressed level of consciousness and depressed gag and laryngeal reflexes is often difficult. Silent aspirations of repeated small quantities during neurologic recovery are common; they are minimized by frequent oral suctioning and management of the patients in the 30° to 45° head-up position. The clinical impact of aspiration is determined by the general medical status of the patient, the quantity of the aspirate, and the acidity of the aspiration (264).

The inflammatory effect of gastric aspiration occurs in the tracheobronchal tree and damages the mucosa on contact. A period of significant bronchospasm can immediately follow the aspiration and increase respiratory failure. The parenchymal effects of aspiration are maximal on the metabolic activities of the type II alveolar cells. A decrease in surfactant production is followed by an increase in interstitial edema. The compliance of the lung is thus decreased and an obligatory increase in the work of breathing occurs (299, 300).

Aspiration pneumonia produces interstitial edema, pulmonary consolidation, hypoxic respiratory failure, a reduction in FRC, and ARDS unless the pathologic progression is therapeutically aborted. Aspiration pneumonia is treated with supportive ventilatory therapy as required. Pulmonary therapy includes oxygen therapy, airway protection, bronchial hygiene, and PEEP when elements of ARDS appear. Prophylactic antibiotics for prevention of aspiration pneumonia following aspiration are not effective and may lead to the selection of resistant organisms. Chest films are followed on a daily basis and transtracheal suction cultures are obtained. When a pathologic organism is isolated, appropriate antibiotic therapy is instituted (189, 194).

Steroid therapy in aspiration pneumonia remains controversial. Advocates of steroid therapy point out that high doses of steroids can be administered for 2 days without undesirable systemic effects; steroids can theoretically decrease the inflammatory response; and the administration of steroids prior to the onset of a chemical inflammatory process is beneficial (194, 265, 299).

PULMONARY THROMBOEMBOLISM

Deep vein thrombosis with secondary pulmonary embolism is common in neurosurgical patients. Postoperative neurosurgical patients have been shown to have rates of pulmonary embolism that cannot be explained by immobilization secondary to hemiparesis or other neurologic deficits. Complications include embolization producing hypoxic respiratory failure. Venous thrombi that embolize to the pulmonary arterial circulation either partially or completely block blood flow to a portion of the pulmonary arterial tree. Secondary bronchoconstriction is one pathophysiologic response to regional occlusion of the pulmonary arteries. Blockage of pulmonary blood flow to regions of the lung results in areas that are ventilated and not perfused. The bronchoconstriction effect in adjacent areas produces additional ventilation/perfusion mismatch. Both of these effects contribute to a hypoxic respiratory failure with respiratory alkalosis. However, a normal arterial blood gas does not rule out subclinical pulmonary emboli (286, 292, 293).

Pulmonary thromboembolism arises almost exclusively from deep venous thrombosis in the lower extremities or in deep pelvic vessels. The risk factors for developing deep venous thrombosis and secondary pulmonary emboli include prolonged immobilization or direct trauma to the region. Neurologically compromised patients and head-injured patients in particular have been shown to be at high risk for the development of deep venous thrombosis. The risk of thromboembolism is especially great in patients with pituitary tumors and other intracranial neoplasms (272). Overall, the incidence of deep venous thrombosis in neurologic patients is between 23% and 40%. As much as half of the incidence is assigned to neurosurgical operative intervention (145, 268). A 15% incidence of pulmonary emboli has been reported in an autopsy series of patients with nervous system dysfunction (51).

The clinical diagnosis of pulmonary emboli in neurosurgical patients is often difficult because of the patient's inability to communicate early symptoms and is often delayed until irreversable symptoms appear. A massive pulmonary embolism presents with dyspnea, tachypnea, localized chest pain, hemoptysis, hypotension, and cardiovascular collapse. Blood gas analysis reveals hypoxemia with a normal carbon dioxide tension or mild respiratory alkalosis. Chest films are initially normal but progress to show a unilateral pleural infusion, infiltrates with atelectasis, or an elevated hemidiaphragm (39, 190). Diminished pulmonary vascular markings or pulmonary vascular congestion is sometimes also visualized on chest films. In a small percentage of patients the electrocardiogram demonstrates right heart strain. Fever is also common and temperatures from 38° to 40° C are typical. Pulmonary thromboembolism should be included in the differential of any fever of unknown origin in a debilitated patient (22, 178, 193).

Noninvasive studies on a serial basis remain the cornerstone of assessing unresponsive patients. Three separate modalities are used for the noninvasive diagnosis of deep venous thrombosis and subsequent pulmonary thromboembolism: measurement of the calves and thighs of the patients on a daily basis; Doppler and impedance plethysmography (IPG) on a weekly basis; and perfusion scan of the lung on a weekly basis with a ventilation scan when indicated. IPG measures the blood volume in the lower extremity. Venous occlusion with a tourniquet on the leg results in a large increase in the venous volume; when the tourniquet is released there is normally a rapid decrease in the venous blood volume due to venous outflow. The IPG utilizes the high electrical conductivity of blood to estimate the volume of blood in the limb. A venous function index is defined as the ratio of the venous outflow to the venous capacitance and is a sensitive indicator of deep venous thrombosis with a 90% to 95% accuracy of detecting occluding thrombi in the popliteal, femoral, or iliac veins. This test does not, however, detect nonoccluding thrombi higher in the venous system, superficial thrombi, or thrombi in the internal iliac veins. Furthermore, it may not be positive in the presence of good collateral circulation. The Doppler ultrasound investigation is performed in conjunction with the IPG. The ultrasound wave is reflected back from the moving red blood cells in the venous circuit with a shift in frequency proportional to the velocity of flow. The Doppler shifted signal is then transformed into an audible sound to assess presence of flow, variation of flow with respiration, and changes in flow with distal compression or release of compression. The test is operator-dependent but when performed by an experienced technician and combined with the IPG provides a high degree of accuracy and specificity for detecting deep venous thrombosis and is available at the bedside (43, 146, 268).

A nuclear medicine lung perfusion scan is the major diagnostic tool for evaluating pulmonary blood flow to diagnose pulmonary embolism. A normal perfusion scan is associated with a low probability of pulmonary embolism. However, despite high sensitivity the perfusion scan lacks specificity. The study rates only the probability of pulmonary embolism as being low, intermediate, or high. The low probability scan demonstrates single or multiple small matching defects on the ventilation study. The intermediate probability perfusion scan correlates with a 40% to 50% incidence of pulmonary embolism and demonstrates a single segmental defect or perfusion defect with some areas clearly identified on a ventilation scan. A high probability perfusion scan correlated with an 80% chance of pulmonary embolism and has multiple segmental defects with at least one of the defects greater than the size of a lung segment (25, 179, 180).

In patients with intermediate or high probability lung perfusion scans pulmonary arteriography is used to confirm the diagnosis (40, 54, 224). When the pulmonary arteriogram is positive, inferior venacavography is done at the same time to measure the size of the vena cava and visualize the position of the renal veins. A Kim-Ray Greenfield filter is inserted in the inferior vena cava below the renal veins under local anesthesia for protection from large pulmonary emboli when anticoagulation is contraindicated or when there is clinical evidence of continued embolization on anticoagulation (46, 295). Anticoagulation for deep venous thrombosis is delayed 2 weeks after head injury and at least a week after cranial surgery. Anticoagulation is started with heparin sodium for 7 days and then converted to warfarin sodium. Serial neurologic examinations and at least one CT scan after starting anticoagulation are used for early detection of intracranial bleeding (146, 268).

Although prophylaxis with low dose heparin has been reported to reduce the incidence of deep venous thrombosis in neurosurgical patients with minimum risk, the prophylactic use of low-dose heparin has produced complications in other patient groups that have been studied (50, 96, 246, 282). Low-dose heparin would appear to have no place in the early management of the multitrauma head-injured patient for fear of potentially fatal hemorrhagic complications. Pulsating boots of several types are reported to decrease the incidence of deep venous thrombosis and pulmonary emboli. It has been suggested that pulsating boots be used in neurologically impaired patients without spontaneous movement in their lower extremities and during all surgical procedures for effective prophylaxis against venous thrombosis and pulmonary embolism (146, 268).

PNEUMONIA

Pneumonia is the most common cause of acute respiratory failure and acute respiratory failure is the most common complication of pneumonia. The onset of bronchopulmonary infection is a potentially life-threatening event in patients with concurrent respiratory failure. Pneumonia occurs in 25% of patients with respiratory failure. The mortality rate of patients in respiratory failure with pneumonia is said to be 50% whereas without pneumonia it is only 3.8%. Nosocomial pneumonias with sepsis occurred in 70% of the fatal cases (263). Acute respiratory failure develops in 90% of patients with the onset of sepsis. In 45% of these cases sepsis originates from a pneumonia and in 55% an extrapulmonary source originated the sepsis (95).

Over 50% of nosocomial pneumonias are caused by Gram-negative bacilli (207). Staphylococci are the second most common bacteria associated with acute respiratory failure. In one series, Gram-positive organisms were isolated as the infective agent for pneumonia in 13% of cases while Gram-negative bacilli were identified in 87% of the cases. The mortality of Gram-negative pneumonias is reported from between 33% and 70%, while the mortality for pneumonia caused by Gram-positive organisms is around 5% (207, 263).

Colonization of the upper respiratory tract and oral pharynx by Gram-negative bacilli precedes Gram-negative pneumonia in over 90% of the cases. This colonization is caused by contaminated respiratory therapy equipment or hand transfer contamination. Even when these causative agents are eliminated, a high incidence of Gram-negative pneumonias persists since the principal reservoir for these organisms is the patient's own flora with contamination of the upper respiratory tract by organisms from the gut. Hand contact by medical personnel remains a significant source for the Gram-negative bacilli and can be decreased with hand washing between patient contact and strict sterile technique for endotracheal suctioning (127).

Gram-negative bacilli in normal individuals are only infrequently cultured from the oropharynx. Furthermore, when Gram-negative bacilli are inoculated into healthy subjects, persistent colonization does not occur. When the normal flora of the pharyngeal cavity is altered with antibiotic therapy, especially by obliteration of alpha-hemolytic streptococci, the growth of Gram-negative bacilli seems to be enhanced. Gram-negative bacilli are more adherent to oropharyngeal cells in the presence of an endotracheal tube.

The primary event in nosocomial pneumonias appears to be colonization of the upper respiratory tract. The colonized organisms then gain entry to the lung by aspiration of small quantities of pharyngeal secretions rather than the inhalation of airborne organisms. The clinical development of pneumonia depends upon the interaction between the bacterial inoculum and host defenses. Multiple factors may compromise the bacterial defenses of the lung in seriously ill patients: ARDS, hypoxia, hyperoxia, and pulmonary edema. The primary bacterial defense in the normal parenchyma is the macrophage. After macrophages ingest bacteria, polymorphonuclear chemotactic factor is released and attracts polymorphonuclear cells from the blood stream to aid in the pulmonary defense.

The diagnosis of pneumonia in the setting of acute respiratory failure is often difficult. Trauma and debilitated neurologic patients in the intensive care unit often have many underlying medical or surgical illnesses that can account for fever and leukocytosis. A daily chest film aids in the diagnosis of pneumonia by early detection and noting progression of pulmonary infiltrates. Since the upper respiratory tract is frequently colonized with Gram-negative organisms, even quantitative culture of respiratory secretions is not universally successful in identifying the causative organism of pneumonias. The technique of fiberoptic bronchoscopy with selective protected brush culture is useful in establishing the agent of bacterial pneumonia in many patients with acute respiratory failure.

Pneumonia is a presumptive diagnosis when a new infiltrate appears on a chest film with the concomitant onset of new signs and symptoms of infection. Plug atelectasis is differentiated from pneumonia on serial chest films with the aid of physical therapy since atelectasis clears, but pneumonia does not. A Gram stain of the tracheal secretions identifying bacteria and inflammatory polymorphonuclear cells favors pneumonia. An improving or stable blood gas analysis suggests an atelectatic process whereas an increase in hypoxic respiratory failure favors an active pulmonary infection (58).

CHRONIC OBSTRUCTIVE PULMONARY DISEASE

Chronic obstructive pulmonary disease (COPD) affects 450,000 new patients each year and has a prevalence of 15 million in the United States. COPD is the second most frequent diagnosis requiring support from the Social Security Disability fund. The recent rise in the prevalence and incidence of patients afflicted with COPD is due to cigarette smoking, air pollution, and increased longevity due to modern medical practice. COPD is a broad group of pulmonary dysfunction syndromes that have in common chronic airflow obstruction within the lungs. The clinical presentation of a typical patient is dominated by a mixture of chronic obstructive bronchitis with centrilobular emphysema. Chronic bronchitis causes inflammation of the mucosal lining of the tracheobroncheal tree and in many cases permanent colonization of the lower respiratory tract. Centrilobular emphysema is an irreversible pulmonary disease. The intralobular septal walls are destroyed along with the connective tissue responsible for the elastic recoil of the lung. Large alveolar sacs with little elastic recoil result in an increase in the FRC and the airway resistance.

COPD is a progressive process consisting of some combination of emphysema, bronchitis, asthma, right heart failure, and left heart failure (118, 206, 255, 270).

Arterial blood gases provide an accurate assessment of respiratory failure in these patients. A patient with severe COPD has an elevated Pa_{CO_2}, a significantly decreased Pa_{O_2}, and a $(A\text{-}a)O_2$ gradient greater than 40 torr. The high $(A\text{-}a)O_2$ gradient with an increased Pa_{CO_2} results from the severe ventilation/perfusion mismatch of ineffective ventilation in the large distended alveolar sacs. The work of breathing in these individuals is so high that hyperventilation is eliminated as a physiologic method to correct the abnormalities (27, 284, 287).

Pulmonary treatment of patients with decompensated COPD starts with oxygen therapy. An increased inspired oxygen concentration increases the alveolar oxygen partial pressure which relaxes pulmonary artery vasoconstriction. The work required by the right side of the heart is decreased and right-sided heart failure improves. Beta-adrenergic antagonists and theophylline are useful therapeutically as bronchodilators and mucociliary escalators. Theophylline has the added value of increasing central nervous system respiratory drive, of having positive inotropic properties, and of increasing the diaphragmatic contractility. COPD patients in acute respiratory failure can have elevated systemic blood pressures, decreased renal blood flow, and right-sided heart failure. All of these effects favor extravasation of water into the tissues of the body. The increased edema in both the lung parenchyma and the brain is responsive to diuretics (41, 44, 80, 174, 206, 241).

BRONCHIAL ASTHMA

Bronchial asthma afflicts an estimated 3% to 6% of the United States population. Narrowing of the airways can be triggered by pharmacologic challenge or allergic response. Bronchial asthma has the potential for increasing the airway resistance with a reversible partial airway obstruction. Although an increase in the eosinophil count is commonly seen in asthmatics, the count is not helpful for diagnosis in acutely ill or traumatized patients. Diagnosis is based on two factors: a reversible airway obstruction quantified clinically as a decrease in the FEV_1 on pulmonary function testing and an above normal increase in airway responsiveness to drug challenge with an inhaled bronchodilator on FEV_1 tests. Flow-volume-pressure analysis of the ventilator delivered breaths can be analyzed to infer the resistance of the airway and to quantify treatment. A computer analysis scheme, as shown in Figure 1.2*B*, can harvest the signals from the respirator to provide flow-volume-pressure analysis of the respiratory dynamics and compliance to aid as a guide in the therapeutic management of these patients (172, 177, 228, 280, 282, 290).

Acute asthmatic attacks can be triggered in the intensive care unit environment by exposure to allergens such as drugs or linens; by the hyperdynamic state caused by sepsis; by histamine release from pulmonary tissue damage; by cholinergic medications used for inotropic therapy; by beta-blocking drugs used for cardiovascular therapy or diencephalic fits; and by emotional upset during disorientation, waking up, or ICU psychosis.

The arterial blood gas of an acute asthmatic attack demonstrates hypoxic respiratory insufficiency with respiratory alkalosis in contrast to COPD where CO_2 retention is common. Retention of CO_2 is seen only in asthma patients when severe airflow obstruction occurs. The FEV_1 in these cases is less than 20% and in many cases less than 10% of predicted normal values. Elevation in the Pa_{CO_2} during an acute asthma attack indicates a severe degree of airway flow obstruction requiring mechanical ventilation and pharmaceutical intravenous therapy (172, 176, 177, 287).

Asthma is associated with wheezing and chest rales. A prolonged expiratory phase suggests functional airway impairment. Conscious patients experience cough, shortness of breath, and a feeling of chest tightness. Although pulmonary wheezing is often caused by asthma other causes must be investigated and include: (*a*) pulmonary embolism; (*b*) passive congestion produced by left ventricular failure; (*c*) central airway obstruction in the thorax of a major bronchus due to a mucous plug; (*d*) extrathoracic upper airway obstruction such as a hematoma in the neck compressing the trachea; (*e*) aspiration of gastric contents; (*f*) COPD; and (*g*) bronchiolitis. The cause of pulmonary wheezing needs to be elucidated before specific therapy for bronchial asthma is instituted (172).

The treatment of an acute bronchial asthma attack is based on pharmacologic manipulation with one or a combination of the three main groups of drugs: adrenergic drugs, aminophylline, and corticosteroids. Beta-adrenergic agents and aminophylline act to reverse the bronchoconstrictive pathology of bronchial asthma. Subcutaneous injections of epinephrine or terbutaline provide rapid onset of bronchodilator activity. Metaproterenol can be administered by inhalation and has a predominant beta-2 adrenergic action (204, 220, 256). A loading dose of intravenous aminophylline is given initially followed by constant infusion. Blood levels are followed daily to assure the clinically optimal range of 15 to 18 μg/ml (126, 212, 289). Adverse reactions of aminophylline include nausea, vomiting, reflex cardiovascular changes, arrhythmia, hypotension, and seizures (172, 174). These drugs can complicate the cardiovascular management of critically ill patients.

Corticosteroids enhance the rate of improvement in airflow and are indicated when the obstruction is severe (5). They are utilized in combination with aminophylline or adrenergic drugs. Supplemental oxygen is used to correct the arterial hypoxemia produced by the ventilation-perfusion mismatch in asthma. The application of PEEP does not usually benefit patients with an increase in airway resistance. Chest percussion and postural drainage are not indicated when asthma is the predominant disease process; however, they are often useful in clearing secretions when bronchial asthma is superimposed on other pulmonary diseases (172).

THE FAT EMBOLI SYNDROME

Respiratory failure can occur secondary to the fat emboli syndrome. This is a rare clinical syndrome usually manifested after long bone fractures. Many other etiologies are hypothesized to initiate the fat emboli syndrome: blast injuries, external cardiac massage, burns, seizures, acute fatty liver syndromes, steroid therapy, renal transplantation, and simulated high altitude. The hypoxic respiratory failure can range from a subclinical reduction in the Pa_{O_2} to severe ARDS. The clinical onset of the pulmonary dysfunction is generally delayed from 1 to 3 days in the fat emboli syndrome with resolution in approximately 1 week. Symptoms include mental change, cough, and dyspnea. Fat globules enter the circulation from either the fracture site or by release of chylomicrons from fat stores in response to circulating catecholamine levels. The circulating fat globules are then filtered in the pulmonary capillaries where serum lipases hydrolize them. The hydrolized products cause direct damage to the pulmonary endothelium and are capable of triggering the kinin cascade causing additional endothelial damage. When respiratory failure is severe, supportive care similar to ARDS therapy is utilized. A characteristic petechial rash appears on the upper torso, axillae, conjunctiva, and retina and aids in the diagnosis. The chest film demonstrates pulmonary edema. Laboratory examination of the serum discloses abnormalities in the serum and urinary lipase, elevation in the blood urea nitrogen and bilirubin, and hypocalcemia. Fat globules can be visualized in either the urine or sputum. Pulmonary function testing reveals a decrease in both diffusion capacity and compliance (20, 34, 82, 107, 116, 233, 250a, 281).

PULMONARY EFFECTS OF SPINAL CORD INJURY

Physiologic transection of the cervical spine cord interrupts the sympathetic outflow to the body and results in hypotension and brachycardia. Additionally, the innervation of the intercostal muscles is lost. Thus, these patients are dependent on the phrenic nerve innervating the diaphragm and the cranial nerves innervating the accessory muscles for respiration. In high cervical spinal cord injuries the outflow to the phrenic nerve can be damaged either directly or as a result of ascending vasculitis or edema. In the past, patients with injuries at or above C3 rarely survived, but with rapid institution of cardiopulmonary resuscitation by paramedic teams these patients are reaching the emergency room. Similarly, removal of intramedullary cord tumors in the high cervical region has become a not infrequent microsurgical exercise and these patients often need temporary respiratory support (6, 241).

Hypoxemia from compromised muscular effort occurs in up to 50% of cord-injured patients at C5 and above (252). Cervical cord-injured patients can be assessed at the bedside with a forced vital capacity (FVC) and a measurement of the peak NIF. These values are followed on a daily basis to serve as an early warning of respiratory failure or upward progression of the cord lesion in a C5 quadriplegic. The weaning of all high quadriplegics is difficult after an operation when some postoperative atelectasis is present or when the vital capacity is less than 1 liter. After an anterior cervical fusion, local edema or hematoma in the anterior neck can compromise the function of auxiliary muscles and hence decrease respiratory function. Tracheal suctioning in spinal injury patients may induce reflex brachycardia and cardiac arrest from the severe vagovagal response in the sympathectomized state. Attempts at intubation can also trigger bradycardia; intravenous atropine effectively prevents these complications (6, 23, 93).

The establishment of an airway in a patient with compromised pulmonary function and a spinal cord injury requires special consideration. The intubation can be performed safely with the patient in Gardner-Wells tongs and the neck aligned except in the most unstable fractures. Fiberoptic laryngoscope intubation eliminates all neck motion but is more time consuming and hence not useful in emergencies. Tracheostomy is to be avoided because its presence compromises the performance of an anterior cervical fusion. Muscle relaxants are not used for intubation without radiographic verification that the fracture is reduced and that the fragments will not move compromising the neural canal during the intubation procedure. Spasm of the neck muscles sometimes splints the fracture and provides the only acute stabilization preventing further cord damage. Extreme caution is used during intubation because muscle paralysis and neck manipulation can result in irrepairable damage to the spinal cord. In some instances, transtracheal ventilation with intermittant jets of O_2 under high pressure is a useful lifesaving maneuver while preparing for a definitive airway (48).

Hypotension following cervical spinal cord injury results from a loss of sympathetic tone in the venous circuit with pooling of blood. When the hypotension is reversed with intravascular volume expansion, pulmonary edema often results. The use of low dose dopamine (3 to 5 μg/kg/min) will restore the blood pressure to normal and eliminates the need for large volumes of fluids to reverse the hypotension. Pulmonary edema with hypoxic respiratory failure is prevented in the large majority of cord-injured patients (93, 296).

The respiratory function in spinal-cord-injured patients is also compromised by other factors. The abdominal distention secondary to loss of abdominal motor tone and decreased gut mobility effectively elevates the diaphragms and further compromises the respiratory effort. Many patients require nursing with cervical traction for many days or weeks and dependent atelectasis forms from the inability to fully mobilize the patient. Pulmonary infections can occur in atelectatic areas when they persist for many days. Interruption of normal respiration with a decrease in the vital capacity and impaired coughing prevent periodic expansion of the alveoli in the atelectatic regions. The use of a rocking bed, resisted diaphragmatic breathing to gradually increase vital capacity, postural drainage on a turning frame, and incentive spirometry are all respiratory therapies that aid in the prevention of pulmonary complications (6).

A phrenic pacemaker may help some spinal-cord-injured patients above C3 without sufficient respiratory drive. The phrenic nerves need to be intact from the anterior horn-cell through the neuromuscular junction in the diaphragm for the use of such devices. In selected cases, phrenic nerve stimulation is superior to long-term positive pressure respiratory maintenance (303).

NONPENETRATING CHEST WALL TRAUMA

Nonpenetrating trauma to the chest is commonly associated with head trauma in motor vehicle accidents. The driver is typically not wearing a seatbelt and is thrown forward against the steering wheel. Penetrating injuries of the chest have immediate and severe consequences secondary to intrapulmonary hemorrhage or pneumothorax (297). However, nonpenetrating injuries to the chest can result in severe pulmonary injuries that are also life-threatening. Initial laboratory data may underestimate the severity of these injuries. A chest film is the single most useful test in determining pulmonary injury. Repeat films can detect delayed consolidations or fluid accumulation.

The most common injury to the thoracic region is a rib fracture with the ribs near the middle of the thoracic cage being most frequently fractured. The fractures usually occur along the posterior axillary line. Rib fractures can be discovered on physical examination by localized tenderness or pain on pressure of the chest in either the anterior/posterior or lateral planes. Some rib fractures may not be disclosed on the initial films but are visualized on subsequent studies. Atelectasis and pneumonia commonly occur following rib fracture due to splinting of respiration and an ineffective cough secondary to the pain. There is a local decrease in surfactant generation secondary to diminished ventilation and secretions are poorly cleared. Alveolar collapse and subsequent secondary infections in patients are common. Other complications of rib fractures include: flail chest syndrome, pneumothorax, pneumomediastinum, hemothorax, pulmonary contusion, pulmonary hematoma, traumatic pulmonary thrombosis, bronchial fracture, diaphragmatic injury, esophageal injury, and aortic rupture. Treatment typically includes respiratory support with PEEP until resolution (117, 151, 208).

DIAPHRAGMATIC DISORDERS

Traumatic diaphragmatic ruptures occur following direct penetration or blunt nonpenetrating trauma to the abdomen or chest. Ninety-five percent of all traumatic diaphragmatic hernias occur on the left side. It is believed that the liver on the right side provides some protection from the transmitted forces secondary to abdominal compression. The typical diaphragmatic injury is a tear in the radial direction of the posterior lateral section on the left side of the diaphragm. This represents a massive injury to the body and the multiple trauma injury aspects usually dominate the initial clinical presentation. Physical signs of traumatic diaphragmatic rupture include respiratory distress, cyanosis, and hypotension. Patients who are conscious complain of pain in the left upper quadrant, left lower thorax, or left shoulder. Suggestive signs on the chest films include: gas densities above the level of the diaphragm; atelectasis adjacent to an arch-like shadow; presence of air fluid levels in the left hemithorax; and displacement of the mediastinal structures to the right. The abdominal contents that herniate into the chest cavity often produce respiratory distress by preventing full expansion of the lung (151).

Diaphragmatic dysfunction can also result from diaphragmatic paralysis. The phrenic nerve can be interrupted anywhere from its origin in the cervical spinal cord to its termination at the neuromuscular junctions of the diaphragm. Diaphragmatic paralysis following trauma occurs from surgical section of the phrenic nerve during urgent chest surgery or directly from thoracic trauma. Bilateral diaphragmatic paralysis is rare except in spinal cord injuries with a high cervical lesion. Patients with bilateral paralysis require assisted ventilation. The accessory muscles of inspiration all show hyperactivity with bilateral diaphragmatic paralysis. Pulmonary function testing reveals a reduction in TLC and VC. Fluoroscopic examination of the diaphragm can be used to observe motion and diagnose paralysis (165, 175, 241, 287).

ACKNOWLEDGMENTS

The authors thank Dr. Stuart Mirvis for the x-rays; Joan Stoklosa for the respiratory graphics; Diana Ruhling for typing the manuscript; and Robin Pollard for assistance with references.

REFERENCES

1. Abdulmajid, O. A., Abdelmomen, M. E., Motaweh, M. M., *et al.* Aspirated foreign bodies in the tracheobronchial tree: Report of 250 cases. Thorax, *31:* 635, 1976.
2. Acres, J. C., and Kryger, M. H. Clinical significance of pulmonary function tests: Upper airway obstruction. Chest, *80:* 207, 1981.
3. Adorato, D. C., Gildenberg, P. L., Ferrarro, C. M., *et al.* Pathophysiology of intravenous air embolism in dogs. Anesthesiology, *49:* 120–127, 1978.
4. Aidinis, S. J., Lafferty, J., and Shapiro, H. M. Intracranial responses to PEEP. Anesthesiology, *45:* 275–286, 1976.
5. Albert, R. K., Martin, T. R., and Lewis, S. W. Controlled clinical trial of methylprednisolone in patients with chronic bronchitis and acute respiratory insufficiency. Ann. Intern. Med., *92:* 753, 1980.
6. Albin, M. S. Acute spinal cord trauma. In: *Textbook of Critical Care*, edited by W. C. Shoemaker, W. L. Thompson, and P. R. Holbrook, pp. 928–936. W. B. Saunders, Philadelphia, 1984.
7. Alper, J. S., Irwin, R. S., and Dalen, J. E. Pulmonary hypertension. Curr. Probl. Cardiol., *5:* 1, 1981.
8. Anderson, F. L., McDonnell, M. A., Tsagaris, T. J., *et al.* Absence of clinical pulmonary edema de-

spite elevated wedge pressures. Arch. Intern. Med., *141:* 1207, 1981.

9. Anderson, W. H., Dossett, B. E., and Hamilton, G. L. Prevention of postoperative pulmonary complications. J.A.M.A., *186:* 763, 1963.
10. Andrews, J. C., Jr. The clinical roles of pulmonary function testing. Med. Clin. North Am., *63:* 355–377, 1979.
11. Apuzzo, M. L. J., Weiss, M. H., Petersons, V., *et al.* Effect of positive end expiratory pressure ventilation on intracranial pressure in man. J. Neurosurg., *46:* 227–232, 1977.
12. Argov, Z., and Mastaglia, F. L. Disorders of neuromuscular transmission caused by drugs. N. Engl. J. Med., *301:* 409, 1979.
13. Asch, M. J., Dell, R. B., and Williams, G. S. Time course for development of respiratory compensation in metabolic acidosis. J. Lab. Clin. Med., *73:* 610–615, 1969.
14. Ashbaugh, D. G., Bigelow, D. B., Petty, T. L., *et al.* Acute respiratory distress in adults. Lancet, *2:* 319, 1967.
15. Aubier, M., Troyer, A. D., Sampson, M., Macklem, P. T., *et al.* Aminophylline improves diaphragm contraction. N. Engl. J. Med., *305:* 249, 1981.
16. Auffant, R. A., Shuptrine, J. R., Hotchkiss, R. S., *et al.* Effects of HFV vs IPPV on cerebral perfusion pressure and cardiopulmonary function. Anesthesiology, *57:* A88, 1982.
17. Bachofen, M., and Weibel, E. R. Structural alterations of lung parenchyma in the adult respiratory distress syndrome. Clin. Chest. Med., *3:* 35–56, 1982.
18. Baehreniltz, S., and Hedenstierna, G. Differential ventilation and selective positive end-expiratory pressure: Effects on patients with acute bilateral lung disease. Anesthesiology, *61:* 511–517, 1984.
19. Baigelman, W., and O'Brien, J. C. Pulmonary effect of head trauma. Neurosurgery, *9:* 729–740, 1981.
20. Banyai, A. L. Fat embolism. Chest, *69:* 355, 1976.
21. Bartlett, J. G., and Gorbach, S. L. The triple threat of aspiration pneumonia. Chest, *68:* 560, 1975.
22. Bell, W. R., Simon, T. L., and Demetts, D. L. The clinical features of submassive and massive pulmonary emboli. Am. J. Med., *62:* 355, 1977.
23. Bellamy, R., Potts, F., and Stauffer, E. Respiratory complications in traumatic quadriplegia. J. Neurosurg., *39:* 596, 1973.
24. Berger, A. J., Mitchell, R. A., and Severinghaus, J. W. Regulation of respiration. N. Engl. J. Med., *297:* 92–97, 138–143, 194–201, 1977.
25. Biello, D. R., *et al.* Interpretation of indeterminate lung scintigrams. Radiology, *133:* 189, 1979.
26. Bone, R. C. Pressure-volume measurements in detection of bronchospasm and mucus plugging in acute respiratory failure. Respir. Care, *21:* 620, 1976.
27. Bone, R. C., and Pierce, A. K., and Johnson, R. L., Jr. Controlled oxygen administration in acute respiratory failure in chronic obstructive pulmonary disease: A reappraisal. Am. J. Med., *65:* 896, 1978.
28. Bowers, R. E., McKeen, C. R., Park, B. E., *et al.* Increased pulmonary vascular permeability follows intracranial hypertension in sheep. Am. Rev. Respir. Dis., *119:* 637–641, 1979.
29. Boysen, P. G., and Modell, J. H. Pulmonary edema. In: *Textbook of Critical Care*, edited by W. C. Shoemaker, W. L. Thompson, and P. R. Holbrook, pp. 238–241. W. B. Saunders, Philadelphia, 1984.
30. Brackett, C. E., and Bone, R. C. Pulmonary care and complications. In: *Neurological Surgery*, Ed. 2, edited by J. R. Youmans, pp. 1004–1030. W. B. Saunders, Philadelphia, 1982.
31. Bradley, R. D., Spencer, G. T., and Semple, S. J. G. Rate of change of CSF PCO2 and (HCO3) in acid-base disturbances in man. In: *Symposium on Cerebrospinal Fluid and the Regulation of Ventilation*, edited by C. M. Brooks, F. F. Kao, B. B. Lloyd, pp. 281–292. Davis, Philadelphia, 1965.
32. Brantigan, C. O., and Grow, J. B. Cricothyroidotomy: Elective use in respiratory problems requiring tracheotomy. J. Thorac. Cardiovasc. Surg., *71:* 72–81, 1976.
33. Bryan-Brown, C. W. Gas transport and delivery. In: *Textbook of Critical Care*, edited by W. C. Shoemaker, W. L. Thompson, and P. R. Holbrook, pp. 210–218. W. B. Saunders, Philadelphia, 1984.
34. Burgher, L. W., *et al.* Fat embolism and the adult respiratory distress syndrome. Mayo Clin. Proc., *49:* 107, 1974.
35. Burrows, B., Knudson, R. J., Quan, S. F., *et al.* *Respiratory Disorders: A Pathophysiologic Approach*, 209 pp. Year Book Medical Publishers, Chicago, 1983.
36. Butler, P. M., Fairley, H. B., and Isenberg, M. D. Optimum end-expiratory airway pressure in patients with acute pulmonary failure. N. Engl. J. Med., *292:* 284, 1975.
37. Butler, W. J., Bohn, D. J., Bryan, A. C., *et al.* Ventilation by high frequency oscillation in humans. Anesth. Analg., *59:* 577–584, 1980.
38. Bynum, L. J., and Pierce, A. K. Pulmonary aspiration of gastric contents. Am. Rev. Respir. Dis., *114:* 1129, 1976.
39. Bynum, L. J., and Wilson, J. E. Radiographic features of pleural effusions in pulmonary embolism. Am. Rev. Respir. Dis., *117:* 829, 1978.
40. Bynum, L. J., Wilson, J. E., Christensen, E., *et al.* Radiographic techniques for balloon-occlusion pulmonary angiography. Radiology, *133:* 518, 1979.
41. Campbell, E. J. M. The management of acute respiratory failure in chronic bronchitis and emphysema. Am. Rev. Respir. Dis., *96:* 626–639, 1967.
42. Carroll, R. G., *et al.* Recommended performance specifications for cutted endotracheal and tracheostomy tubes. Crit. Care Med., *1:* 155, 1973.
43. Cheely, R., *et al.* The role of noninvasive tests versus pulmonary angiography in the diagnosis of pulmonary embolism. Am. J. Med., *70:* 17–22, 1981.
44. Chester, E. H., Racz, I. Barlow, P. B., and Baum, G. L. Bronchodilator therapy: Comparison of acute response to three methods of administration. Chest, *62:* 394–399, 1972.
45. Christensen, M. S. Acid-base changes in CSF and blood, and blood volume changes following prolonged hyperventilation in man. Br. J. Anaesth., *46:* 348–357, 1974.
46. Cimochowski, G. E., *et al.* Greenfield filter versus Mobin-Uddin umbrella: The continuing quest for

the ideal method of vena caval interruption. J. Thorac. Cardiovasc. Surg., *79:* 358–365, 1980.
47. Civetta, J. M. A new look at the starling equation. Crit. Care Med., *7:* 84–91, 1979.
48. Collicott, P. E. *Advanced Trauma Life Support Course for Physicians*, 525 pp. American College of Surgeons, Chicago, 1984.
49. Comroe, J. J. *Physiology of Respiration*, 316 pp. Year Book Medical Publishers, Chicago, 1965.
50. Coon, W. W., and Willis, P. W. Hemorrhagic complications of anticoagulation therapy. Arch. Intern. Med., *133:* 386, 1974.
51. Coon, W. W. Risk factors in pulmonary embolism. Surg. Gynecol. Obstet., *143:* 385–390, 1976.
52. Crockard, H. A., Coppel, D. L., and Morrow, W. F. K. Evaluation of hyperventilation in treatment of head injuries. Br. Med. J., *4:* 634–640, 1973.
53. Cullen, D. J., and Caldera, D. L. Incidence of ventilator-induced pulmonary barotrauma in critically ill patients. Anesthesiology, *50:* 185–190, 1979.
54. Dalen, J. E., *et al.* Pulmonary angiography in acute pulmonary embolism: Indications, techniques, and results in 367 patients. Am. Heart. J., *81:* 175–185, 1971.
55. DaLuz, P. L., Shubin, H., Weil, M. H., *et al.* Pulmonary edema related to changes in colloid osmotic pulmonary artery wedge pressure in patients after acute myocardial infarction. Circulation, *51:* 350, 1975.
56. Dantzker, D. R. Gas exchange in the adult respiratory distress syndrome. Clin. Chest Med., *3:* 56–67, 1982.
57. Davenport, H. W. *The ABC of Acid-Base Chemistry: The Elements of Physiological Blood Gas Chemistry for Medical Students and Physicians*, 124 pp. University of Chicago Press, Chicago, 1974.
58. deJongh, C. A., Caplan, E. S., and Schimptt, S. C. Infection in the critical care patient. In: *Textbook of Critical Care*, edited by W. C. Shoemaker, W. L. Thompson, and P. R. Holbrook, pp. 505–517. W. B. Saunders, Philadelphia, 1984.
59. Demers, R. R., and Saklad, M. Mechanical aspiration: A reappraisal of its hazards. Respir. Care, *20:* 661, 1975.
60. Demers, R. R., Irwin, R. S., and Braman, S. S. Criteria for optimum PEEP. Respir. Care, *22:* 596–601, 1977.
61. Demers, R. R., Sullivan, J. J., and Paliotta, J. Airflow resistances of endotrachael tubes. J.A.M.A., *237:* 1362, 1977.
62. Demers, R. R., and Irwin, R. S. Management of hypercapnic respiratory failure: A systematic approach. Respir. Care, *24:* 328–335, 1979.
63. Demers, R. R., Pratter, M. R., and Irwin, R. S. Use of the concept of ventilator compliance in the determination of static total compliance. Respir. Care, *26:* 644–648, 1981.
64. Demers, R. R. Complications of respiratory therapy: Complications of endotracheal suctioning procedures. Respir. Care, *27:* 453–457, 1982.
65. Demers, R. R., and Irwin, R. S. Positive end-expiratory pressure. In: *Manual of Intensive Care Medicine*, edited by J. M. Rippe and M. E. Csete, pp. 142–145. Little, Brown, Boston, 1983.
66. Deming, M. V., *et al.* Steroid and antihistaminic therapy for post intubation subglottic edema in infants and children. Anesthesiology, *22:* 933, 1961.
67. Deutschman, C. W., Wilton, P. B., Sinow, J., *et al.* Paranasal sinusitis: A common complication of nasotracheal intubation in neurosurgical patients. Neurosurgery, *17:* 296–299, 1985.
68. Didier, E. P. Principles in the management of assisted ventilation. Chest *58:* 423–426, 1970.
69. Donegan, J. Physiology and metabolism of the brain and spinal cord. In: *Handbook of Neuroanesthesia: Clinical and Physiologic Essentials*, edited by P. Newfield, and J. E. Cottrell, pp. 2–15. Little, Brown, Boston, 1983.
70. Donegan, M. F., and Bedford, R. R. Intravenously administered lidocaine prevents intracranial hypertension during endotrachael suctioning. Anesthesiology, *52:* 516–518, 1980.
71. Douglas, M. E., and Downs, J. B. Applied physiology and respiratory care. In: *Critical Care State of the Art*, edited by W. C. Shoemaker, pp. III(E) 1–35. The Society of Critical Care Medicine, Fullerton, 1982.
72. Douglas, M. E., and Downs, J. B. Respiratory therapy for ventilatory failure. In: *Textbook of Critical Care*, edited by W. C. Shoemaker, W. L. Thompson and P. R. Holbrook, pp. 301-310. W. B. Saunders, Philadelphia, 1984.
73. Ducker, T. B. Central nervous system pressure and pulmonary edema. Trans. Am. Neurol. Assoc., *92:* 225–227, 1967.
74. Ducker, T. B. Increased intracranial pressure and pulmonary edema. Part I: Clinical study of 11 patients. J. Neurosurg., *28:* 112–117, 1968.
75. Ducker, T. B., and Simmons, R. L. Increased intracranial pressure and pulmonary edema. Part 2: The hemodynamic response of dogs and monkeys to increased intracranial pressure. J. Neurosurg., *28:* 118–123, 1968.
76. Ducker, T. B., Simmons, R. L., and Anderson, R. W. Increased intracranial pressure and pulmonary edema. Part 3: The effect of increased intracranial pressure on the cardiovascular hemodynamics of chimpanzees. J. Neurosurg, *29:* 475–483, 1968.
77. Ducker, T. B., and Redding, J. S. Pulmonary complications in neurosurgery. Clin. Neurosurg., *23:* 483–493, 1976.
78. Dunham, C. M., and LaMonica, C. Prolonged trachael intubation in the trauma patient. J. Trauma, *24:* 120–124, 1984.
79. Dunn, C. R., Dunn, D. L., and Moser, K. M. Determinants of tracheal injury by cuffed tracheostomy tubes. Chest, *65:* 128–135, 1974.
80. Eaton, M. L., Green, B. A., Church, T. R., *et al.* Efficacy of theophylline in "irreversible" airflow obstruction. Ann. Intern. Med., *92:* 758–761, 1980.
81. Enevoldsen, E. J., and Jensen, F. T. Autoregulation and CO_2 responses of cerebral blood flow in patients with acute severe head injury. J. Neurosurg., *48:* 689–703, 1978.
82. Evarts, C. M. The fat embolism syndrome: A review. Surg. Clin. North Am., *50:* 493–507, 1970.
83. Fairley, H. B. Physiology of mechanical ventilation. In: *Scientific Foundations of Anaesthesia*, edited

by C. Scurr and S. Feldman, pp. 243-248. Year Book Medical Publishers, Chicago, 1982.

84. Falke, K. J., *et al.* Ventilation with end-expiratory pressure in acute lung disease. J. Clin. Invest., *51:* 2315-2323, 1972.

85. Feeley, T. W., and Hedley-Whyte, J. Weaning from controlled ventilation and supplemental oxygen. N. Engl. J. Med., *292:* 903-906, 1975.

86. Fisher, V. J., and Christianson, L. C. Cerebrospinal fluid acid-base balance during a changing ventilatory state in man. J. Appl. Physiol. *18:* 712-716, 1963.

87. Francis, P. B. Spirometry in office practice: Getting full measure from a useful tool. Postgrad. Med., *63:* 72-81, 1978.

88. Friedman, I., and Stoklosa, J. C. Preoperative clinical evaluation and management of chronic respiratory disease in the aged surgical patient. In: *The Aged and High Risk Surgical Patient: Medical, Surgical, Anesthetic Management*, edited by J. H. Siegel and P. C. Chodoff, pp. 185-192. Grune & Stratton, New York, 1976.

89. Froese, A. B., and Bryan, A. C. High-frequency oscillation in humans. Anesth. Analg., *59:* 577-584, 1980.

90. Froese, A. B. High-frequency ventilation: A critical assessment. In: *Critical Care State of the Art*, edited by W. C. Shoemaker, pp. 2-55. Society of Critical Care Medicine, Fullerton, 1984.

91. Frost, E. A. M. Effects of positive end-expiratory pressure on intracranial pressure and compliance in brain-injured patients. J. Neurosurg., *47:* 195-200, 1977.

92. Frost, E. A. M. Respiratory problems associated with head trauma. Neurosurgery, *1:* 300-306, 1977.

93. Frost, E. A. M. The physiopathology of respiration in neurosurgical patients. J. Neurosurg, *50:* 699-714, 1979.

94. Frost, E. A. M., Arancibia, C. U., and Shulman, K. Pulmonary shunt as a prognostic indicator in head injury. J. Neurosurg., *50:* 768-772, 1979.

95. Fulton, R. L., and Jones, D. E. The case of post traumatic pulmonary insufficiencies in man. Surg. Gynecol. Obstet., *140:* 179, 1975.

96. Gallus, A. S., *et al.* Small subcutaneous doses of heparin in prevention of venous thrombosis. N. Engl. J. Med., *288:* 545-551, 1973.

97. Garcia-Uria, J., Hoff, J. T., Miranda, S., and Nishimura, M. Experimental neurogenic pulmonary edema. Part 2: The role of cardiopulmonary pressure change. J. Neurosurg., *54:* 632-636, 1981.

98. Geiger, K. Differential lung ventilation. Int. Anesth. Clin., *21:* 83-98, 1983.

99. Geisler, F. H., Farrell, E. J., and Siegel, J. H. A new non-invasive method for the simultaneous determination of cardiac outpatient VA/QC disparity and the magnitude of peripheral perfusion, suitable for use in the critically ill patient. J. Trauma, *18:* 751, 1978.

100. Geisler, F. H., Siegel, J. H., Shetye, M., *et al.* A non-invasive method utilizing non-linear computer analysis of respiratory tracer gases to obtain cardiac output, lung tissue volume and the effective volume of perfused peripheral tissues. IEEE Proc. 78CH1391-2C, Computers in Cardiology, 1978.

101. Geisler, F. H., and Siegel, J. H. Clinical evaluation of a non-invasive inert gas washout method to quantify cardiopulmonary abnormalities in critically ill patients. IEEE 80CH157-1, Computer Applications in Medical Care, November, Vol. III, 1980.

102. Gilbert, R., Auchincloss, J. H., Jr., Peppi, D., *et al.* The first few hours off a respirator. Chest, *65:* 152-157, 1974.

103. Gildenberg, P. L., O'Brien, P., Britt, W. J., *et al.* The efficacy of Doppler monitoring for the detection of venous air embolism. J. Neurosurg, *54:* 75-78, 1981.

104. Glauser, F. L. Differentiating noncardiogenic from cardiogenic pulmonary edema. Hosp. Physician, 41-46, December, 1984.

105. Goldman, A. L., Morrison, D., and Foster, L. J. Oral progesterone therapy: Oxygen in a pill. Arch. Intern. Med., *141:* 574, 1981.

106. Goodman, L. R., and Putman, C. E. Radiological evaluation of patients receiving assisted ventilation. J.A.M.A., *245:* 858-860, 1981.

107. Gossling, H. R., and Donahue, T. A. The fat embolism syndrome. J.A.M.A., *241:* 2740-2742, 1979.

108. Gothard, J. W. Thoracic anaesthesia. In: *A Practice of Anaesthesia*, edited by H. C. Churchill-Davidson, Ed. 5, pp. 374-404. Year Book Medical Publishers, Chicago, 1984.

109. Graf, C. J., and Rossi, N. P. Pulmonary edema and the central nervous system: A clinico-pathological study. Surg. Neurol., *4:* 319-325, 1975.

110. Grasberger, R. C., Spatz, E. L., Mortara, R. W., *et al.* Effect of high-frequency ventilation versus conventional mechanical ventilation on ICP in head-injured dogs. J. Neurosurg., *60:* 1214-1218, 1984.

111. Greenbaum, D. M., and Marshall, K. E. The value of routine daily chest x-rays in intubated patients in the medical intensive care unit. Crit. Care Med., 10: 29-30, 1982.

112. Greenberg, J. H., Alavi, A., Reivich, M., *et al.* Local cerebral blood volume response to carbon dioxide in man. Circ. Res., *43:* 324-331, 1978.

113. Grillo, H. C., Cooper, J. D., Gettin, B., *et al.* A low-pressure cuff for tracheostomy tubes to minimize tracheal injury: A comparative clinical trial. J. Thorac. Cardiovasc. Surg., *62:* 898-906, 1971.

114. Grimes, C. A., and Hanes, B. Influence of cigarette smoking on the spirometric evaluation of employees of a large insurance company. Am. Rev. Respir. Dis., *108:* 273-282, 1973.

115. Grubb, R. L., Jr., Raichle, M. E., Eichling, J. O., *et al.* The effects of changes in Pa_{CO_2} on cerebral blood volume, blood flow, and vascular mean transit time. Stroke, *5:* 630-639, 1974.

116. Guenter, C. A., and Braun, T. E. Fat embolism syndrome: Changing prognosis. Chest, *79:* 143-145, 1981.

117. Guenter, C. A. Chest trauma. edited by C. A. Guenter and M. H. Welch, In: *Pulmonary Medicine*, ed. 2, Philadelphia, Lippincott, 1982, 511-533, 535-537.

118. Gump, D. W., Phillips, C. A., Forsyth, B. R., *et al.* Role of infection in chronic bronchitis. Am. Rev. Respir. Dis., *113:* 465-474, 1976.

119. Guyton, A. C. *Textbook of Medical Physiology*, 1074 pp. W. B. Saunders, Philadelphia, 1981.
120. Hammerschmidt, D. E., White, J. G., and Craddock, D. R. Corticosteroids inhibit complement-induced granulocyte aggregation: Possible mechanism for their efficacy in shock states. J. Clin. Invest., *63:* 798-803, 1979.
121. Harley, H. P. S. Laryngotracheal obstruction complicating tracheostomy or endotracheal intubation with assisted respiration: A critical review. Thorax, *26:* 493-533, 1971.
122. Havill, J. H. Prolonged hyperventilation and intracranial pressure. Crit. Care Med., *12:* 72-74, 1984.
123. Hayes, G. J., and Slocum, H. C. The achievement of optimal brain relaxation by hyperventilation technics of anesthesia. J. Neurosurg., *19:* 65-70, 1961.
124. Head, J. M. Tracheostomy in the management of respiratory problems. N. Engl. J. Med., *264:* 587, 1961.
125. Heffner J. E., and Sahn, S. A. Controlled hyperventilation in patients with intracranial hypertension: Application and management. Intern. Med., *143:* 765-769, 1983.
126. Hendeles, L., Weinberger, M., and Bighley, L. Disposition of theophylline after a single intravenous infusion of aminophylline. Am. Rev. Respir. Dis., *118:* 97-103, 1978.
127. Higuchi, J. H., and Johanson, W. G. Colonization and bronchopulmonary infection. Clin. Chest Med., *3:* 133-142, 1982.
128. Hobelmann, C. F., Smith, D. E., Virgilio, R. W., *et al.* Mechanics of ventilation with positive end-expiratory pressure. Ann. Thorac. Surg., *24:* 68-76, 1977.
129. Hoff, J. T., Nishimura, M., Garcia-Uria, J., *et al.* Experimental neurogenic pulmonary edema. Part 1: The role of systemic hypertension. J. Neurosurg. *54:* 617-631, 1981.
130. Hosea, S., Brown, E., Hammer, C., and Frank, M. Role of complement activation in a model of adult respiratory distress syndrome. J. Clin. Invest., *66:* 375-382, 1980.
131. Huseby, J. S., Pavlin, E. G., and Butler, J. Effect of positive end-expiratory pressure on intracranial pressure in dogs. J. Appl. Physiol.: Respir. Environ. Excercise Physiol., *44:* 25-27, 1978.
132. Huxley, E. J., Viroslav, J., Gray, W. R., *et al.* Pharyngeal aspiration in normal adults and patients with depressed consciousness. Am. J. Med., *64:* 564-568, 1978.
133. Ingram, R. H., Jr. Mechanical aids to lung expansion. Am. Rev. Respir. Dis., *122:* 23-24, 1980.
134. Iverson, R. L. Airway and ventilator management of the head injured patient. J. Indiana State Med. Assoc., *76:* 824-827, 1983.
135. Iwabuchi, T., Sobata, E., Suzuki, M., Suzuki, S., *et al.* Dural sinus pressure as related to neurosurgical positions. Neurosurgery, *12:* 203-207, 1983.
136. Jacob, H. S., Craddock, P. H., Hammerschmidt, D. E., *et al.* Complement-induced granulocyte aggregation. N. Engl. J. Med., *302:* 789-794, 1980.
137. Jacquez, J. A. *Respiratory Physiology*, 442 pp. McGraw-Hill, New York, 1979.
138. James, H. E., Langfitt, T. W., and Kumar, V. S. Analysis of the response to therapeutic measures to reduce intracranial pressure in headinjured patients. J. Trauma, *16:* 437-441, 1976.
139. Johanson, W. G., Jr. Complications of respiratory therapy. Infectious complications of respiratory therapy. Respir. Care, *27:* 445-452, 1982.
140. Jon Euler, C. On the central generator for the basic breathing rhythmicity. J. Appl. Physiol., Respir. Environ. Exercise Physiol., *55:* 1647-1659, 1983.
141. Joorhies, R. M., Fraser, R. A. R, and Poznak, A. V. Prevention of an embolism with positive end-expiratory pressure. Neurosurgery, *12:* 503-506, 1983.
142. Jordan, W. S., *et al.* New therapy for post intubation laryngeal edema and tracheitis in children. J.A.M.A., *212:* 585, 1970.
143. Juhl, J. H. (ed.) *Essentials of Roentgen Interpretation.* p. 933. Harper & Row, Hagerstown, Md., 1981.
144. Jung, R. C. Respiratory management in head injury. In: *Clinical Neurosurgery*, edited by J. G. Galbraith, pp. 300-311. Williams & Wilkins, Baltimore, 1982.
145. Kanak, R., Fahey, P. J., and Vanderwarf, C. Oxygen cost of breathing: Changes dependent upon mode of mechanical ventilation. Chest, *87:* 126-127, 1985.
146. Kaufman, H. H., Satterwhite, T., McConnell, B. J., *et al.* Deep vein thrombosis and pulmonary embolism in head injured patients. Angiology, *34:* 627-638, 1983.
147. Kazemi, H. Pulmonary function tests. J.A.M.A., *206:* 2302-2304, 1968.
148. Kelman, G. R., and Nunn, J. F. Normogram for the correction of blood PO_2, PCO_2, pH, and base excess for time and temperature. J. Appl. Physiol., *21:* 1484-1490, 1966.
149. Kennedy, S. K. Airway management and respiratory support. In: *Neurological and Neurosurgical Intensive Care*, Chap 5, edited by A. H. Ropper, S. K. Kennedy, and N. T. Zervas, University Park Press, Baltimore, 1983.
150. Kirby, R. R., Downs, J. A., Civetta, J. M., *et al.* High level positive end-expiratory pressure (PEEP) in acute respiratory insufficiency. Chest, *67:* 156-163, 1975.
151. Kirsh, M. M. *Blunt Chest Trauma: General Principles of Management*, 247 pp. Little, Brown, Boston, 1977.
152. Klain, M. High-frequency ventilation. In: *Textbook of Critical Care*, edited by W. C. Shoemaker, W. L. Thompson, P. R. Holbrook, pp. 323-327. W. B. Saunders, Philadelphia, 1984.
153. Kogure, K., Sheinberg, P. Reinmuth, O.M., *et al.* Mechanism of cerebral vasodilation in hypoxia. J. Appl. Physiol., *29:* 223-229, 1970.
154. Kress, T. D., *et al.* "Cricothyroidotomy." Ann. Emerg. Med., *11:* 197, 1982.
155. Kumar, A. Continuous positive-pressure ventilation in acute respiratory failure. Effects on hemodynamics and lung function. N. Engl. J. Med., *283:* 1430-1436, 1970.

156. Kumar, A., Pontoppidan, H., Falke, K.J., *et al.* Pulmonary barotrauma during mechanical ventilation. Crit. Care Med., *1:* 181–186, 1973.
157. Kurzweg, F. T. Pulmonary complications following upper abdominal surgery. Am. Surg., *19:* 967–974, 1953.
158. Langfitt, T. W. Increased intracranial pressure and the cerebral circulation. In: *Neurological Surgery*, Vol. II, Chap. 29, ed. by J. R. Youmans. W.B. Saunders, Philadelphia, 1982.
159. Lassen, N. A. The luxury-perfusion syndrome and its possible relation to acute metabolic acidosis localised within the brain. Lancet, *2:* 1113–1115., 1966.
160. Latimer, R. G., Dickman, M., Day, W.C., *et al.* Ventilatory patterns and pulmonary complications after upper abdominal surgery determined by preoperative and postoperative computerized spirometry and blood gas analysis. Am. J. Surg., *122:* 622–632, 1971.
161. Lee, M. C., Klassen, A. C., Heaney, L. M. *et al.* Respiratory rate and pattern disturbances in acute brain stem infarction. Stroke, *7:* 382–385, 1976.
162. Leeming, B. W. Gravitational edema of the lungs observed during assisted respiration. Chest, *64:* 719–722, 1973.
163. Leich, J. M. Oxygen therapy. In: *Scientific Foundations of Anaesthesia*, edited by C. Scurr and S. Feldman, pp.235–243. Year Book Medical Publishers, Chicago, 1982.
164. Leitch, A. G., McLennan, J. E., Balkenhol, S., Loudon, R. G., *et al.* Mechanisms of hyperventilation in head injury: Case report and review. Neurosurgery, *5:* 701–707, 1979.
165. Loh, L., Goldman, M., and Newsom-Davis, J. The assessment of diaphragmatic function. Medicine, *56:* 165, 1977.
166. Luce, J. M., Pierson, D. J., and Hudson, L. D. Intermittent mandatory ventilation. Chest, *79:* 678–685, 1981.
167. Luce, J. M. The cardiovascular effects of mechanical ventilation and postive end-expiratory pressure. J.A.M.A., *252:* 807–811, 1984.
168. Luce, J. M., Tyler, M. L., and Pierson, D. J. *Intensive Respiratory Care*, 345 pp. W. B. Saunders, Philadelphia, 1984.
169. Mackay, E. M. Experimental pulmonary edema. IV. Pulmonary edema accompanying trauma to the brain. Proc. Soc. Exp. Biol. Med., *74:* 695–697, 1950.
170. Mackenzie, C. F., Ciesla, N., Imle, P. C., *et al.* *Chest Physiotherapy in the Intensive Care Unit*, 260 pp. Williams & Wilkins, Baltimore, 1981.
171. Marini, J. J., Pierson, D. J., and Hudson, L. D. Acute lobar atelectasis: A prospective comparison of fiberoptic bronchoscopy and respiratory therapy. Am. Rev. Respir. Dis. *119:* 971–978, 1979.
172. Marquardt, D. L., and Wasserman, S. I. Asthma in the adult. In: *Textbook of Critical Care*, edited by W. C. Shoemaker, W. L. Thompson, and P. R. Holbrook, pp. 258–264, W. B. Saunders, Philadelphia, 1984.
173. Matjasko, J. Cardiorespiratory management in neurologic emergencies. In: *Neurologic Emergencies: Recognition and Management*, edited by M. Salcman, pp. 35–64. Raven Press, New York, 1980.
174. Matthewson, H. S. *Pharmacology for Respiratory Therapists*, 97 pp. C. V. Mosby, St. Louis, 1981.
175. McCredia, M., Lovejoy, F. W., and Kudtreider, N. L. Pulmonary function in diaphramatic paralysis. Thorax, *17:* 213, 1962.
176. McFadden, E. R., Jr., and Lyons, H. A. Arterial blood gas tension in asthma. N. Engl. J. Med., *278:* 1027–1032, 1968.
177. McFadden, E. R., Jr., Kiser, R., and DeGroot, W. J. Acute bronchial asthma: Relations between clinical and physiologic manifestations. N. Engl. J. Med., *288:* 221–225, 1973.
178. McIntyre, K. M., and Sasahara, A. A. Hemodynamic and ventricular responses to pulmonary embolism. Prog. Cardiovasc. Med., *42:* 175, 1974.
179. McNeil, B. J. A diagnostic strategy using ventilation-perfusion studies in patients suspect for pulmonary embolism. J. Nucl. Med., *17:* 613–616, 1976.
180. McNeil, B. J. Ventilation-perfusion studies and the diagnosis of pulmonary embolism: Concise communication. J. Nucl. Med., *21:* 319–323, 1980.
181. McPherson, S. P. *Respiratory Therapy Equipment*, 514 pp. C. V. Mosby, St. Louis, 1981.
182. Meade, J. W. Tracheotomy: Its complications and their management: A study of 212 cases. N. Engl. J. Med., *265:* 519–523, 1961.
183. Meneely, G. R., and Ferguson, J. L. Pulmonary evaluation and risk in patient's preparation for anaesthesia and surgery. J.A.M.A., *175:* 1074–1080, 1961.
184. Menn, S. J. Mechanical ventilation: Devices and methods. In: *Manual of Clinical Problems in Pulmonary Medicine*, edited by R. A. Bordow, E. W. Stool, and K. M. Moser, pp. 259-264, Little Brown, Boston, 1980.
185. Menn, S. J., and Stool, E. W. Mechanical ventilation: Weaning and complications. In: *Manual of Clinical Problems in Pulmonary Medicine*, edited by R. A. Bordow, E. W. Stool, and K. M. Moser, pp. 264-269, Little, Brown, Boston, 1980.
186. Meszaros, W. T. Lung changes in left heart failure. Circulation, *47:* 859–871, 1973.
187. Michenfelder, J. D., Granert, G. A., and Rehder, K. Neuroanesthesia. Anesthesiology, *30:* 65–100, 1969.
188. Miller, J. D., Becker, D. P., Ward, J. D., Sullivan, H. G., *et al.* Significance of intracranial hypertension in severe head injury. J. Neurosurg., *47:* 503–516, 1977.
189. Modell, J. H., and Boysen, P. G. Pulmonary aspiration of stomach contents. In: *Textbook of Critical Care*, edited by W. C. Shoemaker, W. L. Thompson, and P. R. Holbrook, pp. 272–275, W. B. Saunders, Philadelphia, 1984.
190. Moses, D. C., Silver, T. M., and Bookstein, J. J. The complementary roles of chest radiography, lung scanning, and selective pulmonary angiography in the diagnosis of pulmonary embolism. Circulation, *49:* 179–188, 1974.
191. Moss, E., Gibson, S., McDowall, D. G., and Gibson, R. M. Intensive management of severe head injuries: A scheme of intensive management of se-

vere head injuries. Anaesthesia, *38:* 214–225, 1983.

192. Mulder, D. A., *et al.* Complication of tracheostomy: Relationships to long-term ventilatory assistance. J. Trauma, *9:* 389, 1969.
193. Murray, J. F. Mechanisms of acute respiratory failure. Am. Rev. Respir. Dis., *115:* 1071–1080, 1977.
194. Murray, H. W. Antimicrobial therapy and pulmonary aspiration. Am. J. Med., *66:* 188–190, 1979.
195. Murray, H. W., *et al.* Fever and pulmonary thromboembolism. Am. J. Med., *67:* 232–235, 1979.
196. Narins, R. G., and Emmett, M. Simple and mixed acid-base disorders: A practical approach. Medicine, *59:* 161–187, 1980.
197. Natanson, C., Shelhamer, J. H., and Parrillo, J. E. Intubation of the trachea in the critical care setting. J.A.M.A., *253:* 1160–1165, 1985.
198. National Heart, Lung, and Blood Institute 1979. Extracorporeal support for respiratory insufficiency at collaborative study in response to RFP NHLI, 73-20, p.10, NHLBI DLD, December 1979.
199. Neely, W. A., Robinson, W. T., McMullen, W. H., *et al.* Postoperative respiratory insufficiency: Physiological studies with therapeutic implications. Ann. Surg., *171:* 679–685, 1970.
200. North, J. B., and Jennett, S. Abnormal breathing patterns associated with acute brain damage. Arch. Neurol., *31:* 338–344, 1974.
201. O'Donnell, J. M., Thompson, D. R., and Layton, T. R. The effect of high-frequency jet ventilation on intracranial pressure in patients with closed head injuries. J. Trauma, *24:* 73–75, 1984.
202. O'Rourke, P. P., and Crone, R. K. High-frequency ventilation. A new approach to respiratory support. J.A.M.A., *250:* 2845–2847, 1983.
203. Parsons, L. C., and Shogan, J. S. The effects of the endotracheal tube suctioning/manual hyperventilation procedure on patients with severe closed head injuries. Heart Lung, *13:* 372–380, 1984.
204. Paterson, J. W., Woolcook, A. J., and Shenfield, G. M. Bronchodilator drugs. Am. Rev. Respir. Dis., *120:* 1149–1188, 1979.
205. Petty, T. L. Adult respiratory distress syndrome: Definition and historical perspective. In: *Clinics in Chest Medicine*, Vol. 3, No. 1, edited by R. C. Bone, pp. 3–7, W. B. Saunders, Philadelphia, 1982.
206. Petty, T. L. Acute respiratory failure in chronic obstructive pulmonary disease. In: *Textbook of Critical Care*, edited by W. C. Shoemaker, W. L. Thompson, and P. R. Holbrook, pp. 264–272, W. B. Saunders, Philadelphia, 1984.
207. Pierce, A. K., and Sanford, J. P. Gram-negative pneumonias. Am. Rev. Respir. Dis., *110:* 647, 1974.
208. Pinilla, J. C. Acute respiratory failure in severe blunt chest trauma. J. Trauma, *22:* 221–226, 1982.
209. Plum, F., and Posner, J. B. *The Diagnosis of Stupor and Coma*, 373 pp. F. A. Davis, Philadelphia, 1980.
210. Pontoppidan, H., Geffin B., and Lowenstein, E. Acute respiratory failure in the adult (1 of 3). N. Engl. J. Med., *287:* 690–698, 743, 799, 1972.
211. Poulton, T. J., and James, F. M. Cough suppression by lidocaine. Anesthesiology, *50:* 470–472, 1979.
212. Powell, J. R., *et al.* Theophylline disposition in acutely ill hospitalized patients: The effect of smoking, heart failure, severe airway obstruction, and pneumonia. Am. Rev. Respir. Dis., *118:* 229, 1978.
213. Powner, D. J. Eross, B., and Grenvik, A. Differential lung ventilation with PEEP in the treatment of unilateral pneumonia. Crit. Care Med., *5:* 170–172, 1977.
214. Pratter, M. R., Corwin, R. W., and Irwin, R.S. An integrated analysis of lung and respiratory muscle dysfunction in the pathogenesis of hypercapnic respiratory failure. Respir. Care, *27:* 55, 1982.
215. Price, K. A. Neurogenic pulmonary oedema. Anaesthesia, *39:* 1254–1255, 1984.
216. Qvist, J., Pontoppidan, H., Wilson, R. S., *et al.* Hemodynamic responses to mechanical ventilation with PEEP: The effect of hypervolemia. Anesthesiology, *42:* 45–55, 1975.
217. Rackow, E. C., Fein, I. A., and Leppo, J. Colloid osmotic pressure as a prognostic indicator of pulmonary edema and mortality in the critically ill. Chest, *72:* 709–713, 1977.
218. Reynolds, R. W. Pulmonary edema as a consequence of hypothalamic lesions in rats. Science, *141:* 930–932, 1963.
219. Rick, J. J., and Burke, S. S. Respirator paradox. South. Med. J., *71:* 1376–1378, 1978.
220. Riker, J. F., and Cacace, L. G. Double-blind comparison of metaproterenol and isoetharine phenylephrine solutions in intermittent positive pressure breathing in bronchospastic conditions. Chest, *78:* 723–725, 1980.
221. Rinaldo, J. E., and Rogers, R. M. Adult respiratory distress syndrome; changing concepts of lung injury and repair. N. Engl. J. Med., *306:* 900, 1982.
222. Robin, E. D., Carey, L. C., Grenvik, A., Glauser, F., *et al.* Capillary leak syndrome with pulmonary edema. Arch. Intern. Med., *130:* 66–71, 1972.
223. Robin, E. D., Cross, C. E., and Zelis, R. Pulmonary edema. N. Engl. J. Med., *288:* 292–304, 1973.
224. Robin, E. D. Overdiagnosis and overtreatment of pulmonary embolism: The emperor may have no clothes. Ann. Intern. Med., *87:* 775–781, 1977.
225. Robin, E. D. *et al.* A shunt is (not) a shunt is (not) a shunt. Am. Rev. Respir. Dis., *115:* 553–557, 1977.
226. Rose, B. D. *Clinical Physiology of Acid-Base and Electrolyte Disorders,* p. 548. McGraw-Hill, New York, 1977.
227. Rossi, N. P., and Graf, C. J. Physiological and pathological effects of neurologic disturbances and increased intracranial pressure on the lung. A review. Surg. Neurol., *5:* 366–372, 1976.
228. Rubinfeld, A. R., and Pain, M. C. F. Perception of asthma. Lancet, *1:* 882–884, 1976.
229. Sackner, M. A., *et al.* Pathogenesis and prevention of tracheobronchial damage with suction procedures. Chest, *64:* 284, 1973.
230. Sahn, S. A., Lakshminarayan, S., and Petty, T. L. Weaning from mechanical ventilation. J.A.M.A., *235:* 2208–2212, 1976.

231. Salcman, M. *Neurologic Emergencies: Recognition and Management*, 248 pp. Raven Press, New York, 1980.
232. Sarnoff, S. J., and Sarnoff, L. C. Neurohemodynamics of pulmonary edema. II. The role of sympathetic pathways in the elevation of pulmonary and systemic vascular pressures following the intracisternal injection of fibrin. Circulation, *6:* 51–62, 1952.
233. Schneider, R. C. Fat embolism—A problem in the differential diagnosis of cranio-cerebral trauma. J. Neurosurg., *9:* 1–14, 1952.
234. Schumacker, P. T., Rhodes, G. R., Newell, J. C., Dutton, R. E., *et al.* Ventilation-perfusion imbalance after head trauma. Am. Rev. Respir. Dis., *119:* 33–43, 1979.
235. Selecky, P. A. Tracheostomy: A review of present-day indications, complications, and care. Heart Lung, *3:* 272, 1974.
236. Severinghaus, J. W., Mitchell, R. A., Richardson, B. W., *et al.* Respiratory control at high altitude suggesting active transport regulation of CSF pH. J. Appl. Physiol., *18:* 1155–1166, 1963.
237. Severinghaus, J. W. The role of cerebrospinal fluid pH in normalization of cerebral blood flow in chronic hypocapnia. Acta. Neurol. Scand. (Suppl.), *14:* 116–120, 1965.
238. Shalit, M. N., Reinmuth, O. M., Shimojyo, S., and Scheinberg, P. Carbon dioxide and cerebral circulatory control. I. The extravascular effect. Arch. Neurol., *17:* 298-303, 1967.
239. Shalit, M. N., Reinmuth, O. M., Shimojyo, S., and Scheinberg, P. Carbon dioxide and cerebral circulatory control. II. The intravascular effect. Arch. Neurol., *17:* 337-341, 1967.
240. Shapiro, B. A., Harrison, R. A., and Walton, J. R. *Clinical Application of Blood Gases*, 316 pp. Year Book Medical Publishers, Chicago, 1973.
241. Shapiro, B. A., Harrison, R. A., and Trout, C. A. *Clinical Application of Respiratory Care*, 578 pp. Year Book Medical Publishers, Chicago, 1979.
242. Shapiro, B. A. Airway pressure therapy for acute restrictive pulmonary pathology. In: *Critical Care State of the Art*, edited by W. C. Shoemaker, pp. II(C):1–53. The Society of Critical Care Medicine, Fullerton, 1981.
243. Shapiro, B. A. Airway pressure therapy for acute restrictive pulmonary pathology. In: *Textbook of Critical Care*, edited by W. C. Shoemaker, W. L. Thompson, and P. R. Holbrook, pp. 224–238, W. B. Saunders, Philadelphia, 1984.
244. Shapiro, H. M. Intracranial hypertension: Therapeutic and anesthetic considerations. Anesthesiology, *43:* 445-471, 1975.
245. Shapiro, H. M., and Marshall, L. F. Intracranial pressure responses to PEEP in head-injured patients. J. Trauma, *18:* 254–256, 1978.
246. Sherry, S. Low-dose heparin for the prophylaxis of pulmonary embolism. Am. Rev. Respir. Dis., *114:* 661-666, 1976.
247. Shoemaker, W. C. Fluids and electrolytes in the adult. In: *Critical Care State of the Art*, edited by W. C. Shoemaker, pp. III(N):1–96. The Society of Critical Care Medicine, Fullerton, 1982.
248. Shoemaker, W. C. Circulatory pathophysiology of ARDS and its fluid management. In: *Textbook of Critical Care*, edited by W. L. Thompson and P. R. Holbrook, pp. 310-318. W. B. Saunders, Philadelphia, 1984.
249. Siegel, J. H., and Chodoff, P. The assessment of respiratory function. In: *The Aged and High Risk Surgical Patient: Medical, Surgical, and Anesthetic Management*, edited by J. H. Siegel and P. C. Chodoff, pp. 99–192. Grune & Stratton, New York, 1976.
250. Siegel, J. H., Stoklosa, J., Geisler, F. H., *et al.* Computer-based evaluation of cardiopulmonary function for the optimization of ventilatory therapy in the adult respiratory distress syndrome. Int. J. Clin. Monitoring and Computing, *1:* 107–126, 1984.
250a. Silverstein, A. Significance of cerebral fat embolism. Neurology, *2:* 292–310, 1984.
251. Simmons, R. L., Martin, A. M., Jr., Heisterkamp, C. A., *et al.* Respiratory insufficiency in combat casual ties: Part II. Pulmonary edema following head injury. Ann. Surg., *170:* 39–44, 1969.
252. Sinha, R. P., Dacker, T. B., and Perot, P. L., Jr. Arterial oxygenation: Findings and its significance in central nervous system trauma patients. J.A.M.A. *224:* 1258–1260, 1973.
253. Sjostraud, V. H. High-frequency positive-pressure ventilation (HFPPV): A review. Crit. Care Med., *8:* 345–363, 1980.
254. Skatrud, J. B., Dempsey, J. A., and Kaiser, D. G. Ventilatory response to medroxyprogesterone acetate in normal subjects: Time course and mechanism. J. Appl. Physiol., *44:* 939–944, 1978.
255. Smith, C. B., Golden, C. A., Kanner, R. E. *et al.* Association of viral and mycoplasma pneumoniae infections with acute respiratory illness in patients with chronic obstructive pulmonary diseases. Am. Rev. Respir. Dis., *121:* 225–232, 1980.
256. Smith, P. R., Heurich, A. E., Leffler, C. T., *et al.* A comparative study of subcutaneously administered terbutaline and epinephrine in the treatment of acute bronchial asthma. Chest, *71:* 129–134, 1977.
257. Sprung, C. L., Rackow, E. C., Fein, I. A., *et al.* The spectrum of pulmonary edema: Differentiation of cardiogenic, intermediate and noncardiogenic forms of pulmonary edema mortality in the critically ill. Am. Rev. Respir. Dis., *124:* 718, 1981.
258. Standefer, M., Bay, J. W., and Trusso, R. The sitting position neurosurgery: A retrospective analysis of 488 cases. Neurosurgery, *14:* 649–658, 198X.
259. Staub, N. C. Pulmonary edema. Physiol. Rev., *54:* 679–811, 1974.
260. Staub, N. C. "State of the art" review. Pathogenesis of pulmonary edema. Am. Rev. Respir. Dis., *109:* 358–372, 1974.
261. Stauffer, J. L., Olsen, D. E., and Petty, T. L. Complications and consequences of endotracheal intubation and tracheostomy: A prospective study of 150 critically ill adult patients. Am. J. Med., *70:* 65–76, 1981.

262. Stein, M., and Cassara, E. L. Preoperative pulmonary evaluation and therapy for surgery patients. J.A.M.A., *211:* 787-790, 1970.
263. Stevens, R. M., *et al.* Pneumonia in an intensive care unit. Arch. Intern. Med., *134:* 106, 1974.
264. Stewardson, R. H., and Nyhus, L. M. Pulmonary aspiration. Arch. Surg., *112:* 1192-1197, 1977.
265. Sukumaran, M., Granada, M. J., Berger, H. W., Lee, M., *et al.* Evaluation of corticosteroid treatment in aspiration of gastric contents: A controlled clinical trial. Mt. Sinai J. Med., *47:* 335-340, 1980.
266. Sullivan, M., Paliotta, J., and Saklad, M. Endotracheal tube as a factor in measurement of respiratory mechanics. J. Appl. Physiol., *41:* 590-592, 1976.
267. Suter, P. M., Fairley, H. B., and Isenberg, M. D. Optimum end-expiratory airway pressure in patients with acute pulmonary failure. N. Engl. J. Med., *292:* 284-289, 1975.
268. Swann, K. W., and Black, P. Deep vein thrombosis and pulmonary emboli in neurosurgical patients: A review. J. Neurosurg., *61:* 1055-1062, 1984.
269. Theodore, J., and Robin, E. D. Speculations on neurogenic pulmonary edema. Am. Rev. Respir. Dis., *113:* 405-411, 1976.
270. Thurlbeck, W. M., Henderson, J. A., Fraser, R. G., *et al.* Chronic obstructive lung disease. Medicine, *49:* 81, 1970.
271. Tisi, G. M. *Pulmonary Physiology in Clinical Medicine*, pp. 207. Williams & Wilkins, Baltimore, 1980.
272. Tomita, T., and Raimondi, A. J. Brain tumors in the elderly. J.A.M.A., *246:* 53-55, 1981.
273. Tyler, M. L. Complications of positioning and chest physiotherapy. Respir. Care, *27:* 458, 1982.
274. Unger, K. M., Shibel, E. M., and Moser, K. M. Detection of left ventricular failure in patients with adult respiratory distress syndrome. Chest, *67:* 8-13, 1975.
275. Uzawa, T., and Ashbaugh, D. G. Continuous positive-pressure breathing in acute hemorrhagic pulmonary edema. J. Appl. Physiol., *26:* 427, 1969.
276. Valtin, H. *Renal Function-Mechanisms Preserving Fluid and Solute Balance in Health*, Ed. 2, p. 316. Little, Brown, Boston, 1983.
277. Wauchob, T. D., Brooks, R. J., and Harrison, K. M. Neurogenic pulmonary oedema. Anaesthesia, *39:* 529-534, 1984.
278. Webb, W. R. Postoperative pulmonary complications: Including complications of bronchoscopy. In: *Management of Surgical Complications*, edited by C. P. Artz and J. D. Hardy, Ed. 3, pp. 93-107. W.B. Saunders, Philadelphia, 1975.
279. Webb, W. R., and Moulder, P. V. Postoperative pulmonary complications. In: *Complications in Surgery and Their Management*, edited by J.D. Hardy, Ed. 4, pp. 98-113. W.B. Saunders, Philadelphia, 1981.
280. Weiss, E. B. Bronchial asthma. CIBA Clin. Symp., *27:* 3-72, 1979.
281. Weisz, G. Fat embolism. Curr. Probl. Surg., pp. 1-54, Nov. 1974.
282. Wessler, S., and Gitel, S.N. Low-dose heparin: Is the risk worth the benefit? Am. Heart. J., *98:* 94-101, 1979.
283. West, J. B. *Ventilation/Blood Flow and Gas Exchange*, 117 pp. Blackwell, Philadelphia, Oxford, 1965.
284. West, J. B. Causes of carbon dioxide retention in lung disease. N. Engl. J. Med., *284:* 1232-1236, 1971.
285. West, J. B. Ventilation-perfusion relationships. Am. Rev. Respir. Dis., *116:* 919-943, 1977.
286. West, J. B. Ventilation-perfusion relationships. In: *Scientific Foundations of Anaesthesia*, edited by C. Scurr and S. Feldman, pp. 217-222. Year Book Medical Publishers, Inc., Chicago, 1982.
287. West, J. B. *Pulmonary Pathophysiology: The Essentials*, Ed. 2, 229 pp. Williams & Wilkins, Baltimore, 1982.
288. West, J. B. *Respiratory Physiology: The Essentials*, Ed. 3, 183 pp. Williams & Wilkins, Baltimore, 1985.
289. Westerfield, B. T., Carder, A. J., and Light, R. W. The relationship between arterial blood gases and serum theophylline. Am. Rev. Respir. Dis., *124:* 17-20, 1981.
290. Westerman, D. E., Benatar, S. R., Potgieter, P. D., *et al.* Identification of the high-risk asthmatic patient: Experience with 39 patients undergoing ventilation for status asthmaticus. Am. J. Med., *66:* 565-572, 1979.
291. Wightman, J. A. K. A prospective survey of the incidence of postoperative pulmonary complications. Br. J. Surg., *55:* 85-91, 1968.
292. Wilson, J. E. Pulmonary embolism—diagnosis and treatment. Part I. Clin. Notes Respir. Dis., *19:* 3-13, 1981.
293. Wilson, J. E. Pulmonary embolism-diagnosis and treatment. Part II. Clin. Notes Respir. Dis., *20:* 3-11, 1981.
294. Wilson, R. S., Henning Pontoppidan, and Rie, M. A. Acute respiratory failure. In: *Neurological and Neurosurgical Intensive Care*, Chap. 6, edited by A. H. Ropper, S. K. Kennedy, and N. T. Zervas, University Park Press, Baltimore, 1983.
295. Wingerd, M., *et al.* Comparisons of caval filters in the management of venous thromboembolism. Arch. Surg., *113:* 1264-1271, 1978.
296. Wolman, L. The disturbance of circulation in traumatic paraplegia in acute and late stages: A pathologic study. Paraplegia, *2:* 213-226, 1965.
297. Worth, M. H. Managing penetrating chest trauma. Hosp. Med., 53, 1982.
298. Wray, N. P., and Nicotra, M. B. Pathogenesis of neurogenic pulmonary edema. Am. Rev. Respir. Dis., *118:* 783-786, 1978.
299. Wynne, J. W., and Modell, J. H. Respiratory aspiration of stomach contents. Ann. Intern. Med., *87:* 466-474, 1977.
300. Wynne, J. W., Ramphal, R., and Hood, C. I. Tracheal mucosal damage after aspiration: A scanning electron microscope study. Am. Rev. Respir. Dis., *124:* 728-732, 1981.

301. Wynne, J. W. Aspiration pneumonitis: Correlation of experimental models with clinical disease. Clin. Chest Med., *3:* 25–34, 1982.

302. Youmans, J. R. Cerebral blood flow in clinical problems. In: *Neurological Surgery*, Vol. II, edited by J. R. Youmans, pp. 786–845. W. B. Saunders, Philadelphia, 1982.

303. Young, R. F. Diaphragm pacing. In: *Neurosurgery*, edited by R. H. Wilkins and S.S. Rengachary, pp. 1733–1734. McGraw-Hill, New York, 1985.

304. Zimmerman, J. E., Goodman, L. R., and Shahvari, M. B. G. Effect of mechanical ventilation and positive end-expiratory pressure (PEEP) on chest radiograph. Am. J. Radiol., *133:* 811–815, 1979.

CHAPTER 2

Cardiovascular System: Physiology, Pathophysiology and Management

MARTIN I. GRIFFEL, M.D.,
MAX HARRY WEIL, M.D., PH.D.,
and ERIC C. RACKOW, M.D.

INTRODUCTION

In the critical care setting, the ability to maintain cardiovascular homeostasis is of utmost importance for the continued function of each individual organ system and for the patient as a whole. This concept is of no less importance in the neurosurgical intensive care unit. The proper function of the cardiovascular system allows for adequate blood flow to all organ beds including the central nervous system. Optimum cardiovascular performance is dependent upon the co-ordinated function of five components of the cardiovascular system: (*a*) the heart, serving as a pump; (*b*) the high pressure resistance circuit, the arterial bed, which transports blood to tissues; (*c*) the capillary network, which allows for exchange of nutrients and metabolic products; (*d*) the low pressure, capacitance circuit, the venous bed, which returns blood to the pump; and (*e*) the circulating blood volume. Circulatory failure reflects a defect in the proper function of one or more of these components, disrupting the normal perfusion of tissues. The capability of the clinician to rapidly diagnose circulatory failure, assess the specific defect, intervene appropriately to correct the problem, and document a return of homeostasis is the goal of cardiovascular management in the critical care unit.

CARDIAC PHYSIOLOGY

The determinants of cardiac performance are alteration in muscle length or preload, muscle tension or afterload, contractile state of the myocardium, and the frequency of contraction of the heart.

Normal myocardial cells contain myofibrils, which are composed of repeating sarcomeres. Each sarcomere is made up of overlapping, parallel myofilaments. The thicker filaments are composed of myosin and the thinner filaments are of actin. It is the interaction between these two filaments that cause contraction with shortening of the myocardial fiber.

There are also specialized myocardial cells which initiate intrinsic electrical activity in the heart, the so-called pacemaker cells as well as other cells which are specialized for conduction of impulses throughout the myocardium, i.e. Purkinje cells. Details of the ultrastructure and function of myocardial cells are deferred to more comprehensive discussions of this subject (7).

The action potential of cardiac cells is generated by ionic movement of sodium and calcium across the cell membrane. Na^+ enters the cell, followed by entry of Ca^{++}. It is the slower Ca^{++} entrance which is blocked by calcium entry channel blocking agents like verapamil, nifedipine, and diltiazem and increased by

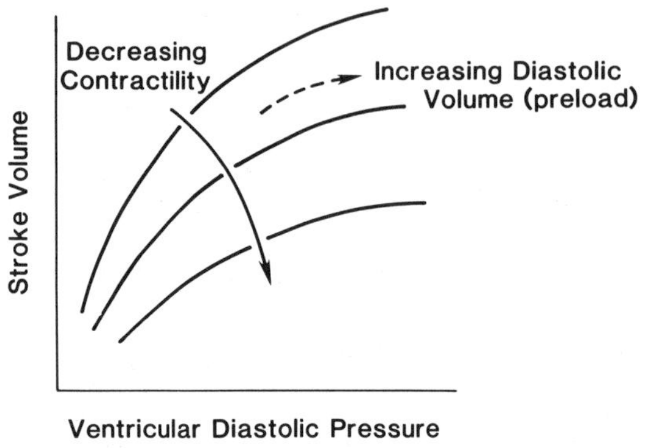

Figure 2.1. The ventricular function curve best describes the relationships of cardiac output and ventricular filling as initially enunciated by Starling. For practical purposes, when ventricular diastolic pressure is increased, stroke output is increased (*dashed arrow*). When myocardial contractility is increased (*solid arrow*) stroke output is increased at relatively lower diastolic pressures.

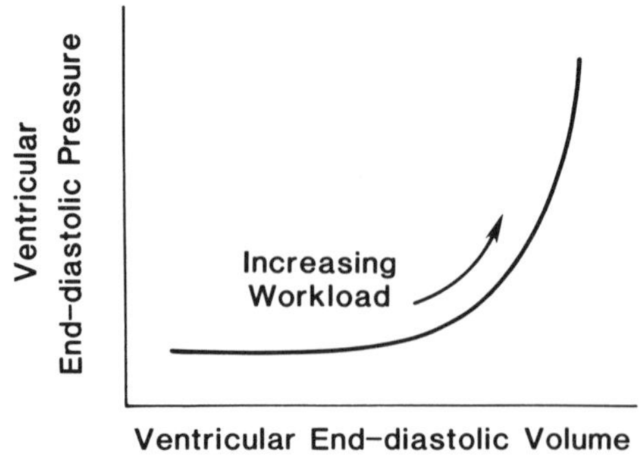

Figure 2.2. With small increments in preload or afterload and therefore diastolic volume, there is little change in ventricular diastolic pressure. When ventricular diastolic volume is greatly increased, there is a disproportionate increase in diastolic pressure.

catecholamines like epinephrine, dopamine, and dobutamine. The concentration of intracellular calcium moderates the force of contraction. During relaxation, calcium is taken up by the sarcoplasmic reticulum, thereby inhibiting the interaction of actin and myosin.

Cardiac function has been extensively studied in isolated muscle preparations (102). Despite many limitations, the concepts pertaining to isolated muscle can be applied to the intact heart (127). The Frank-Starling principle indicates the relationship between initial myocardial fiber length and the force of contraction of that fiber. If the stretch of the fiber is greater due to increases in ventricular diastolic volume, then that fiber will contract to a greater extent during systole. Consequently, more blood is expelled before the fiber returns to its usual end-systolic length. There is a curvilinear relationship between left ventricular end-diastolic pressure and stroke volume (Fig. 2.1). When ventricular diastolic volume is very moderately increased, there is a little change in ventricular diastolic pressure; with greater increases in diastolic volume, disproportionate increases in ventricular diastolic pressure are observed (Fig. 2.2). This has important clinical implications.

In the normal heart, increases in diastolic volume by the administration of fluid may substantially augment cardiac output (i.e. stroke volume × heart rate) with little increase in ventricular diastolic pressure. With excessive volumes, and especially in the failing heart, increases in diastolic volume produce substantial and deleterious increases in ventricular diastolic pressure.

Large increases in ventricular diastolic pressure have adverse effects on ventricular compliance. When the ventricular myocardium is stretched, it becomes stiffer, i.e. there is a reduction in compliance. Such a loss of compliance further increases the pressure within the ventricular chamber and reduces the capability of the heart to maintain cardiac output. Drugs which increase compliance and therefore decrease intraventricular pressure like the arterial vasodilator agent, nitroprusside, may therefore increase cardiac output.

Afterload is defined as the tension developed within the ventricle after the onset of fiber shortening. It is a major determinant of the workload on the heart and ventricular compliance and therefore of cardiac output. In the clinical setting, increases in aortic pressure, due to increases in systemic vascular resistance, impede the ejection of blood from the left ventricle and thereby increase cardiac work. When the heart has limited contractile capability, stroke volume is reduced (8). The more severely depressed the inotropic state of the heart, the greater the benefit of decreasing afterload (14, 88). This is shown in Figure 2.3. The normal heart also compensates for increases in afterload, by increasing preload and end-diastolic volume which serve to increase stroke volume.

The venous blood volume that is returned to the heart constitutes the preload. When preload is increased, the velocity and extent of fiber shortening is usually increased and this accounts for increases in stroke volume and therefore in cardiac output. However, there is a critical limit to the preload that can be accommodated (8). These concepts provide the basis for fluid challenge techniques in which the clinician monitors the relationship between filling pressures (central venous or pulmonary artery occlusive or wedge pressure) and cardiac output. As such, the clinician utilizes the Starling concept of ventricular function as he infuses volume to augment preload and therefore cardiac output at the bedside, minimizing the risk of ventricular failure.

Contractility is best defined as cardiac performance independent of preload or afterload. Many authors have studied contractility in the intact heart in an attempt to define a parameter for measurement useful at the bedside. However, no single parameter for such assessment of contractility at the bedside has been forthcoming (34, 71). Inotropic agents such as dobutamine and amrinone increase the contractile state of the heart (8) with increases in velocity of fiber shortening, stroke volume, and ventricular emptying (ejection fraction).

Heart rate also affects myocardial performance by increasing the frequency of contraction. In the normal heart, reflex adjustments in preload are such that there are no net changes in cardiac output within the physiologic range of heart rate. During exercise, increases in heart rate account for increases in cardiac output with increased preload and decreased afterload (36). At very rapid heart rates and especially in the absence of exercise (paroxysmal tachycardia), a decrease in diastolic filling time may account for decreases in cardiac output.

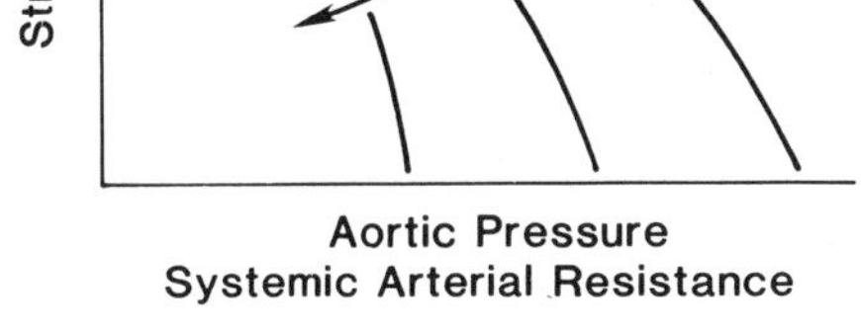

Figure 2.3. The relationship between systemic vascular resistance (afterload) and stroke output. Decreases in afterload result in increases in stroke output. Note that this effect is magnified in the failing heart.

Accordingly, control of cardiac performance is regulated primarily by changes in preload and afterload and, to a lesser extent, contractility and heart rate. The primary responses to increased demands for cardiac output are an increase in venous return and decrease in systemic resistance. The mechanisms by which cardiac output is augmented by increases in cardiac contractility and heart rate are primarily related to reflex neurologic and humoral responses acting through adrenergic mechanisms.

PATHOPHYSIOLOGY OF HEART FAILURE

Myocardial failure is the state in which an abnormality of intrinsic cardiac function accounts for inadequate cardiac output such that the demands of the systemic tissues for blood flow are incompletely met. We will distinguish between intrinsic myocardial disease from valvular or obstructive defects, hypo- or hypervolemia, anemia, hypoxia, and primary vasomotor disorders, all of which may account for hemodynamic deficits in the absence of impaired myocardial function.

When myocardial failure is due to excessive ventricular workloads or impaired muscle function, three compensatory mechanisms are in evidence: (a) increases in preload; (b) increases in catecholamine production; and (c) myocardial hypertrophy and/or dilation. When these options are exhausted, cardiac output declines. Typically, ventricular diastolic pressure is increased. In the case of left ventricular failure, this increase in ventricular diastolic pressure is the cause of increased pulmonary venous pressure and capillary pressure accounting for pulmonary edema. With right ventricular failure, increases in venous pressure account for visceral congestion and progressive systemic edema.

The etiologic mechanisms that account for low output failure include coronary artery disease, hypertension, and primary myocardial disease. High output failure is most often due to anemia, increases in metabolic rate due to hyperthyroidism, nutritional heart disease due to thiamin deficiency (beriberi), or arteriovenous shunts. The pathophysiology of acute myocardial infarction will be addressed separately.

More chronic states of congestive heart failure result in an overall increase in total blood volume and body water. In low cardiac output states, the circulatory system is driven by endocrine mechanisms that are much like those that appear during hypovolemia. Renin, angiotensin, and aldosterone are increased and there is increased sodium and water reabsorption in the kidneys. Increases in neurogenic and endocrine-generated catecholamines increase pre- and postcapillary sphincter tone. Predominant increases in venous pressure account for losses of volume from the vascular space and increased fluid transfer to the interstitium, accentuating renal stimuli for water retention. There also appears to be a redistribution of blood flow to vital organs, away from skin and muscle.

Chronic pressure overload leads to myocardial hypertrophy and fibrosis, which reduces the maximal velocity of fiber shortening and therefore myocardial contractility (104). For any level of tension generated, a higher than normal pressure and/or volume are required in accordance with Starling's law of the heart. Increases in arterial resistance (afterload) generate concentric ventricular hypertrophy (hypertrophic cardiomyopathy) and increases in diastolic ventricular pressure account for ventricular dilatation (congestive cardiomyopathy) (35).

During cardiac failure, catecholamine production is increased (15). Increases in plasma norepinephrine correlate directly with the severity of failure (119). Adrenergic support by beta-adrenergic actions on the failing heart usually serves to maintain cardiac output. However, the peripheral alpha-adrenergic effects of catecholamines by which they increase afterload may intensify heart failure. It is in this setting that vasodilator drugs may be especially useful (14).

HEMODYNAMIC MONITORING

Recent technologic advances have enabled the clinician to rapidly assess changes in cardiovascular function at the bedside. Peripheral arterial and pulmonary artery catheterization with continuous electrocardiographic recording have become routine for management of the critically ill patient with hemodynamic instability. The data obtained from such serve to establish hemodynamic diagnoses, allow more precise selection of one or more pharmacologic or physical interventions, and permit evaluation of efficacy and hemodynamic detriments of therapy. Clinical evaluation alone may be misleading in critically ill or injured patients with cardiac and multisystem failure. When hemodynamic measurements are available, it may alter the plan of therapy in as many as 60% of cases (17, 22, 47).

Hemodynamic monitoring has provided the clinician with practical options by which the principles of circulatory physiology may be applied to the management of circulatory disorders in the critically ill or injured patient (131, 132). Conventional hemodynamic monitoring includes continuous or intermittent measurement of heart rate, systemic and pulmonary arterial pressures, right and left heart filling pressures, and cardiac output. Measurements of cardiac output and computation of cardiac index provide an indication of systemic blood flow. The average volume of blood ejected with each beat, i.e. stroke volume (SV), and the work performed by both the right and left heart, i.e. stroke work (SW), can be calculated for any given heart rate. SW incorporates arterial pressure such that it represents the combined volume and pressure work performed by the heart at a given preload and afterload. By convention, normal values are determined according to body surface area (BSA) and the terms cardiac index (CI), stroke volume index (SVI) and stroke work index (SWI) are used to denote values which are normalized to BSA. The computation of systemic and pulmonary vascular resistance provides an estimate of impedance to ejection of blood flow from the left and right ventricles and the relative state of constriction of systemic and pulmonary resistance vessels, i.e., arteries and arterioles.

With this data, the clinician may estimate preload, afterload, and myocardial contractility, and plan hemodynamic interventions with reference thereto. Knowledge of the left atrial filling pressure by measurement of pulmonary capillary wedge (occlusive) pressure (PAO) and determination of plasma colloid osmotic pressure indicates the likelihood of fluid flux across the pulmonary capillary microvascular membrane and therefore the risk of pulmonary edema (9, 37, 78, 82, 109).

In addition, the catheters provide access for direct sampling of arterial and mixed venous blood, which can be analyzed for blood gases, hemoglobin, and related biochemical measurements. One can then calculate arterial and venous oxygen content (CaO_2 and $C\bar{v}O_2$), arterial-venous content difference ($Ca\text{-}\bar{v}O_2$), and the extraction of oxygen between arterial and mixed venous blood. With this information, the amount of oxygen in arterial and venous blood may be quantified. Inadequate arterial content may be corrected by increasing the concentration of inspired oxygen, augmenting ventilation by mechanical means, or by increasing hemoglobin by red cell transfusion. Low venous content or a large a-$\bar{v}$ oxygen difference suggests inadequate delivery of oxygen to tissues because of inadequate blood flow (cardiac output). High venous oxygen content or a narrow a-$\bar{v}$ difference in oxygen content implies poor tissue utilization of oxygen, a condition which is most often observed during sepsis (45, 56). Calculation of oxygen delivery ($\dot{D}o_2$) and consumption ($\dot{V}o_2$) provide the clinician with an estimate of oxygen availability to tissues and its consumption by tissues over time. Inadequate oxygen delivery has been shown to correlate with lactic acidosis and poor outcome (6, 83). Once these data are available, the clinician is able to assess cardiovascular performance, tissue requirements for oxygen, and the adequacy of both the delivery system and compensatory mechanisms. In the patient whose demands exceed the supply of oxygen which is delivered, interventions by which oxygen delivery is augmented are utilized (27, 51, 60, 67, 80, 83).

Indications for Hemodynamic Monitoring

Hemodynamic monitoring and measurements are, for practical purposes, of little benefit without the conventional clinical examination and especially the history, physical examination, and routine laboratory studies (112). Therapy may be started at times of life-threatening circulatory crises if either practical restraints that would significantly delay insertion of catheters are encountered and especially so if the intervention is of itself unequivocally life-saving, e.g. volume and red cell replacement during massive hemorrhage. However, hemodynamic monitoring may be instituted within 20 minutes by well trained clinicians and this usually provides substantial refinement and safety of therapy.

One of the indications for vascular catheterization that emerged early during introduction of hemodynamic monitoring was the optimal management of shock after acute myocardial infarction (29, 30, 113). It is now apparent that for management of patients in whom myocardial infarction is complicated by shock, severe congestive heart failure, prolonged ischemia, hypotension, or tachycardia, hemodynamic monitoring is uniquely helpful (76). In addition, unstable patients, patients who are unresponsive to conservative therapy, and patients who require titration of vasopressors or vasodilators may benefit from hemodynamic monitoring after myocardial infarction (66).

Patients may be in clinical shock from many causes unrelated to myocardial infarction. Among these etiologies are hypovolemic, distributive, or obstructive shock (130). Pulmonary artery catheterization may be useful both for differentiating these causes of shock and for optimum cardiovascular management. Right heart catheterization may also be helpful for the management of acute respiratory failure, especially if mechanical ventilation with positive end-expiratory pressure is utilized. Acute respiratory failure may be due to decompensation of chronic obstructive pulmonary disease (31), cardiogenic or noncardiogenic pulmonary edema (adult respiratory distress syndrome) (81, 98, 107), or ventilatory failure due to cerebral depression after anesthesia or drug intoxication. Hemodynamic monitoring may prove to be beneficial for those patients at risk for cardiopulmonary complications who undergo major surgery (5, 94, 96, 97). In addition, a recent study suggests that routine pulmonary artery catheterization may be useful during the course of high risk surgery in patients with impaired myocardial function (125).

Techniques of Hemodynamic Monitoring

The essential components for hemodynamic monitoring include vascular access introducer devices; intravascular catheters; noncompliant pressure tubing; transducers and electrical cables; pressurized, heparinized flush solutions;

automatic, continuous and manual flush devices; and a bedside monitor. The availability of digital displays has been of advantage but both waveform display and recording should not be compromised. The system is arranged such that pressure is transmitted via a continuous column of fluid from the intravascular catheter, through the connecting tubing and to the diaphragm of the transducer. This diaphragm is physically imprinted by the pressure wave such that an electrical signal is created which is transmitted to the bedside processor. The signal is amplified, related to a preset zero, and calibrated. It is then displayed as an analog signal and quantified for presentation as a digital measurement or on an analog meter. In the clinical setting, the system is referenced to atmospheric pressure, and the zero reference point is standardized. The midchest in the third interspace is conventionally identified as the reference point approximating the right atrium. To ensure accurate calibration of the entire system, mercury standards are used. Accordingly, the transducer is calibrated by using a pressure calibrator which represents a refined mercury manometer.

Balloon-tipped pulmonary artery catheters may be inserted rapidly at the bedside by flotation techniques without fluoroscopy (93, 113). Currently available pulmonary artery catheters have a distal lumen for measuring pulmonary artery systolic, diastolic, and mean pressures and for obtaining blood samples that represent mixed venous blood. A proximal lumen is in a position corresponding to the right atrium or superior vena cava for measurement of right-sided pressures. There may be an additional port just proximal to the right atrial port for fluid or drug infusion and an additional port for balloon inflation. Finally, there is a lumen which accommodates the leads to a thermistor at the tip of the catheter which is used for thermodilution measurements of cardiac output. We prefer to set up all bedside equipment, including transducers and monitors prior to catheterization. We prepare a sterile tray with all of the instruments required for insertion of the catheter. It is necessary to assure access to the airway during the procedure for endotracheal intubation. Advanced cardiac life support equipment and medication are kept near the bedside. The electrocardiogram should be continuously monitored. Sterility must be maintained, and the operator and assistants should wear gowns, masks, hair covers, and sterile gloves. An adequately large sterile field should be prepared, and the skin well-cleansed.

The choice of access site is largely contingent on the skill of the operator. Sites available include the internal jugular, subclavian, and femoral veins for the percutaneous insertion and the basilic vein for surgical insertion. In our experience, the posterior approach to the right internal jugular vein affords the easiest, fastest, and most direct route to the right ventricle with minimal risk of pneumothorax (16, 52, 70). The percutaneous guidewire technique enables the operator to catheterize the vein with minimal trauma and blood loss. After venous access has been established with an 18-g to 20-g needle, a guidewire is advanced into the vein. The vein is then dilated by advancing a tapered obturator over the guide wire together with a thin-walled sheath (3). The catheter is then checked carefully for defects. Each lumen is flushed and capped with a fluid-filled syringe to prevent inadvertent air embolism (18, 77, 103). The balloon is observed for air leaks and symmetric inflation. The guidewire and obturator are then removed and the flotation catheter is advanced through the sheath into the vein for a distance of 10 cm. The balloon is then inflated and, with continuous pressure monitoring, allowed to float through the right atrium and ventricle into the pulmonary artery. The central venous pressure (CVP) tracing has characteristic a, c, and v waves. CVP should be recorded as a mean, with normal pressure being 0 to 10 mm Hg. From the posterior approach to the right internal jugular vein, the CVP position is reached within 15 to 20 cm. from the skin entry point. Careful electrocardiogram (ECG) and waveform monitoring during transit of the catheter through the right atrium (RA) and right ventricle (RV) and into the pulmonary artery (PA) is important for detection of potentially dangerous dysrhythmias (10, 94, 106). Characteristic waveform changes are noted during transit through the right heart and into the pulmonary artery. Normal PA pressures are 15 to 25/8 to 16 mm Hg with a mean of 10 to 20 mm Hg. Pressures during transit are recorded. With the balloon still inflated, the catheter is allowed to advance into the pulmonary capillary or wedge position. This makes it possible to record reflected left-sided pressures which approximate left atrial pressure. As the catheter maneuvers from the pulmonary artery to the occluded (wedge) position, the pressure pulse gives way to a lower pressure with atrial pulse morphology. Characteristic a, c, and v waves of an atrial pressure pulse are observed. The normal occlusive pressure is 6 to 15 mm Hg. After balloon deflation, there is a return of the pulmonary artery pressure pulse because the catheter floats back from a distal occluded position to a more proximal pulmonary artery position. When the tip of the catheter remains distal after balloon inflation, there is substantial risk of prolonged occlusion with great risk of pulmonary infarction. Typically, the catheter will be inserted for a distance of between 45 to 55 cm from the jugular vein entry site. Each lumen is then attached to appropriate intravenous flush solutions, syringe for balloon inflation, or electrically connected to a cardiac output computer. The catheter is then secured. A chest radiograph should be taken to confirm position and exclude malposition and complications, especially pneumothorax or perforation of a major vessel or the heart itself.

Complication of PA Catheterizations

Complications of PA catheterizations have been well studied (24, 69, 79, 94, 99) and may be separated into two groups, i.e., those related to vascular access and those related more specifically to the pathway of the catheter itself. Access to the central circuit is complicated most commonly by infection, pneumothorax, hemorrhage, and thrombosis; and less often by damage to the trachea, thoracic duct, carotid or subclavian arteries, and recurrent laryngeal nerve. Infection with bacteremia may occur in as many as 20% of catheterized patients (89). Endocardial lesions appear to be common, in as many as 53% of catheterized patients at autopsy. True infective endocarditis occurred in only 7% of all catheterized patients, but in 36% of those with positive blood cultures. Infection is diagnosed on the basis of local tissue invasion, signs of systemic sepsis, and recovery of pathogenic organisms on wound and blood cultures. The risks of infection are closely related to the duration of catheter insertion, the extent of the manipulations that were performed during and following catheter insertion, breaks in sterile technique during insertion, and procedures in which breaks of technique with contamination of stopcocks, transducers, and syringes are not rigorously controlled. To minimize infectious complications, catheters should be inserted aseptically, manipulations minimized, and impeccable nursing care continued both for care of the insertion site and the manipulation of the catheter. In addition, we recommend catheter and site changes after a maximum of 4 days. New disposable transducer domes, closed cardiac output injection systems and sterile external sleeves may provide additional protection.

Venous thrombosis secondary to jugular vein cannulation by guidewire technique may occur in as many as 66% of patients. Remarkably, there are no major complications attributable thereto (13). Whether heparin bonding of catheters decreases the incidence of thrombotic embolization is still unsettled (46).

Complications unique to pulmonary artery catheters include dysrhythmias, pulmonary artery rupture, pulmonary infarction, and catheter knotting (28, 38, 64, 75, 105, 106, 114, 124). The incidence of each of these appears to be acceptably low, and most are preventable. Nevertheless, there is potential for fatal complications. In the immediately life-threatened patient with limited cardiovascular reserve, however, pulmonary artery catheterization is a valuable and redeeming adjunct for clinical assessment and for monitoring of the effects of interventions in the critically ill.

Intra-arterial Monitoring

Arterial catheterization is equally important for the management of the critically ill patient and especially for management of shock states. Conventional indirect (cuff) techniques are inaccurate during circulatory shock regardless of whether these are automated. Excessive vasoconstriction in the brachial artery with reduced blood flow leads to underestimations of true intra-arterial pressure by as much as 60 mm Hg (136). Access to the arterial circuit by way of the femoral, radial, or brachial arteries is technically feasible. However, smaller arteries such as the dorsalis pedis artery have been used. The femoral artery is, in our experience, most accessable and complication rates are comparable to those observed with other sites (2, 79, 90, 101). As with venous catheters, use of a guidewire technique as well as meticulous catheter care appear to decrease the incidence of complications.

Cardiac Output

Cardiac output (CO) is measured by the thermodilution technique. A bolus of 10 ml of iced 5% dextrose in water is injected rapidly into the proximal port of the pulmonary artery catheter such that the tracer is delivered to the right atrium. Triplicate measurements are typically performed with the aid of a CO computer. The normal CI ranges from 2.3 to 3.5 liters/min/M^2. The CI is preferred to cardiac output because the value is normalized to body surface area. The thermodilution method provides accuracy comparable to that of dye-dilution and the Fick (oxygen consumption) techniques (32). It is relatively independent of catheter position (41). It may be performed with injections of either smaller amounts of iced tracer or larger amounts of room temperature solution (23, 95).

Other Variables

Routines of monitoring also include the measurement of body temperatures, heart rate, and respiratory rate. Laboratory studies include arterial and mixed venous blood gases, arterial blood lactate, and colloid osmotic pressure and hemoglobin. The chest radiograph is also routinely ordered to assess presence and magnitude of congestive or infiltrative pulmonary changes, pulmonary barotrauma, and cardiac size. The pulmonary artery wedge pressure measurement may be hampered by respiratory variations (11, 65, 85). If the patient is maintained on positive pressure ventilation, the apparent occlusive (wedge) pressure may be increased and this is especially true with positive end-expiratory pressure breathing (PEEP). Breath-holding or disconnection of the ventilator from the airway does not resolve the problem (85); however, when readings are obtained at end-expiration (85) or after neuromuscular paralysis, accuracy of readings may be improved (92).

Indices of Perfusion Failure

Over the last 20 years, the focus on management of circulatory shock has been shifted from blood pressure to blood flow. More specifically, it is the adequacy of tissue perfusion and oxygenation which are now recognized as the primary determinants of outcome (100). Both systemic and regional or local perfusion are addressed. Systemic measurements include lactic acid, mixed venous oxygen tension and saturation, oxygen consumption, and oxygen delivery. Local indices include toe temperature, transcutaneous oxygen, subcutaneous oxygen, and tissue oxygen.

The arterial blood concentrations of lactic acid correlate highly with outcome in critically ill patients with circulatory shock (43, 123, 129). Arterial blood lactate quantifies anaerobic metabolism. In the absence of adequate tissue concentrations of oxygen, glucose is preferentially metabolized to lactate. Accordingly, increases in lactate are closely related to decreases in oxygen transport or utilization (129). The lactate concentration increases after body reserves of oxygen have been exhausted. A rapid, technically simple technique has recently been developed for bedside measurement of lactate with excellent accuracy (57).

Mixed venous oxygen tension or saturation is a reflection of tissue oxygen levels (100). For practical purposes, mixed venous blood represents a weighted mean of the effluent of all tissue beds (115). If tissue oxygen supply is reduced or if demands for oxygen are increased, additional quantities of oxygen are extracted from capillary blood and the oxygen content (tension, saturation) of mixed venous blood is correspondingly reduced. The other major compensatory mechanism is an increase in oxygen delivery by increases in cardiac output and therefore oxygen delivery. When these mechanisms are exhausted, oxygen deficits are created and lactic acidosis appears (20, 50). In patients with adult respiratory distress syndrome, septic shock, and drug-induced coma including general anesthesia, there may be critical decreases in tissue perfusion, lactic acidosis, and fatal oxygen deficits even though mixed venous oxygen tension or saturation remains at normal levels (20, 45, 56, 72). This apparent lack of correlation between mixed venous tension and tissue oxygen levels may be explained by redistribution of blood flow, e.g. arteriovenous shunts with selective reduction in capillary blood flow or impairment in oxygen uptake due to metabolic block, e.g. cyanide intoxication. In our opinion, monitoring of mixed venous oxygen tension or saturation may be useful but only in select clinical settings for diagnosis and management.

Oxygen delivery and consumption also may discriminate between survival and death, especially in surgical patients (6, 83, 133). Oxygen delivery reflects supply and consumption reflects utilization. The essential issue is whether the supply matches the demand for oxygen to fulfill the metabolic requirements. For practical purposes, this is resolved by measurement of arterial blood lactate. It is technically much more formidable to measure oxygen consumption as an indicator of adequacy of tissue perfusion and this is more often reserved for experimental or teaching applications.

Measurements of peripheral (local or regional) perfusion have been advocated by several authors, especially since these provide noninvasive options for monitoring and may be cost redeeming (4, 12, 54, 126). These assessments primarily reflect regional perfusion. Blood is usually redistributed away from muscle, skin, and subcutaneous tissues during circulatory shock and changing indices of peripheral blood flow serve as indicators of the direction of systemic changes during therapy. Transcutaneous oxygen sensors have been utilized as a noninvasive measurement of tissue oxygenation (120, 126). With normal flow, transcutaneous oxygen tension approximates systemic arterial oxygen tension. During regional low flow states, transcutaneous oxygen tension is reduced such that there is a decrease in the ratio of transcutaneous to arterial oxygen tension at the site of measurement. This may be used to assess the onset and the severity of the low flow (shock) state (120, 126).

Subcutaneous oxygen tension and muscle oxygen tension histograms are invasive measurements that have been utilized for experimental study of tissue perfusion (12, 54). Both methods are clinically less useful because of the need for surgical invasion of the patient. For measurement of subcutaneous oxygen tension, a small catheter is inserted into the subcutaneous fat under local anesthesia. Muscle oxygen tension histograms are obtained after a multiwire surface electrode is implanted on the surface of striated muscle.

Measurement of toe temperature is a disarmingly simple, noninvasive monitor which has been advocated for quantifying severity of acute circulatory failure (42). In patients who present with circulatory shock, the temperature gradient between the great toe and ambient air is reduced to less than 2°C whereas it normally exceeds 2°C. Decreases in the toe-ambient temperature gradient have been closely correlated with lactate concentration and survival (48).

ACUTE MYOCARDIAL INFARCTION

When blood flow to the myocardium is critically reduced, myocardial ischemia is likely to occur. In the normal heart, there is a balance between oxygen supply and demand. When myocardial oxygen demands increase, coronary blood flow increases to meet this demand. When demands outstrip supply, ischemia appears. Prolonged ischemia accounts for tissue necrosis and therefore myocardial infarction. Myocardial blood flow may be impaired because of fixed coronary obstruction due to atheromata as a primary cause; this is followed by platelet adhesion and thrombosis (26). In a small minority of patients, vascular spasm may be the primary cause of ischemia and acute infarction (1, 33). In general terms, the primary goal of therapy is to restore coronary blood flow to levels that will sustain the myocardial oxygen demands.

Myocardial oxygen consumption is determined by heart rate, afterload, preload, and state of contractility. Agents which decrease myocardial oxygen requirements may be beneficial; heart rate may be reduced by treatment with beta-adrenergic blocking agents. Agents that decrease arterial blood pressure, i.e. afterload, may be utilized such as nitroprusside. Drugs may be administered to decrease the venous return, i.e. the preload, such as nitroglycerin. Finally, agents may be used that decrease contractility such as beta-adrenergic or calcium channel blockers. Each reduces myocardial oxygen requirements (63).

Nitrates are coronary vasodilators and may improve flow in patients who have fixed lesions or when ischemia is due to coronary spasm (44, 49). Calcium channel blockers act in a similar fashion to improve coronary blood flow (1, 25, 91). Newer thrombolytic agents such as streptokinase, urokinase, and tissue plasminogen activator appear to improve coronary blood flow via clot lysis in the initial 3 hours after thrombosis (53, 55, 84, 118, 121, 122). Mechanical relief of fixed obstructions with transluminal angioplasty may also improve coronary blood flow (21, 40, 74). The exact role of these newer modalities remains to be elucidated in ongoing trials.

Typically, the patient who has acute coronary obstruction presents with substernal chest pain or pressure with radiation to one or both arms and associated dyspnea, nausea, or diaphoresis. Acute myocardial infarction may occur in a surgical setting. Occasionally, such patients present with abdominal, back, and/or neck pain, rather than chest pain; less commonly there may be loss of consciousness due to cardiac dysrhythmias, conduction defects, or very low output states. The clinician must be alert for subtle clues such as unexplained hypertension, hypotension, tachycardia, tachypnea, or oliguria. Routine preoperative and postoperative ECGs are likely to be useful, especially in the elderly. Diagnosis of infarction is based on clinical history, electrocardiographic changes, and serial cardiac enzyme studies. ECG findings include acute ST segment elevation, subsequent T wave inversion, and the development of Q waves. Serial increases in serum creatine phosphokinase (MB fraction) or lactate dehydrogenase with inversion of isoenzyme fractions 1 and 2 corroborate the diagnosis.

The majority of patients are likely to be hemodynamically stable (68) and then do not require invasive monitoring. The patients with acute myocardial infarction should be observed with continuous ECG monitoring for dysrhythmias with awareness of recurrent chest pain, congestive heart failure, or signs of hypoperfusion. They are maintained at bed rest and well-sedated. Antacid and anti-emetic therapy may be administered. Pulmonary embolism prophylaxis should be provided with subcutaneous mini-heparin in the absence of contraindications. Lidocaine is injected or infused intravenously to prevent spontaneous life-threatening ventricular ectopic rhythms (39, 59).

Persistent pain should be aggressively treated, initially with coronary vasodilator drugs and especially nitrates, preferably by the intravenous administration of nitroglycerin. The dose is titrated to the point of pain relief or hypotension. As much as 400 μg/min may be required until pain is relieved. In the higher dose ranges, increased venous pooling and arterial vasodilation occur; arterial blood pressure may therefore be reduced. For refined management, direct intra-arterial pressure monitoring may be required, guided by measurements of left-sided filling pressure with a balloon-tipped pulmonary artery catheter. A fluid challenge may be appropriate such as to increase cardiac output. Beta-blockade may be strikingly effective for relief of ischemic pain. Propanolol may be given either by mouth in amounts of 20 to 80 mg or, preferably, by intravenous injection in divided doses of 1 mg, slowly, to a maximum of 0.1 mg/kg. Heart rate must be carefully monitored to avoid symptomatic brady- or tachydysrhythmias. However, there is a relative contraindication to beta-adrenergic blocking agents in the presence of bradydysrhythmias, congestive heart failure, and bronchospastic pulmonary disease (63). Intravenous injection or infusion of morphine sulfate in doses of 2 to 5 mg may be utilized to decrease pain, anxiety, and therefore hyperactivity (hypermetabolism). However, morphine is a venodilator which, like nitroglycerin, increases venous capacitance (87). It may therefore reduce preload and cardiac output and thereby reduce blood pressure and coronary perfusion. If pain is not relieved, calcium channel blocking agents such as nifedipine, 10 to 20 mg orally every 8 hours, may be used. Hemodynamic measurements are used to guide medical therapy with nitrates, beta-adrenergic blocking agents and calcium channel blocking agents. If ischemia persists despite maximal medical therapy, arrangements may be made for more invasive studies and interventions including intra-aortic balloon counterpulsation, coronary and left heart catheterization with angiography, and urgent coronary angioplasty or coronary artery bypass surgery.

Myocardial dysfunction manifested by congestive heart failure and/or cardiogenic shock occurs when a critical mass of myocardium is impaired by ischemia or infarction. When clinical examination demonstrates signs of mild congestive heart failure, including basilar lung crepitations, increased jugular venous pressure, and a ventricular gallop rhythm, supplementing oxygen, maintaining a head-up body position, administration of morphine as a venodilator and calming agent, and the intravenous injection of a loop diuretic, e.g. 40 mg of furosemide, are usually effective. If there is evidence of hypoperfusion with clinical signs of shock including cool clammy extremities, peripheral cyanosis, hypotension, and progressive lactic acidemia, hemodynamic monitoring is mandatory. This enables the clinician to optimize preload (filling pressure), afterload (arterial resistance), and flow (cardiac output) (29, 30, 128). Our preference is for titrated therapy, especially when nitroglycerin or nitroprusside are used. This has the aim of reducing filling pressures of the heart or reducing arterial resistance (14). Nitroglycerin is predominately a venodilator and nitroprusside has dual arterial and venodilator actions. It has been shown that an increased left ventricular filling, i.e. pulmonary artery occlusive (wedge) pressure of about 16 mm Hg provides for more optimum cardiac output in the acutely infarcted patient (19). It must be emphasized, however, that single measurements of pulmonary artery occlusion pressure may be misleading because the estimate of zero reference, calibration of the transducer, and catheter position have substantial variability not infrequently exceeding ± 4 mm Hg. Fluid challenge is therefore used in an attempt to maximize cardiac output without disproportionate increase in pulmonary occlusive pressure and the high risk of pulmonary edema. The coronary perfusion pressure is also of import. With obstructive lesions, it appears that the minimal mean arterial pressure which will maintain adequate coronary perfusion is approximately 65 mm Hg (66).

Patients have been divided into hemodynamic subsets (29, 30, 128). When the PAO exceeds 18 mm HG and CI is less than 2.2 liters/min/m^2, this is characteristic of cardiogenic shock. With PAO pressure substantially less than 14 mm Hg and CI less than 2.2 liters/min/m^2, the features are those of relative hypovolemia and fluid challenge is indicated. When the CI is within normal levels but PAO pressure is greater than 18, the features are those of congestive heart failure. These patients often do well with preload and/or afterload reduction with nitroglycerin and/or nitroprusside. When the patient presents with substantial increases in PAO pressure to levels exceeding 18 mm Hg, a low CI (less than 2.2 liters/min/m^2 and hypotension, the features are diagnostic of cardiogenic shock. Afterload reduction is hazardous when hypotension predominates. Inotropic support is often attempted but with the risk of increasing oxygen requirements of poorly perfused myocardium; digitalis glycosides are weak inotropic agents but not contraindicated. Adrenergic agonists may be transiently effective in increasing cardiac index and arterial pressure but at the expense of greatly increasing myocardial oxygen demands (66, 67). Although dobutamine and nonadrenergic amrinone have become available as more rational inotropic drugs which have higher efficacy with lower oxygen demands, their ultimate benefit is unproven in this setting. Intraortic balloon counterpulsation has been attempted but it has not altered mortality unless a specific surgical intervention, such as mitral valve replacement for reversal of valvular insufficiency after papillary muscle infarction or closure of an acquired septal defect after septal infarction, restores hemodynamic stability. Mortality in patients with cardiogenic shock is uniformly high, typically greater than 90%. With the exception of a few patients for whom surgical repairs are life-saving, no definitive therapy is currently available for patients who are in shock when more than 40% of cardiac muscle is infarcted.

In patients with uncomplicated myocardial infarction, recovery is likely. However, in the surgical setting, the options of management are more restrictive; pain and stress increase myocardial and systemic oxygen demands and increase both the risk of a coronary catastrophe and adversely affect outcome. For instance, the option of manipulating the hemodynamic status in patients with cerebral edema is constrained. Above all, cerebral perfusion pressures must be maintained at levels of greater than 50 mm Hg regardless of adverse effects on preload and afterload. Intracranial pressure monitoring in this setting is even more important and should be utilized in conjunction with routine hemodynamic monitoring. When cerebral edema is suspected in patients with acute coronary crises, agents which decrease intracranial pressure, such as osmolar diuretics, may be hazardous because they expand intravascular volume and intensify heart failure. Hyperventilation with respiratory alkalosis may increase the frequency and severity of ectopic atrial and ventricular rhythms (134, 135). Antiarrhythmic therapy including lidocaine, procainamide, or bretylium tosylate may be administered for the treatment of ectopic ventricular rhythms.

Ventricular tachycardia may present with or without evidence of hemodynamic compromise. It should be treated very promptly with antiarrhythmic therapy. In the case of pulselessness due to ventricular tachycardia or ventricular fibrillation, immediate electrical cardioversion is indicated (58, 61).

Atrial tachydysrhythmias result in diminished ventricular diastolic filling with decreases in cardiac output. This may be hazardous if cerebral perfusion is compromised. Paroxysmal supraventricular tachycardia is best managed with intravenous boluses of verapamil, 5 to 10 mg, and this is usually followed by conversion to sinus rhythm. Alternatively, propanolol or digoxin may be used. Atrial fibrillation with rapid rates can be controlled with repeated intravenous doses of 0.25 mg of digoxin at intervals of 1 to 2 hours until the rate is reduced to less than 100. Conversion to sinus rhythm is often spontaneous following digitalis administration. Occasionally quinidine may be added to the regimen in an attempt to facilitate cardioversion. The electrocardiogram and preferably blood levels of drugs are monitored. When supraventricular tachydysrhythmias cause hemodynamic compromise, low voltage synchronized cardioversion is indicated after sedation with a tranquilizing drug such as intravenous diazepam. Isolated premature atrial beats do not usually require therapy.

If bradydysrhythmias are due to heart block, the option of pharmacologic therapy with intravenous atropine and/or isoproterenol infusion and/or temporary transvenous electrical pacing are utilized.

In the event of cardiac arrest, conventional cardiopulmonary resuscitation should be performed with ventilation, external cardiac com pressions, and administration of medications according to current standards of cardiopulmonary resuscitation (CPR) (108). Asystole should be treated primarily with epinephrine. Electromechanical dissociation may be an agonal rhythm, but may be due to a physical cause and especially cardiac tamponade.

HYPERTENSION

The most common cause of hypertension in the hospitalized patient is that of an exacerbation of essential hypertension. Though it is uncontrolled hypertension that may lead to intracranial hemorrhage, hypertension may be due to central nervous system (CNS) damage itself and represent an adaptive response that may sustain cerebral perfusion.

Hypertensive emergencies include hypertension associated with encephalopathy, intracerebral bleed, pulmonary edema, and aortic dissection. Both pheochromocytoma and eclampsia represent unique causes. However, the goal of therapy is to lower arterial pressure to a level consistent with maintaining organ perfusion including cerebral perfusion but minimizing the immediate risks of the hypertensive state. In the chronically hypertensive patient with encephalopathy, there may a shift of autoregulation such that high blood pressure does not necessarily affect cerebral blood flow (111). Sudden decreases in arterial pressure may therefore compromise cerebral blood flow. These patients typically present with headaches, visual complaints, and decreases in mental acuity. Focal deficits tend to be transient. Systolic blood pressure may not exceed 200 mm systolic, yet profound fundoscopic changes characteristic of hypertensive retinopathy may be present. Structural CNS lesions must be excluded. Arterial blood pressure monitoring should be instituted in preparation for antihypertension treatment with nitroprusside or alternatively trimethophan. We prefer to lower pressure progressively (and gently) with nitroprusside to near normal levels as long as there is no evidence of hypoperfusion. Patients usually improve promptly and dramatically.

After intracerebral hemorrhage or infarction, therapy is similar. As a rule, systolic pressure of approximately 140 to 160 mm Hg and diastolic pressures of 90 to 110 mm Hg suffice for adequate systemic, cerebral, and coronary perfusion. In the patient with traumatic head injury, we prefer to monitor both mean arterial and intracranial pressure such that cerebral perfusion pressure may be quantified.

Sodium nitroprusside is a potent vasodilator with rapid onset and short duration of action (73). Dose is gradually increased from 0.5 μg/kg/min to 15 μg/kg/min. After 24 hours, the dose may be tapered and oral therapy may be initiated. Two prominent side effects of nitroprusside are hypotension, and thiocyanate toxicity. Hypotension is avoidable with routine arterial pressure monitoring. Thiocyanate toxicity is very uncommon and occurs more often in patients with renal failure after protracted therapy. Headaches, confusion, fatigue and nausea are the predominant symptoms. The diagnosis is confirmed by measurement of thiocyanate blood levels (86).

There is concern based on controversial data lest nitroprusside may produce unfavorable cerebral vasodilation and increases in intracranial pressure in the brain-injured patient (110). Intracranial pressure monitoring resolves this issue.

Trimethophan camsylate is a potent ganglionic blocking agent which effectively lowers blood pressure. It also has rapid onset and short duration of action. Disadvantages include orthostatic effects and parasympathetic blockade.

Agents such as furosemide, labetalol, diazoxide, or hydralazine are not ideal for hypertensive emergencies. Effects cannot be titrated with ease.

NEUROGENIC PULMONARY EDEMA

For purposes of completeness, we will refer to neurogenic pulmonary edema and its hemodynamic significance. After acute central nervous system injury, arterial pressure may be elevated, together with intracardiac pressures. In addition, clinical signs of tachypnea, tachycardia, pulmonary edema with fulminant frothy edema fluid, and hypoxemia may appear. Onset of the syndrome is often rapid.

The mechanism by which neurogenic pulmonary edema occurs remain controversial (62, 116, 117). There appear to be marked centrally mediated increases in sympathetic tone, which result in severe transient left atrial and consequently pulmonary capillary hypertension. This leads to extravasation of plasma water into the pulmonary interstitium and subsequently into alveoli. There are also instances in which there is increased pulmonary capillary permeability attributed to vasoactive mediators such as thromboxane, pulmonary microembolization, and lymphatic obstruction.

In spite of its striking clinical features, patients tend to tolerate the syndrome well. The course is typically self-limited, requiring supplemental oxygen as the only therapeutic intervention. Pulmonary pressures are transiently elevated and return to normal rapidly, with more delayed clearing of pulmonary edema (116). Prognosis is contingent on the natural history and reversibility of the underlying neurologic injury.

CONCLUSION

The availability and wide use of newer techniques of hemodynamic study have substantially improved the understanding of the pathophysiology of cardiovascular crises in the critical care setting. Though invasive techniques of hemodynamic monitoring together with measurements of blood gases and related parameters have come into wide use, we now recognize that they are best reserved for diagnosis, monitoring, and management when refined decision-making cannot be otherwise accomplished. The very fact that understanding of hemodynamic mechanisms has been improved has allowed the clinician to be more discriminating in the application of such techniques. However, when survival is immediately threatened by acute circulatory failure for which the cause is not identified with reasonable certainty, such techniques are invaluable for decision-making. In instances in which potentially high risk interventions with fluids, vasoactive drugs, or cardiorespiratory support devices are utilized, monitoring techniques are likely to provide substantial safety. Finally, routines of monitoring may in other settings be the best option for identifying the specific need for high risk interventions and thereby avoid the premature use of interventions which of themselves carry substantial iatrogenic risks.

REFERENCES

1. Antman, E., Muller, J., Goldberg, S., MacAlpin, R., Rubentire, M., Tabatznik, B., Liang, C., *et al.* Nifedipine therapy for coronary artery spasm. N. Engl. J. Med., *302:* 1269–1273, 1980.
2. Baud, J. D., and Maki, D. G. Infections caused by arterial catheters used for hemodynamic monitoring. Am. J. Med., *67:* 735–741, 1979.
3. Benumof, J. L., Wyte, S. R., and Rogers, S. N. A large catheter sheath introducer with an increased side-port functional gauge. Crit. Care Med., *11:* 660–662, 1983.
4. Bisera, J., Weil, M. H., and Rackow, E. C. The perfusometer: An instrument for assessing the condition of critically ill patients. Med. Instrum., *18:* 134–136, 1984.
5. Bland, R. D., Shoemaker, W. C., Abraham, E., and Cobo, J. C. Hemodynamic and oxygen transport patterns in surviving and nonsurviving postoperative patients. Crit. Care Med., *13:* 85–90, 1985.

6. Bland, R., Shoemaker, W. C., and Shabot, M. M. Physiologic monitoring goals for the critically ill patient. Surg. Gynecol. Obstet., *174:* 833–841, 1978.
7. Braunwald, E., Sonnenblick, E. M., and Ross, J. Contraction of the normal heart. In: *Heart Disease: A Textbook of Cardiovascular Medicine,* pp 413–430, edited by E. Braunwald. W. B. Saunders, Philadelphia, 1980.
8. Burns, J. W., Covell, J. W., and Ross, J. Mechanics of isotonic left ventricular contractions. Am. J. Physiol., *224:* 725–732, 1973.
9. Carlson, R. W., and Haupt, M. T. Colloid-hydrostatic gradients and pulmonary edema. Chest, *82:* 398–400, 1982.
10. Castellanos, A., Ramirez, A. V. Mayorgo-Cortes, A., Petkaros, K., Rozanski, J. J., Sprung, C. L., and Myerburg, R. J. Left fascicular blocks during right-heart catheterization using the Swan-Ganz catheter. Circulation, *64:* 1271–1276, 1981.
11. Cengiz, M., Crapo, R. O., and Gardner, R. M. The effect of ventilation on the accuracy of pulmonary artery and wedge pressure measurements. Crit. Care Med., *11:* 502–507, 1983.
12. Chang, N., Goodson, W., Gottrup, F., and Hunt, T. Direct measurement of wound and tissue oxygen tension in postoperative patients. Ann. Surg., *197:* 470–478, 1983.
13. Chastre, J., Cornud, F., Bochama, A., Viau, F., Benacerraf, R., and Gilbert, C. Thrombosis as a complication of pulmonary artery catheterization via the internal jugular vein. N. Engl. J. Med., *306:* 278–281, 1982.
14. Chatterjee, K., Parmley, W. M., Ganz, W., Forrester, J., Walinsky, P., Crexells, C., and Swan, H. J. C. Hemodynamic and metabolic responses to vasodilator therapy in acute myocardial infarction. Circulation, *48:* 1183–1193, 1973.
15. Chidsey, C. A., Braunwald, E., and Morrow, A. G. Catecholamine excretion and cardiac stores of norepinephrine in congestive heart failure. Am. J. Med., *39:* 442–451, 1965.
16. Civetta, J. M., and Gabel, J. C. Flow directed pulmonary artery catheterization in surgical patients: Indication and modifications of technique. Ann. Surg., *176:* 753–756, 1972.
17. Connors, A. F., McCaffree, D. R., and Gray, B. A. Evaluation of right heart catheterization in the critically ill patient without acute myocardial infarction. N. Engl. J. Med., *308:* 263–267, 1983.
18. Coppa, G. F., Gouge, T. H., and Hofstetter, S. R. Air embolism: A lethal but preventable complication of subclavian vein catheterization. J.P.E.N. *5:* 166–68, 1981.
19. Crexells, C., Chatterjie, K., Forrester, J. S. *et al.* Optimal level of filling pressure in the left side of the heart in acute myocardial infarction. N. Engl. J. Med. *289:* 1263–1266, 1973.
20. Danek, S., Lynch, J., Weg, J., and Dantzker, D. The dependence of oxygen uptake on oxygen delivery in the adult respiratory distress syndrome. Am. Rev. Respir. Dis. *122:* 387–395, 1980.
21. DeFeyter, P. J., Serruys, P. W., VandenBrand, M., Balakumaran, K., Mochtar, B., Soward, A. L., Arnold, A. E. R., and Hugenholtz, P. G. Emergency coronary and angioplasty in refractory unstable angina. N. Engl. J. Med., *313:* 342–346, 1985.
22. Eisenberg, P. R., Jaffe, A. S., and Schuster, D. P. Clinical evaluation compared to pulmonary artery catheterization in the hemodynamic assessment of critically ill patients. Crit. Care Med., *12:* 549–53, 1984.
23. Elkayam, V., Berkley, R., Azen, S., Weber, L., Geva, B., and Henry W. L. Cardiac output by thermodilution technique. Chest, *84:* 418–27, 1983.
24. Elliot, C. G., Zimmerman, G. A., and Clemmer, T. P. Complications of pulmonary artery catheterization in the care of critically ill patients. Chest, *76:* 647–52, 1979.
25. Engel, H., and Lichtlen, P. R. Beneficial enhancement of coronary blood flow by nifedipine. Am. J. Med., *71:* 658–666, 1981.
26. Epstein, S. E., and Palmeri, S. T. Mechanisms contributing to precipitation of unstable angina and acute myocardial infarction: Implications regarding therapy. Am. J. Cardiol., *54:* 1245–1252, 1984.
27. Finch, C. A., and Lenfant, C. Oxygen transport in man. N. Engl. J. Med. *286:* 407–415, 1982.
28. Foote, G. A., Schabel, S. I., and Hodges, M. Pulmonary complications of the flow-directed balloon-tipped catheter. N. Engl. J. Med., *290:* 927–931, 1974.
29. Forrester, J. S., Diamond, G., Chatterjee, K., and Swan, H. J. C. Medical therapy of acute myocardial infarction by application of hemodynamic subsets (Part I). N. Engl. J. Med., *295:* 1356–1362, 1976.
30. Forrester, J. S., Diamond, G., Chatterjee, K., and Swant, H. J. C. Medical therapy of acute myocardial infarction by application of hemodynamic subsets (Part II). N. Engl. J. Med., *296:* 1404–1413, 1976.
31. Francis, P. B. Acute respiratory failure in obstructive lung disease. Med. Clin. North Am., *67:* 657–668, 1983.
32. Ganz, W., and Swan, H. J. C. Measurement of blood flow by thermodilution. Am. J. Cardiol., *29:* 241, 1972.
33. Gersh, B. J., Bassendine, M. F., Forman, R., Walls, R. S., and Beck, W. Coronary artery spasm and myocardial infarction in the absence of antiographically demonstrable obstructive coronary disease. Mayo Clin. Proc., *56:* 700–708, 1981.
34. Glower, D. D., Spratt, J. A., Snow, N. D., Kabas, J. S., Davis, J. W., Olsen, C. O., Tyson, G. S., Sabiston, D. C., and Rankin, J. S. Linearity of the Frank-Starling relationship in the intact heart: The concept of preload recruitable stroke work. Circulation, *71:* 994–1009, 1985.
35. Grossman, W., Jones, D., and McLaurin, L. P. Wall stress and patterns of hypertrophy in the human left ventricle. J. Clin. Invest., *56:* 56–64, 1975.
36. Guyton, A. C., Jones, C. E., and Coleman, T. G. *Circulatory Physiology: Cardiac Output and Its*

Regulation, pp. 436–487. W. B. Saunders, Philadelphia, 1973.
37. Guyton, A. C., and Lindsey, A. W. Effect of elevated left atrial pressure and decreased plasma protein concentration on the development of pulmonary edema. Circ. Res., *7:* 649–57, 1959.
38. Hannon, A. T., Brown, M., and Bigman, O. Pulmonary artery catheter induced hemorrhage. Chest, *85:* 128–131, 1984.
39. Harrison, D. C. Should lidocaine be administered routinely to all patients after acute myocardial infarction. Circulation, *58:* 581–584, 1978.
40. Hartzler, G. O., Rutherford, B. D., McConahay, D. R., Johnson, W. L., McCallister, B. D., Gura, G. M., Conn, R. L., and Crockett, J. E. Percutaneous transluminal coronary angioplasty with and without thrombolytic therapy for treatment of acute myocardial infarction. Am. Heart J., *106:* 965–973, 1983.
41. Hasan, F. M., Malanga, A. Corrao, W. M., and Braman, S. Effect of catheter position on thermodilution cardiac output during continuous positive pressure ventilation. Crit. Care Med., *12:* 387–390, 1984.
42. Henning, R. J., Weiner, F., Valdes, S., and Weil, M. H. Measurement of toe temperature for assessing the severity of acute circulatory failure. Surg. Gynecol. Obstet., *149:*1–7, 1979.
43. Henning, R. J., Weil, M. H., and Weiner, F. Blood lactate as a prognostic indicator of survival in patients with acute myocardial infarction. Circ. Shock, *9:* 307–315, 1982.
44. Herling, I. M. Intravenous nitroglycerin: Clinical pharmacology and therapeutic considerations. Am. Heart J., *108:* 141–149, 1984.
45. Hiller, C., Bone, R., Hill., D., and Wilson, F. Mixed venous oxygen tension compared to tissue oxygen tension as a measure of oxygen delivery in endotoxin shock. Clin. Res., *27:* 399A, 1979.
46. Hoor, P. F., Wilson, R. M., Mangano, D. T., Avery, G. J., Szarnicki, R. J., and Hill, J. D. Heparin bonding reduces thrombogenicity of pulmonary artery catheters. N. Engl. J. Med., *305:* 993–5, 1981.
47. Iberti, T. J., and Fisher, C. J. A prospective study on the use of the pulmonary artery catheter in a medical intensive care unit: Its effect on diagnosis and therapy. Crit. Care Med., *11:* 238, 1983.
48. Joly, H. R., and Weil, M. H. Temperature of the great toe as an indication of the severity of shock. Circulation, *39:* 131–138, 1969.
49. Kaplan, K., Davison, R., Parker, M., Przybylek, J., Teagarden, J. R., and Lesch, M. Intravenous nitroglycerin for the treatment of angina at rest unresponsive to standard nitrate therapy. Am. J. Cardiol., *51:* 694–698, 1983.
50. Kasnitz, P., Druger, G., Yorra, F., and Simmons, D. Mixed venous oxygen tension and hyperlactatemia. J.A.M.A., *236:* 570–574, 1976.
51. Kaufman, B. S., Rackow, E. C., and Falk, J. L. The relationship between oxygen delivery and consumption during fluid resuscitation of hypovolemic and septic shock. Chest, *85:* 336–340, 1984.
52. Kaye, W. Intravenous techniques. In: *Textbook of Advanced Cardiac Life Support,* edited by K. M. McIntyre and A. J. Lewis, pp. 149–162. American Heart Association, Dallas, 1983.
53. Kennedy, J. W., Ritchie, J. L., Davis, K. B., and Fritz, J. K. Western Washington randomized trial of intracoronary streptokinase in acute myocardial infarction. N. Engl. J. Med., *309:* 1477–1481, 1983.
54. Kessler, M., Hopper, J., and Krumme, B. A. Monitoring of tissue perfusion and cellular function. Anesthesiology, *45:* 184–196, 1976.
55. Khaja, F., Walton, J. A., Brymer, J. F., Lo, E., Osterberger, L., O'Neill, W. W., Colfer, H. T., Weiss, R., Lee, T., Kurian, T., Goldberg, A. D., Pitt, B., and Goldstein, S. Intracoronary fibrinolytic therapy in acute myocardial infarction. N. Engl. J. Med., *308:* 1305–1311, 1983.
56. Kruse, J. A., and Puri, V. K. Mixed venous oxygen tension is a poor predictor of lactic acidosis. Chest, *86:* 288, 1984.
57. Leavy, J. A., Weil, M. H., Michaels, S., Astiz, M. E., and Rackow, E. C. A technique for automated measurement of blood lactate at the bedside. Crit. Care Med., *13:* 323, 1985.
58. Lewis, A. J. Monitoring and dysrhythmia recognition in advanced cardiac life support. In: *Textbook of Advanced Cardiac Life Support*, edited by K. M. McIntyre and A. J. Lewis, pp. 57–86. American Heart Association, Dallas, 1983.
59. Lie, K. L., Wellens, H. J., van Cappelle, F. J., and Durrer, D. Lidocaine in the prevention of primary ventricular fibrillation. A double blind randomized study of 212 consecutive patients. N. Engl. J. Med., *291:* 1324–1329, 1974.
60. Loeb, H. S., Winslow, E. B. J., Rahimtoola, S. H., Rosen, K. M., and Gunnar, R. M. Acute hemodynamic effects of dopamine in shock. Circulation, *44:* 163–73, 1971.
61. McIntyre, K. M., Lewis, A. J., Parker, M. R., and Paraskos, J. A. Myocardial infarction. In: *Textbook of Advanced Cardiac Life Support*, edited by K. M. McIntyre and A. J. Lewis, pp. 23–26. American Heart Association, Dallas, 1983.
62. Malik, A. B. Mechanisms of neurogenic pulmonary edema. Circ. Res., *57:* 1–18, 1985.
63. Malek, I., Waagstein, F., Hjalmarson, A., Holmberg, S., and Swedberg, K. Hemodynamic effects of the cardioselective β-blocking agent Metoprolol in acute myocardial infarction. Acta Med. Scand., *204:* 195–201, 1978.
64. Mond, H. G., Clark, D. W., Nesbitt, S. J., and Schlant, R. C. A technique for unknotting an intracardiac flow-directed balloon catheter. Chest, *67:* 731–733, 1975.
65. Morns, A. H., Chapman, R. H., and Gardner, R. M. Frequency of technical problems encountered in the measurement of pulmonary artery wedge pressure. Crit. Care Med., *12:* 164–170, 1984.
66. Mueller, H., Ayres, S. M., Giannelli, S., Conklin, E. F., Mazzara, J. T., and Grace, W. R. Effect of isoproterenol, l-norepinephrine, and intra-aortic counterpulsation on hemodynamics and myocardi-

al metabolism in shock following acute myocardial infarction. Circulation, *45:* 335-351, 1972.

67. Mueller, H. S., Evans, R., and Ayres, S. M. Effect of dopamine on hemodynamics and myocardial metabolism in shock following acute myocardial infarction in man. Circulation, *57:* 361-365, 1978.
68. Mulley, A. G., Thibault, G. E., Hughes, R. A., Barnett, G. O., Reder, V. A., and Sherman, E. L. The course of patients with suspected myocardial infarction. N. Engl. J. Med., *302:* 943–948, 1980.
69. Myers, M. L., Austin, T. W., and Sibbald, W. T. Pulmonary artery catheter infections. Ann. Surg. *201:* 237-241, 1985.
70. Nehme, A. E. Swan-Ganz catheter: Comparison of insertion techniques. Arch. Surg. *115:* 1194–1196, 1970.
71. Noble, M. I. M. Problems concerning the application of concepts of muscle mechanics to the determination of the contractile state of the heart. Circulation, *45:* 252–255, 1972.
72. O'Mara, K., Trevino, R. P., Rackow, E. C., Astiz, M. E., Falk, J. L., and Weil, M. H. Impaired oxygen extraction during anesthesia and high risk surgery. Clin. Res., *33:* 294A, 1985.
73. Palmer, R. F., and Lasseter, K. C. Sodium nitroprusside. N. Engl. J. Med., *292:* 294–297, 1975.
74. Papapietro, S. E., MacLean, W. A. H., Stanley, A. W. H., Hess, R. G., Corley, N., Arciniegas, J. G., and Cooper, T. Percutaneous transluminal coronary angioplasty after intracoronary streptokinase in evolving acute myocardial infarction. Am. J. Cardiol., *55:* 48–53, 1985.
75. Pape, L. A., Hattajee, C. I., Markis, J. E., Ockene, I. S., Paraskos, J. A., Dalen, J. E., Alpert, J. S. Fatal pulmonary hemorrhage after use of the flow-directed balloon-tipped catheter. Am. Intern. Med., *90:* 344–347, 1979.
76. Parmley, W. M. The post-MI role of hemodynamic monitoring. Hosp. Prac., *17:* 169–75, 1982.
77. Peters, J. L., and Armstrong, R. Air embolism as a complication of central venous catheterization. Ann. Surg., *187:* 375–78, 1978.
78. Prewitt, R. M., Matthay, M. A., and Chignone, M. Hemodynamic management in the adult respiratory distress syndrome. Clin. Chest Med., *4:* 251–68, 1983.
79. Puri, V. K., Carlson, R. W., Bander, J. J., and Weil, M. H. Complications of vascular catheterization in the critically ill. Crit. Care Med., *8:* 495–99, 1980.
80. Rackow, E. C., Falk, J. L., Fein, I. A., Siegel, J. S., Packman, M. I., Haupt, M. T., Kaufman, B. S., and Putman, D. Fluid resuscitation in circulatory shock: A comparison of the cardiorespiratory effects of albumin, hetastarch and saline solutions in patients with hypovolemic and septic shock. Crit. Care Med., *11:* 839–850, 1983.
81. Rackow, E. C., and Fein, I. A. Fulminant noncardiogenic pulmonary edema in the critically ill. Crit. Care Med., *6:* 360-363, 1978.
82. Rackow, E. C., Fein, I. A., and Seigel, J. The relationship of the colloid osmotic-pulmonary artery wedge pressure gradient to pulmonary edema and mortality in critically ill patients. Chest, *82:*433-437, 1982.
83. Rashkin, M. C., Bosken, C., and Baughman, R. P. Oxygen delivery in critically ill patients. Chest, *87:* 580–84, 1985.
84. Rentrop, P., Blanke, H., Karsch, K. R., Kaiser, H., Kostering, H., and Leitz, K. Selective intracoronary thrombolysis in acute myocardial infarction and unstable angina pectoris. Circulation, *63:* 307–317, 1981.
85. Riedinger, M. S., Slellock, F. G., and Swan, H. J. C. Reading pulmonary artery and pulmonary capillary wedge pressure waveforms with respiratory variations. Heart and Lung, *10:* 675–78, 1981.
86. Rieves, R. D. Importance of symptoms in recognizing nitroprusside toxicity. South. Med. J., *77:* 1035-1037, 1984.
87. Rouby, J. J., Eurin, B., Glaser, P., Guillosson, J. J., Nafziger, J., Guesde, R., and Viars, P. Hemodynamic and metabolic effects of morphine in the critically ill. Circulation, *64:* 54–59, 1981.
88. Ross, J. Afterload mismatch and preload reserve: A conceptual framework for the analysis of ventricular function. Prog. Cardiovasc. Dis., *18:* 255-264, 1976.
89. Rowley, K. M., Clubbs, K. S., Walker Smith, G. J., and Cabin, H. S. Right sided infective endocarditis as a consequence of flow-directed pulmonary artery catheterization. N. Engl. J. Med., *311:* 1152–1156, 1984.
90. Russell, J. A., Joel, M. Hudson, R. J., Mangano, D. T., and Schlobohm, R. M. Prospective evaluation of radial and femoral artery catheterization sites in critically ill adults. Crit. Care Med., *11:* 936–939, 1983.
91. Schanzenbacher, P., Leibau, G., Deeg, P., and Kochsiek, K. Effect of intravenous and intracoronary nifedipine on coronary blood flow and myocardial oxygen consumption. Am. J. Cardiol., *51:* 712–719, 1983.
92. Schuster, D. P., and Seeman, M. D. Temporary muscle paralysis for accurate measurement of pulmonary artery occlusion pressure. Chest, *84:* 593–597, 1983.
93. Senagore, A., Waller, J. D., Bonnell, B. W., Bursch, L. R., and Scholten, D. J. Pulmonary artery catheterization: A prospective study of internal jugular versus subclavian approaches. Crit. Care Med., *13:* 264, 1985.
94. Shah, K. B., Rao, T. L. K., Laughlin, S., and El-Etr, A. A. A review of pulmonary artery catheterization in 6245 patients. Anesthesiology, *61:* 271–275, 1984.
95. Shellock, F. G., Riedinger, M. S., Bateman, T. M., and Gray, R. J. Thermodilution cardiac output determination in hypothermic postcardiac surgery patients; room versus ice temperature injectate. Crit. Care Med., *11:* 668–670, 1983.
96. Shoemaker, W. C., Appel, P. L., Kram, H. B., and Lee, T. Comparison of two monitoring methods (central venous pressure vs pulmonary artery catheter) and two protocols as therapeutic goals (normal valves versus valves of survivors) in a prospective randomized clinical trial of critically ill surgical patients. Crit. Care Med., *13:* 304, 1985.
97. Sibbald, W. J., Calvin, J. E., Holliday, R. L., and Driedger, A. A. Concepts in the pharmacologic

and nonpharmacologic support of cardiovascular function in critically ill surgical patients. Surg. Clin. North Am., *63:* 455–482, 1983.
98. Sibbald, W. J., Cunningham, D. R., and Chin, D. N. Noncardiac or cardiac pulmonary edema? A practical approach to clinical differentiation in critically ill patients. Chest, *84:* 452–461, 1983.
99. Sise, M. J., Hollingsworth, P., Brimm, J. E., Peters, R. M., Virgilio, R. W., and Shackford, S. R. Complications of the flow directed pulmonary artery catheter: A prospective analysis in 219 patients. Crit. Care Med., *9:* 315–318, 1981.
100. Snyder, J., and Carroll, G. Tissue oxygenation: A physiologic approach to a clinical problem. Curr. Prob. Surg., *18:* 650–720, 1982.
101. Soderstrom, C. A., Wasserman, D. H., Dunham, C. M., Caplan, E. S., and Cowley, R. A. Superiority of the femoral artery for monitoring: A prospective study. Am. J. Surg., *144:* 309–312, 1982.
102. Sonnenblick, E. H. Force velocity relations in mammalian heart muscle. Am. J. Physiol., *202:* 931–939, 1962.
103. Soule, D. T., and Powner, D. J. Air entrapment in pressure monitoring lines. Crit. Care Med., *12:* 520–522, 1984.
104. Spann, J. F., Buccino, R. A., Sonnenblick, E. M., and Braunwald, E. Contractile state of cardiac muscle obtained from cats with experimentally produced ventricular hypertrophy and heart failure. Circ. Res., *21:* 341–354, 1967.
105. Sprung, C. L., Jacobs, L. J., Caralis, P. V., and Karpf, M. Ventricular arrhythmias during Swan-Ganz catheterization of critically ill. Chest, *79:* 413–415, 1981.
106. Sprung, C. L., Pozen, R. G., Rozanski, J. J., Pinero, J. R., Eisler, B. R., and Castellanos A. Advanced ventricular arrhythmias during bedside pulmonary artery catheterization. Am. J. Med., *72:* 203–208, 1982.
107. Sprung, C. L., Rackow, E. C., Fein, I. A., Jacob, A. I, and Isikoff, S. K. The spectrum of pulmonary edema: Differentiation of cardiogenic, intermediate and noncardiogenic forms of pulmonary edema. Am. Rev. Respir. Dis., *124:* 718–722, 1981.
108. Standards and guidelines for cardiopulmonary resuscitation (CPR) and emergency cardiac care (ECC). J.A.M.A., *244* (Suppl.)*:* 453–509, 1980.
109. Staub, N. C. The pathogenesis of pulmonary edema. Prog. Cardiovasc. Dis., *23:* 53–80, 1980.
110. Strandgaard, S. Cerebral blood flow in hypertension. Acta Med. Scand., *678* (Suppl.)*:* 11–25, 1983.
111. Strandgaard, S., Olesen, J., Skinhoj, E., and Lassen, N. A. Autoregulation of brain circulation in severe arterial hypertension. Br. Med. J., *1:* 507–510, 1973.
112. Swan, H. J. C. The role of hemodynamic monitoring in the management of the critically ill. Crit. Care Med., *3:* 83–89, 1975.
113. Swan, H. J. C., Ganz, W., Forrester, J., Marcus, H., Diamond, G., and Chonette, D. Catheterization of the heart in man with use of a flow-directed balloon-tipped catheter. N. Engl. J. Med., *283:* 447–451, 1970.
114. Swan, H. J. C., and Ganz, W. Complications with flow-directed, balloon-tipped catheters. Ann. Intern. Med., *91:* 494, 1979.
115. Tenney, S. A theoretical analysis of the relationship between venous blood and mean tissue oxygen pressures. Respir. Physiol., *20:* 283–296, 1974.
116. Theodore, J., and Robin, Ed. Pathogenesis of neurogenic pulmonary edema. Lancet, *2:* 749–751, 1975.
117. Theodore, J., and Robin, Ed. Speculations of neurogenic pulmonary edema. Am. Rev. Respir. Dis., *113:* 405–411, 1976.
118. The TIMI Study Group. The thrombolysis in myocardial infarction (TIMI) trial: Phase I findings. N. Engl. J. Med., *312:* 932–936, 1985.
119. Thomas, J. A., and Marks, B. H. Plasma norepinephrine in congestive heart failure. Am. J. Cardiol., *41:* 233–243, 1978.
120. Tremper, K. L., and Shoemaker, W. Transcutaneous oxygen monitoring of critically ill patients with and without low flow shock. Crit. Care Med., *9:* 706–709, 1981.
121. Valentine, R. P., Pitts, D. E., Brooks-brunn, J. A., Williams, J. G., Van Hove, E., and Schmidt, P. E. Intravenous versus intracoronary streptokinase in acute myocardial infarction. Am. J. Cardiol., *55:* 309–312, 1985.
122. Van de Werf, F., Ludbrook, P. A., Bergmann, S. R., Tiefenbrunn, A. J., Fox, K. A. A., DeGeest, H., Verstraete, M., Collen, D., and Sobel, B. E. Coronary thrombolysis with tissue type plasminogen activator in patients with evolving myocardial infarction. N. Engl. J. Med., *310:* 609–613, 1984.
123. Vitek, V., and Cowley, R. A. Blood lactate in the prognosis of various forms of shock. Ann. Surg., *175:* 308–313, 1971.
124. Voci, G., Gazek, F. A., Burris, A. C., and Zatuchni, J. Retrieval of entrapped and knotted balloon-tipped catheters from the right heart. Ann. Intern. Med., *92:* 638–639, 1980.
125. Waller, J. L., Johnson, S. P., and Kaplan, J. A. Usefulness of pulmonary artery catheters during aortocoronary bypass surgery. Anesth. Analg., *61:* 221–222, 1982.
126. Waxman, K., Sudler, K., Eisner, M., *et al.* Transcutaneous oxygen monitoring of emergency department patients. Am. J. Surg., *146:* 35–38, 1983.
127. Weber, K. T., and Janicki, J. S. Muscle-pump function of the intact heart. In: *Heart Failure*, edited by A. P. Fishman, pp. 29–42, Hemisphere Publishing Co., Washington, D.C., 1978.
128. Weber, K. T., Janicki, J. S., Russell, R. O., and Rackley, C. E. Identification of high risk subsets of acute myocardial infarction. Am. J. Cardiol., *41:* 197–203, 1978.
129. Weil, M. H., and Afifi, A. A. Experimental and clinical studies on lactate and pyruvate as indicators of the severity of acute circulatory failure (shock). Circulation, *41:* 989–1001, 1970.
130. Weil, M. H., Shubin, H., and Carlson, R. W. Treatment of circulatory shock. J.A.M.A., *231:* 1280–1286, 1975.
131. Wiedemann, H. P., Matthay, M. A., and Matthay, R. A. Cardiovascular pulmonary monitoring in the

intensive care unit (Part I). Chest, *85:* 537–549, 1984.

132. Wiedemann, H. P., Matthay, M. A., and Matthay, R. A. Cardiovascular pulmonary monitoring in the intensive care unit (Part II). Chest, *85:* 656–668, 1984.

133. Wilson, R. F., Christensen, C., and LeBlanc, L. P. Oxygen consumption in critically ill surgical patients. Ann. Surg., *176:* 801–804, 1972.

134. Mokhtar, S., Weil, M. H., and Shubin, H. Risks of alkalosis in critically ill patients and their relationship to ventricular arrhythmias. Chest, *68:* 421A, 1975.

135. Mokhtar, S., Shubin, H., and Weil, M. H. Increased mortality of acute myocardial infarction in patients with alkalosis. Circulation, *52:* II-219A, 1975.

136. Cohn, J. N. Blood pressure measurement in shock. J.A.M.A., *199:* 972–976, 1967.

CHAPTER 3

Fluid and Electrolyte Physiology, Pathophysiology, and Management

PAUL B. NELSON, M.D.

GENERAL CONSIDERATIONS

Body Water

Body water represents about 50% of body weight in males and 49% in females and is estimated to be about 40 liters (27). Newborns have a somewhat higher percentage of water and elderly people may have relatively less water. Body water is divided into intracellular water (ICW), extracellular water (ECW), and transcellular water (TSW). Intracellular water represents about 55% of the total body water. Extracellular water represents both plasma water and interstitial water. The capillary basement membrane divides the ICW and ECW. It is freely permeable to water, but less permeable to electrolytes and low molecular weight crystalloids and barely permeable to high molecular weight colloids such as plasma proteins. Transcellular water is formed by active transport of extracellular water across epithelial cells into such spaces as the gastrointestinal (GI) tracts, cerebrospinal fluid (CSF), biliary tract, and peritoneal cavity.

Blood Volume

Blood volume represents about 7% of the body weight in males and 6% in females. The normal red cell volume is 25 to 30 ml/kg, plasma volume varies from 35 to 40 ml/kg, and the total volume is 60 to 75 ml/kg. If hematocrit is greater than 45% viscosity is increased. If hematocrit is less than 30, however, it may lead to decreased oxygen delivery. The optimum hematocrit is between 30% and 45%.

Distribution of Water and Electrolytes in Body Compartments

A 70-kg male has 3,400 mEq of potassium and 2,800 mEq of sodium ion. Ninety-eight percent of potassium is within the cell (27). Only 2% of potassium is in the extracellular water with a concentration of 3.8 to 5 mEq/liter. The ratio of intracellular to extracellular potassium is 30 to 1. There is a similar concentration gradient in the opposite direction for sodium where the intracellular and extracellular concentrations are 5.5 to 15 mEq/l and 138 to 142 mEq/liter respectively. The sodium gradient is maintained by the active transport sodium pump. Body water and electrolytes are maintained by the renal capacity to excrete excesses. The kidney normally reabsorbs sodium and water and excretes potassium and hydrogen.

Osmotic Pressure

Osmolarity is the number of osmoles or moles of solute per liter of solvent plus solute (2). Osmolality is the solute concentration per kilogram of solvent. Plasma and serum osmolality is usually 286 to 305 mOsm/liter. Normally, body compartments are iso-osmolar with the exception of the renal medulla. When two aqueous solutions of unequal concentration are separated by a membrane permeable only to water, the water migrates through the membrane to equalize the concentrations. Osmotic pressure is determined by the number of molecules in the solvent. Colloidal osmotic pressure or oncotic pressure is the osmotic force exerted by the plasma proteins.

The osmolality can be estimated by the following equation: Osmolality (mOsm/kg) = 2 × (Na^+) + (K^+) + BUN/2.8. The measured osmolality is about 10 m0sm/kg greater than the estimated osmolality because of other minor solutes including calcium, magnesium, protein, amino acids, and glucose. If the measured osmolality is more than 10 m0sm/kg greater than the estimated osmolality, other solutes such as administered mannitol may be present.

Colloids and Crystalloids

The molecular weight of a colloid is greater than 8,000. Colloids have difficulty passing through endothelial cells. Replacement with colloid can be done as 1 part colloid to 1 part of blood loss. Albumin, plasmanate, dextran, and blood are the most commonly used colloids.

Albumin has a molecular weight of 69,000. Sodium concentration in albumin is 100 to 160 mEq/liter. Albumin half-life is about 3 hours and it eventually equilibrates with the extravascular fluid. Its oncotic pressure is high and volume overload is possible. Purified protein fraction (Plasmanate) is another commonly used colloid. Most of the protein in plasmanate is albumin. The sodium concentration is 130 to 160 mEq/liter. Plasmanate has been heat-treated and the risk of hepatitis is extremely low. Occasional episodes of hypertension have been noted with rapid infusion rates (20 to 50 ml/min).

Low molecular weight dextran has a molecular weight of 40,000. It is a hydroglucose polymer. Volume expansion lasts around 1 and 1½ hours after it has been stopped. It has not gained wide acceptance in neurosurgery because of its occasional risk of anaphylaxis, increased bleeding with prolonged use, and occasional nephrotoxicity.

Crystalloids have molecular weights of less than 8,000. They can easily pass through the endothelial cells. Volume replacement with crystalloids must be done at a 3 parts crystalloid to 1 part blood loss. The most commonly used crystalloids include 5% dextrose in water (D/W) with 0.45 normal saline, Ringers lactate, and saline.

Normal Replacement Therapy

The normal adult urine output is 1,000 to 1,500 ml/day (27). Insensible loss is 400 to 800 ml/day. Water release from tissue breakdown during starvation may lead to another 100 to 1,000 ml/day loss. The normal adult fluid requirement is approximately 35 ml/kg or 2,500 ml/day. Older patients and patients in states of fluid retention may require less volume. In obese patients the calculated volume requirement should be based on ideal weight rather than their actual weight. The adult patient sodium requirement is 75 mEq/day plus the extra-renal losses. Potassium requirement is 40 mEq/day and glucose requirement is 150 gm/day. Debilitated patients may require 10 to 15 mEq of magnesium per day. The average daily intake and output of body constituents is shown in Table 3.1.

Nutritional Requirements

A standard of care for the hospitalized patient receiving intravenous (IV) fluids appears to be starvation. The patient who receives 2,000 cc of 5% D/W in a 0.45 normal saline is receiving only 400 calories/day. Mortality and morbidity are increased in the malnourished patient. If the patient's mental status does not allow him to eat, and the GI tract is intact, one should begin tube feedings through a soft bore soft silastic tube as soon as possible. Starting slowly with the head up and using a continuous drip of isotonic preparations, 2,000 calories a day can be given by the fourth day. Paregoric (5 cc/kg) may decrease the 20% incidence of diarrhea. Occasionally, peripheral or central hyperalimentation may be needed in the neurosurgical patient.

Body Response to Stress

The body's response to stress includes increased autonomic activity with renal vasoconstriction (27). This leads to water and salt retention and decreased urine output. Increased vasopressin secretion also leads to increased water resorption. Cardiac rate and contraction are increased. Adrenocorticotropic hormone

TABLE 3.1.
Average Daily Intake and Output of Important Body Constituents.*

Substance	Intake (Range)		Output (Range)	
Water, ml				
Drinking water:	1,500	(500–300)	Urine:	1,500 (600–3,000)
Water content in food:	1,000	(500–1,500)	Insensible loss†:	800 (400–1,000)
Water of oxidation:	100	(50–200)	Stool:	200 (50–500)
Total:	2,500	(1,000–4,500)	Total:	2,500 (1,000–4,500)
Sodium, mEq	70	(50–100)	Urine:	65 (50–100)
			Stool:	5 (2–20)
Potassium, mEq	100	(50–120)	Urine:	90 (50–120)
			Stool:	10 (2–40)
Magnesium, mEq	30	(5–60)	Urine:	10 (2–20)
			Stool:	20 (2–50)
Calcium, mEq	15	(2–50)	Urine:	3 (0–10)
			Stool:	12 (2–30)
Protein, gm	55	(30–80)		
Nitrogen, gm	8	(4–12)		
Calories	1,800–3,000			

*From W. C. Shoemaker. Fluids and electrolytes in the acutely ill adult. In: *The Society of Critical Care Medicine Textbook of Critical Care*, edited by W. C. Shoemaker, W. L. Thompson, and P. R. Holbrook, Chap. 82, pp. 614–640. W. B. Saunders Company, Philadelphia, 1984.

†Insensible water losses from evaporation through lungs and skin increase with febrile episodes, tachypnea, scalds, burns, high ambient temperatures, and low ambient humidity.

(ACTH) production leads to increased production of glucocorticoids. If blood loss is present, aldosterone production will lead to increased resorption of sodium in the kidneys in exchange for hydrogen and potassium ions. Water retention generally exceeds sodium retention and dilutional hyponatremia may result. Potassium is released from the cell following injury, causing transient hyperkalemia. Increased potassium excretion subsequently, however, leads to decrease in total body potassium. Nitrogen losses may also increase and are aggravated by inadequate nutrition. The sequential changes in sodium and potassium balance following surgery are shown in Table 3.2.

BLOOD LOSS AND SHOCK

Blood Loss

Blood loss of 15% to 25% (750 to 1,250 cc) usually can be treated without blood with colloids and crystalloids. With losses of this magnitude the hematocrit may decrease to 29% to 30%. This is an adequate hemoglobin assuming there is normal oxyhemoglobin dissociation. With a loss greater than 30% (1,500 ml), the patient generally should be treated with blood in addition to other colloids and crystalloids. Blood loss of 40% to 50% (1,800 to 2,250 ml) is usually associated with hypotension and profound shock.

Hypovolemic Shock

Hypovolemic shock should be treated by control of the hemorrhage and volume replacement with blood, colloid, and crystalloid (19, 26). The goals of treatment include good urine output (0.5 to 1.0 ml/kg/hr), normal heart rate, brisk capillary refill, normal sensorium, and restoration of blood pressure. Central filling pressures including central venous pressure (CVP) and pulmonary wedge pressure (PWP) may not reliably predict preload in the critically ill patient. Hematocrit is also not a good indication of blood volume status. Other treatments of hypovolemic shock include maintenance of a Po_2 greater than 70 ml Hg, and correction of associated metabolic acidosis. Mannitol (12.5 to 20 gm) has at times been given to increase the renal parenchymal blood flow. The use of Naloxone and high-dose steroids is controversial. Vasoconstrictors are in general contraindicated since total peripheral resistance is already increased.

TABLE 3.2.
Sequential Changes in Plasma, Sodium and Potassium Concentrations, Body-Balance Values, and Body Composition Values in Idealized Case Subjected to Elective Surgery and Given Normal Daily Requirements of Salt and Water (70 mEq/day of Na^+, 100 mEq/day of K^+, 2,500 ml/day of water).*

	Plasma Concentration		Body Balance		Body Composition	
Normal preoperative state	Na^+	142 mEq/liter	Na^+ intake	70 mEq/day	na^+	2,670 mEq
			Na^+ output	70 mEq/day		
			Balance	0		
	K^+	4 mEq/liter	K^+ intake	100 mEq/day	K^+	3,360 mEq
			K^+ output	100 mEq/day		
			Balance	0		
			Water intake	2,500 ml/day		
			Water output	2,500 ml/day		
			Balance	0		
Day of operation	Na^+	138 mEq/liter	Na^+ intake	70 mEq/day	Na^+	2,700 mEq
			Na^+ output	40 mEq/day		
			Balance	+30		
	K^+	5 mEq/liter	K^+ intake	0 mEq/day	K^+	3,300 mEq
			K^+ output	60 mEq/day		
			Balance	−60		
			Water intake	2,500 ml/day	Water	41 liter
			Water output	1,500 ml/day		
			Balance	+1,000		
Five days postoperative	Na^+	131 mEq/liter	Na^+ intake	70 mEq/day	Na^+	2,850 mEq
			Na^+ output	40 mEq/day		
			Balance	+30		
	K^+	4 mEq/liter	K^+ intake	0 mEq/day	K^+	3,185 mEq
			K^+ output	20 mEq/day		
			Balance	−20		
			Water intake	2,500 ml/day	Water	43.5 liter
			Water output	2,000 ml/day		
			Balance	+500		

*From W. C. Shoemaker. Fluids and electrolytes in the acutely ill adult. In: *The Society of Critical Care Medicine Textbook of Critical Care*, edited by W. C. Shoemaker, W. L. Thompson, and P. R. Holbrook, Chap. 82, pp. 614–640. W. B. Saunders Company, Philadelphia, 1984.

Spinal Shock

Spinal shock results from the loss of sympathetic tone. The clinical picture includes hypotension, slow heart rate, and warm, dry skin. The decrease in cardiac output is due to a decrease in arteriole and venous tone. The primary circulatory problem is that a previously normal blood volume has been placed in an acutely dilated vascular bed. Treatment consists of volume infusion and vasoconstriction with such adrenergic agents such as ephedrine and phenylephrine hydrochloride.

Septic Shock

Septic shock is an infection-induced loss of ability of the vasculature to regulate flow according to metabolic needs. The vascular bed is vasodilated and frequently there is an increase in the cardiac output. The most important treatment of septic shock is control of the septic nidus. Volume infusion and vasoconstriction (dopamine hydrochloride at 8 to 10 mcg/kg/min) may also be helpful. Beta-adrenergic drugs such as isoproterenol hydrochloride are contraindicated because of the high cardiac output. Digitalis may also be needed.

SALT AND WATER BALANCE

Normal Balance

In healthy adults, plasma osmolality and its principal determinant sodium concentrate are maintained within a markedly narrow range (2, 6). This stability is achieved primarily by adjusting total body water to keep it in balance with sodium. Water balance is largely controlled by the posterior pituitary hormone, arginine vasopressin. Arginine vasopressin is a small peptide made in the supraoptic and paraventricular nuclei of the anterior hypothalamus. It is carried down the hypothalamo-hypophyseal tract to the median eminence and posterior lobe of the pituitary gland and secreted in response to an increased osmolality and decreased volume. It is carried in the blood to the kidneys where it allows for retention of free water from the distal convoluted tubules and collecting ducts of the kidneys. Without antidiuretic hormone function, 20 to 30 liters of urine would be lost daily. With maximal vasopressin secretion the urine output is 18 to 36 ml/hr. The osmoreceptors are thought to be located in the anterior hypothalamus and the set point is about 283 m0sm/kg. Volume receptors are located in the heart and aortic arch and are responsive to decreases in blood volume of 7% or more. Water balance is also partly controlled by thirst. The thirst center is thought to be located in the anterolateral hypothalamus and responds to osmolalities greater than 295 mOsm/kg.

Hyponatremia and the Syndrome of Inappropriate Secretion of Antidiuretic Hormone (SIADH)

Hyponatremia is common in neurosurgical patients and is usually thought to represent SIADH (8, 9, 11, 13, 15, 16, 25, 28). Hyponatremia is frequently associated with a deterioration in the patient's neurologic status. This syndrome may be seen in almost any intracranial disorder and from a number of non-neurosurgical disorders including ectopic production from carcinomas of the lung, pancreas, and duodenum and from such drugs as carbamazepine, tricyclic antidepressants, and barbiturates. The syndrome is defined as the continuous secretion of antidiuretic hormones, despite low serum sodium and osmolality and expanded extracellular volume. Serum sodium and osmolality are low, urine sodium is high, and urine osmolality is greater than serum osmolality. Laboratory criteria for SIADH include a serum osmolarity of less than 135 mEq/liter, a serum osmolality of less than 280 m0sm/kg, a high urinary sodium (greater than 25 mEq/liter) and a high urinary osmolality. The diagnosis assumes there is normal hydration and normal renal and adrenal function and that the patient is not taking diuretics.

The presence of high urinary sodium in this syndrome is not clearly understood. The possible causes of the natriuresis includes (*a*) an increased filtration rate with an increased filter load of sodium, (*b*) decreased aldosterone secretion, and (*c*) a decreased reabsorption of sodium in the proximal tubules secondary to an unknown "third factor". All these explanations for high urinary sodium are thought to be secondary to an expanded extracellular volume. Despite the need for a high urinary sodium in making the diagnosis of SIADH, a low urinary sodium may eventually develop with prolongation of the syndrome if sodium intake is low.

Both elevated antidiuretic hormone levels and water intake are necessary for hyponatremia to develop. Increased urinary sodium and water retention are not reflections of increased levels of antidiuretic hormone. In the absence of fluid intake, high levels of antidiuretic hormone may be present, but hyponatremia may not develop. A patient with this combination may be asymptomatic because it is the hyponatremia that causes the morbidity in SIADH. If levels of antidiuretic hormone are extremely high, however, even normal amounts of maintenance fluid may cause water retention and hyponatremia.

The diagnosis of SIADH can be confirmed by testing the patient's response to an oral water load. This test should not be done, however, if the sodium is less than 125 mEq/liter or if the patient is symptomatic from the hyponatremia. An oral load of 20 mg/kg of water is given on an empty stomach. Hourly urine volumes and osmolalities are checked for 5 hours while the patient is in a recumbent position. Normally a patient should excrete more than 80% of the water by the fifth hour and the urine osmolality should be less than 100 m0sm/kg.

Differential Diagnosis of Hyponatremia

Although SIADH is a common cause of hyponatremia in the neurosurgical patient, there are other causes of hyponatremia. Assessing the extracellular volume and studying urinary electrolytes usually allows the physician to determine the etiology. A urine sodium of more than 20 to 25 mEq/liter in association with hyponatremia is considered to be elevated. Urinary sodium of less than 10 mEq/liter is considered to be decreased. Four hyponatremic syndromes are characterized in Table 3.3. In SIADH, the extracellular volume is increased, but the patients are not edematous. They have a decreased serum sodium and an increased urinary sodium. Patients with hyponatremic dehydration may have a decreased extracellular volume and may show clinical evidence of dehydration. If they have water replacement in excess of sodium loss, serum sodium and urine sodium are low. Patients with cardiac failure or cirrhosis may have increased extracellular volume and frequently will be edematous. The serum sodium is decreased as is the urinary sodium. Patients with adrenal insufficiency, salt-losing nephropathy, and those taking diuretics may have a decreased extracellular volume, a decreased serum sodium, and an elevated urinary sodium.

There also appears to be a group of neurologic patients with low serum sodium, elevated levels of urine sodium, and decreased intravascular volume, in the absence of renal or adrenal disease or diuretic use. These patients have what may have been originally referred to as cerebral salt wasting (20). It was thought that patients with hyponatremia and natriuresis had a defect in the proximal tubular reabsorption of sodium in the kidney.

Treatment of Hyponatremia

When the patient becomes hyponatremic (less than 135 mEq/liter) one should obtain serum electrolytes, glucose, blood urea nitrogen (BUN), and osmolality, and urine electrolytes and osmolality daily until the hyponatremia resolves. If urinary sodium is low (less than 25 mEq/liter), it should be treated by volume replacement with saline solutions. If the urinary sodium is high (greater than 25 mEq/liter) and renal and adrenal insufficiency and diuretic therapy have been ruled out, treatment consists of fluid restriction to approximately 600 to 800 cc/day. Generally, with restriction the serum sodium should increase in 2 to 3 days. If the serum sodium level does not improve with fluid restriction and/or if the patient has been at bed rest for a long period of time, one may also obtain a blood and plasma volume. If the blood volume is decreased treatment may consist of volume and salt replacement rather than fluid restriction.

In patients who are markedly hyponatremic (sodium less than 120 mEq/liter) and symptomatic, i.e., seizures, a more rapid elevation of serum sodium may be necessary. Hypertonic or 3% saline may be used in these extreme conditions. Results of hypertonic saline infusion, however, are inconsistent and may result in acute volume overload. A combination of furosemide and hypertonic saline may be a better choice when rapid correction of hyponatremia is needed. Patients are given furosemide, 1 mg/kg of body weight, intravenously. Urinary losses of sodium potassium are measured and replaced with 3% saline over an 8-hour period (15). Demeclocycline hydrochloride (600 to 1,200 mg/day) and lithium (900 mg/day) are used in treating head-injured patients with chronic SIADH but have little value in the rapid correction of hyponatremia. Alcohol and phenytoin are known to inhibit antidiuretic hormone secretion but are therapeutically ineffective and only work acutely and in high doses.

TABLE 3.3.
Changes in Extracellular Volume (ECV) and Urinary Sodium (U-Na$^+$) in Four Hyponatremic States.

Diagnosis	ECV	U-Na+
1. Dehydration	Decreased	Less than 10 mEq/liter
2. Congestive heart failure, cirrhosis	Increased	Less than 10 mEq/liter
3. Renal and adrenal disease, diuretic therapy, and cerebral salt wasting	Decreased	Greater than 25 mEq/liter
4. SIADH	Increased	Greater than 25 mEq/liter

Hypernatremia

Hypernatremia is defined as a serum or plasma sodium greater than 145 mEq/liter (23). The two most common causes of hypernatremia are water depletion secondary to osmotic challenges such as tube feedings or mannitol and water depletion secondary to decreased vasopressin secretion (diabetes insipidus). Hypernatremia may be associated with impaired mental status and seizures.

Diabetes Insipidus

Diabetes insipidus (DI) is a disorder of excessive renal loss of water due to a deficiency in secretion of antidiuretic hormone (22).

Eighty-five percent of the secretory capacity of antidiuretic hormone must be lost to cause permanent diabetes insipidus. Damage to the posterior lobe or to the lower stalk of the pituitary gland seldom gives permanent diabetes insipidus. However, upper pituitary stalk and basal hypothalamus damage are more likely to give a permanent disorder. The patient presents with polyuria, nocturia, polydipsia, and thirst. Urine output may vary from 3 to 15 liters/day depending upon the severity of the syndrome. The urine remains hypertonic as compared to the serum even with water deprivation. The differential diagnosis of polyuria includes psychogenic water drinking, nephrogenic diabetes insipidus, and polyuria secondary to an osmotic load such as mannitol or glucose.

Although the diagnosis is usually obvious, one may confirm the diagnosis and the severity of the antidiuretic hormone deficit by performing a water deprivation test. This is usually done in a clinical research setting and should not be done if the patient cannot tolerate rapid dehydration. The patient is deprived of intake for 6 to 8 hours or until the urine osmolality plateaus. The patient is not allowed to lose more than 3% of the body weight. A normal response is a decrease in the urinary volume with associated increase in the urine osmolality. Normal individuals with 8 to 10 hours of water restriction will concentrate urine to about 600 to 850 mOsm/kg. If the patient fails to decrease his urinary output and concentrate urine maximally, exogenous antidiuretic hormone is given. The normal response to vasopressin is a decrease in the urinary volume and an increase urine osmolality to at least 300 to 350 mOsm/kg.

After stalk section, a triphasic response may be seen. Polyuria and polydipsia and an elevated serum sodium may be present for 4 to 5 days. A second phase of antidiuresis with decreased urinary output and a lower serum sodium may be seen for the next 4 to 5 days. This is eventually followed by permanent diabetes insipidus.

Incomplete DI may be controlled by the patient regulating his own intake and by giving antidiuretic-hormone-enhancing agents such as chlorpropamide, hydrochlorothiazide, and clofibrate. If the patient is on parenteral fluids, the previous hour's urine output may be replaced with IV fluids. Generally hypotonic fluids are used for fluid replacement. When the urine output is ≥ 300 ml/hr repeatedly and the specific gravity is less than 1.003, it becomes inconvenient and difficult to keep up with fluid losses either orally or with parenteral fluids. The initial treatment of DI traditionally has been with aqueous pitressin, 5 units subcutaneously or intramuscularly (IM). The duration of action of aqueous pitressin is usually 6 to 8 hours, which allowed one to see whether polyuria or polydipsia was a temporary or permanent disorder. When the diagnosis of permanent DI was definitely established, treatment was changed to pitressin tannate in oil given as a 5-unit IM injection. Pitressin tannate comes as a brown pellet and a vial must be warmed and shaken vigorously until the pellet is in suspension. Pitressin tannate has a variable duration of action but lasts for approximately 12 hours to 3 days.

Desmopressin acetate is a synthetic analog of vasopressin. Although it is more expensive than pitressin, it has a more reliable antidiuresis. In the initial treatment of DI, parenteral desmopressin acetate (2 μg subcutaneously) may be used if the nasal cavity is packed. If the nasal cavity is open, the route of nasal insufflation of 0.05 to 0.1 ml may be used. The duration of action is usually 8 to 24 hours.

RENAL FAILURE

Acute renal failure has many causes (4, 14, 17, 18). Traditionally, the causes have been divided into prerenal, intrarenal, or postrenal. Prerenal failure is secondary to the normal kidney response to a decrease in perfusion. Removal of the cause should be followed by an improvement in renal function. Postrenal failure due to an obstruction of urinary pathways is also a treatable disease. The most common type of acute intrarenal failure is acute tubular necrosis following ischemic or toxic damage to the kidney.

The patient with acute renal failure may be oliguric which is defined as urine output less than 400 ml in 24 hours. There are many patients, however, with renal failure that are not oliguric. A patient with a BUN ≥ 30 or creatinine ≥ 1.5 mg/dl must be considered as having impaired renal function. If an oliguric phase does occur, it usually lasts about 10 days. This is followed by a diuretic phase and then a phase of variable recovery of renal function.

History and Physical

The cause of acute renal failure can usually be ascertained from the history and physical. Loss of blood and body fluids accompanied by a decrease in body weight suggests prerenal failure. Obstructive uropathy usually occurs in elderly men with prostatic enlargement and women with pelvic malignancies. Acute tubular necrosis (ATN) is likely to occur following major surgery, prolonged hypotension, and nephrotoxic agents. Aminoglycoside antibiotics including neomycin, streptomycin, kanamycin, gentamicin, tobramycin, and amikacin, and radiographic contrast agents are the most common nephrotoxic agents for hospitalized patients. Differential diagnosis of acute renal failure is outlined in Table 3.4. The clinical manifestations of acute failure may include anorexia, nausea and vomiting, gastrointestinal bleeding, volume overload, fatigue, somnolence, confusion, muscle twitching, asterixis, coma, and seizures.

Laboratory Investigations

Urinalysis in prerenal and postrenal failure is often unremarkable. In ATN, however, the urine is often brown and loaded with pigmented granular cast.

The urinary osmolality and urine sodium may also be helpful in differentiating prerenal azotemia from ATN (Table 3.5). Urine osmolality is high and the urine sodium is low in prerenal azotemia, whereas with decreased tubular function in ATN, the urine is isotonic to plasma and the urine sodium is high.

Electrolyte abnormalities and acute renal failure include hyponatremia and hyperkalemia. Decreased secretion of potassium is the major cause of hyperkalemia. Decreased excretion of $H+$ causes metabolic acidosis and a low serum bicarbonate. In early renal failure the serum calcium falls and the phosphorus levels increase.

Treatment

Treatment of early acute renal failure includes volume replacement, if the volume is thought to be low or if the volume status is unknown. From 250 to 500 cc of isotonic saline should be infused over 1 hour with careful monitoring of the central venous pressure or pulmonary wedge pressure. The use of mannitol (12.5 to 25 gm over 5 minutes with a maximum of 100 gm/24 hr) and furosemide (80 to 420 mg) is somewhat more controversial. These drugs have been used in the acute phase of ATN to minimize the oliguric phase.

Once the renal failure has been established, the daily water intake should be limited to approximately 400 ml which is the estimated insensible loss, plus the volume of remaining urine output and GI secretions. The sodium intake is limited to 2 to 3 gm/day. Treatment of moderate potassium elevations include therapy

TABLE 3.4.
Differential Diagnosis of Acute Renal Failure.*

	Prerenal	Postrenal	Intrarenal (Acute Tubular Necrosis)
History	Vomiting Hemorrhage Heart disease	Prostatism Vaginal bleeding Renal stones	Cardiovascular or abdominal surgery Prolonged hypotension Nephrotoxins
Physical	Loss of skin turgor Postural hypotension	Enlarged bladder, prostate; gynecologic malignancy	Underlying disease
Urinalysis	Normal sediment	Normal sediment or red blood cells	Granular casts Epithelial cell casts Red blood cells and red cell casts†
Ultrasound	Normal kidneys and pelvicalyceal system	Dilated pelvicalyceal system; enlarged kidneys	Normal pelvicalyceal system; kidneys normal or enlarged

*(From R. Rault. The patient with acute renal failure. In: *Disorders of Fluid and Electrolyte Balance Diagnosis and Management*, edited by J. B. Puschett, p. 182. Churchill Livingstone, New York, 1985.)

†Often seen in acute renal failure due to glomerulonephritis or vasculitis.

TABLE 3.5.
Urinary Indices in Acute Renal Failure.*

	Prerenal Azotemia	Oliguric Acute Tubular Necrosis
Urine osmolality	> 500 mOsm/kg	< 350 mOsm/kg
Urine sodium	< 20 mEq/liter	> 40 mEq/liter
Fractional excretion of sodium†	< 1	> 1

*From R. Rault. The patient with acute renal failure. In: *Disorders of Fluid and Electrolyte Balance Diagnosis and Management*, edited by J. B. Puschett, p. 123. Churchill Livingstone, New York, 1985.

†$\frac{\text{urinary sodium}}{\text{plasma sodium}} \div \frac{\text{urinary creatinine}}{\text{plasma creatinine}}$

with calcium, bicarbonate, and insulin-glucose infusions. Correction of metabolic acidosis is indicated when the serum bicarbonate is ≤ 15 mEq/liter. Indications for dialysis include BUN > 100 mg/dl, creatinine > 10 mg/dl, uremic seizures and encephalopathy, acute pulmonary edema, hyperkalemia, and profound acidosis that cannot be controlled by medical means. Serum potassiums > 7 mEq/liter may lead to cardiac arrhythmias and death. Potassium elevations > 6 mEq/liter should probably be treated with dialysis.

Renal Failure Secondary to Iodinated Contrast Materials

Renal failure secondary to iodinated contrast materials has become much more common in the last 10 years (1,3,5,7,24). This is in part due to increased awareness of the disorder and also because of the increased use of iodinated agents for such procedures such as angiography and computed tomography (CT scanning). Renal failure secondary to iodinated contrast agents has been estimated to occur in about 1% of healthy individuals and in up to 20% of high risk patients (3). Impaired renal function usually begins within 12 to 48 hours after the contrast exposure (11). Impaired renal function secondary to contrast agents may be associated with oliguria but may also be nonoliguric (12). The creatinine peaks within 7 days but returns to base line in 70% of the cases. Several risk factors have been identified (10,11,12), the most important of which is pre-existing azotemia (BUN ≥ 30 mg/dl, creatine ≥ 1.5 mg/dl). Other risk factors include diabetes mellitus, hypertension, hyperuricemia (≥ 8 mg/dl), dehydration, multiple contrast studies within 3 days, proteinuria, and multiple myeloma. The mechanism of nephropathy is not well known. Preventive measures include avoiding contrast studies unless absolutely necessary in high risk patients, hydrating the patient before the contrast study, and using the lowest possible dose of the iodinated agent (8). One should monitor urine output and creatinine carefully for 3 days after exposure to the contrast agent in the high risk patient.

ACID BASE BALANCE

Cellular metabolism generally produces 1 mEq of acid/kg/day. CO_2 is produced by the body in vast amounts by oxidation of carbohydrates and fats and is excreted by the lungs. Several buffer systems act to maintain pH in a normal range. The carbonic acid-bicarbonate system is, however, most important (10,12,21):

$$H+\ HCO_3^- \rightleftarrows H_2CO_3^- \rightleftarrows CO_2 + H_2O$$

The pH is determined by the Henderson-Hasselbalch equation:

$$pH = 6.1 + \log\ (HCO_3^-)/0.03 \times Pco_2$$

Normal HCO_3^- is 24 mEq/L.

$$\text{Normal pH} = 6.1 + \log\ (24/1.2) = 6.1 + \log\ (20/1) = 7.4$$

The ratio of bicarbonate to dissolved CO_2 must remain at 20 to 1 to ensure normal pH. Acidemia is defined as pH < 7.36 and alkalosis is defined as > 7.44.

This buffer system allows for respiratory compensation for metabolic disturbances and metabolic compensation for respiratory disturbances. In a simple acid base disturbance, only the primary process (metabolic or respiratory) and its expected compensation (respiratory or metabolic) are present. In a mixed acid-base disturbance, two or more processes are present simultaneously. A diagrammatic representation of the expected values of pH, Pco_2, (HCO_3^-), and (H+) in the four primary acid-base disorders is shown in Figure 3.1.

Laboratory Determinations in Acid-Base Disturbances

Venous electrolytes may be used as a first approach to diagnosis. However, the final acid-

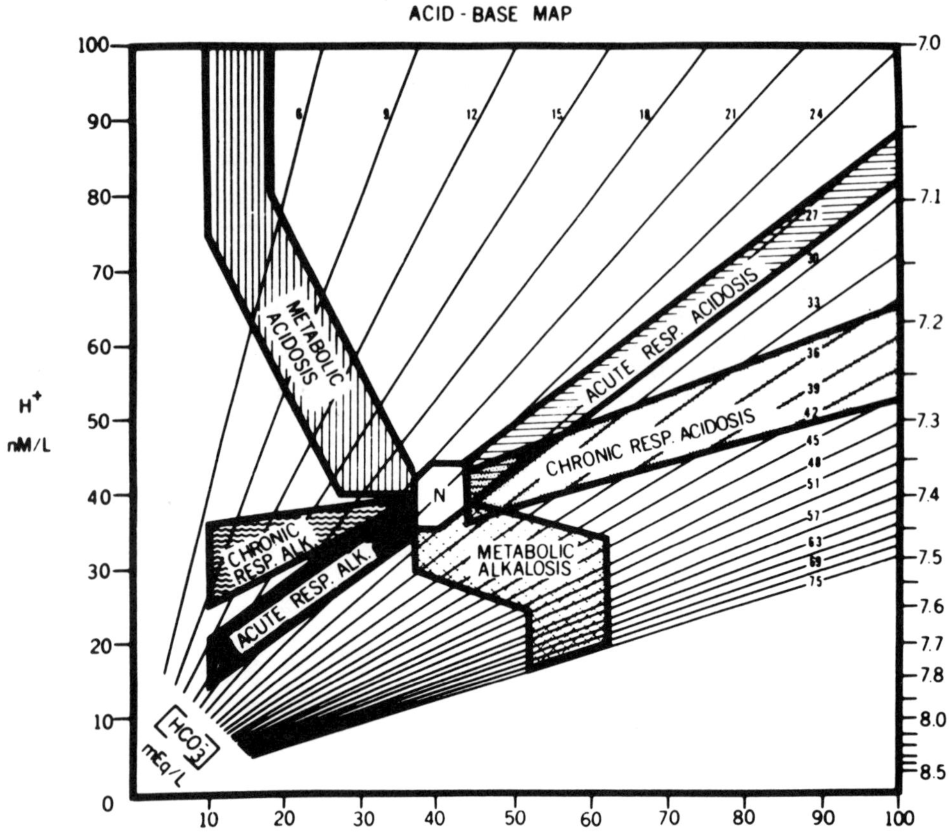

Figure 3.1. Acid-base map. Area of normal values is labled *N*. The map actually extends further up than down (to a pH of 6.6) and further to the right than shown (to a P_{CO_2} of 180 mm Hg). Numbered lines represent isopleths for bicarbonate (mEq/L). (From M. Goldberg *et al.* Computer-based instruction and diagnosis of acid-base disorders. J.A.M.A., *233:* 269–275, 1973.)

base disturbance can be determined only by arterial blood gases. Electrolyte values that may be of value include the "CO_2" which is a sum of all the components of the bicarbonate-carbonic acid system. Quantitatively, however, bicarbonate makes up most of the total CO_2 and can be used as a reflection of the plasma bicarbonate. When the patient has a low CO_2 the possible acid-base diagnoses are metabolic acidosis or chronic respiratory alkalosis or both. If the total CO_2 is high, the patient may have metabolic alkalosis or chronic respiratory acidosis or both. Serum potassium is usually high in acidosis and low in alkalosis.

The anion gap is determined by subtracting the sum of (Cl^-) and (HCO_3^-) from the (Na+). The normal value is 8 to 16 mEq/liter. It represents the negatively charged proteins, sulfates, phosphates, and other unmeasured serum, organic, and inorganic anions whose negative charge is balanced by sodium.

In arterial gases, the pH is determined with a pH meter. The P_{CO_2} is determined by equilibrating the blood with samples of known P_{CO_2} or by using a CO_2 electrode. (HCO_3^-) cannot be determined directly, but can be calculated by the Henderson-Hasselbalch equation or by using nomograms.

Metabolic Acidosis

Metabolic acidosis occurs when (HCO_3^-) falls with an associated fall in pH. Metabolic acidosis can be divided into high and normal ionic gap acidosis. The accumulation of anions of strong acids leads to an increase in the ionic gap. Renal failure, diabetic ketoacidosis, salicylate ingestion, and lactic acidosis are examples of high ionic acidosis. Lactic acidosis is the most severe form of metabolic acidosis and can be seen as a result of impaired tissue oxygenation due to shock, anemia, hypoxia, or malignancy. Lactic levels > 5 mEq/liter are usually associated with a true acid-base emergency. Normal ionic gap acidosis develops from hydrogen ion ingestion or from bicarbonate loss. If there is no accumulation of strong acid anions then hyperchloremic acidosis results. This may be seen in early renal failure and in conditions of diarrhea, laxative abuse, and diuretic use. This form of acidosis is less severe and less likely to require emergency treatment. The respiratory compensation of a metabolic acidosis is an increase in rate and depth of respirations, which leads to a decreased P_{CO_2}. Renal compensations are much slower.

When acidemia is severe, intravenous replacement therapy with sodium bicarbonate may be necessary. It may be given as a bolus (50 mEq/ampule) or as a continuous drip of two to three ampules in 1 liter of 5% D/W. Proper therapy requires frequent measurements of serum bicarbonate and blood gases. The goal of therapy is to return serum bicarbonate to a level out of danger (12 to 15 mEq/liter) and to raise the pH above 7.25. In addition to alkali therapy, treatment of the underlying disorder should be begun at once.

Metabolic Alkalosis

Metabolic alkalosis occurs when the serum bicarbonate concentration rises with an associated increase in pH. Causes include loss of acid from vomiting, nasogastric suction, and gain of alkali from antacids or infusion of organic acids such as lactate, citrate, and plasmanate. A bicarbonate concentrate > 26 mEq/liter suggests this diagnosis. An increase in bicarbonate in response to a chronic respiratory acidosis must be excluded. Volume depletion is the most common maintenance factor in metabolic alkalosis. Potassium depletion is also seen.

Usually a low urine sodium is the laboratory hallmark of volume depletion. In metabolic alkalosis, this relationship may break down. Bicarbonate in the urine causes excretion of sodium to counterbalance the negative charge of bicarbonate. Despite volume depletion, the urine sodium may be high.

Treatment is directed toward eliminating the underlying cause. If it is associated with a volume deficit, the volume deficit should be corrected. Potassium replacement may be also necessary. Because correction of the volume deficit usually leads to urinary loss of bicarbonate in the urine, acid administration is seldom needed.

Respiratory Alkalosis

Acute respiratory alkalosis is characterized by abrupt reduction in P_{CO_2} and elevated pH. It may be caused by hyperventilation associated with anxiety, overventilation by ventilators, hyperthermia, and brain injury. Renal compensation for the respiratory alkalosis takes 12 to 24 hours. Acutely, it may be associated with circumoral and hand paresthesias, tetany, and neuromuscular irritability.

In most cases respiratory alkalosis is not life-threatening. Mild sedation and CO_2 breathing with a paper bag is useful in psychogenic hyperventilation. If the patient is on a ventilator, respiratory rate and volume may be decreased and the dead space increased.

Respiratory Acidosis

Respiratory acidosis is caused by alveolar hypoventilation with resultant increase in P_{CO_2} and lowering of pH. This condition is associated with airway obstruction, inadequate tidal volume, atelectasis, pneumonia, shock, fractured ribs, chest pain, abdominal distention, paralysis of the diaphragm, and over-administration of narcotics. Respiratory acidosis is a true emergency. The patient must be given an adequate airway. Flail chest and pneumothorax should be considered and treated if necessary. Airway obstruction from secretions or bronchospasm should be treated with chest physical therapy and bronchodilators. The threshold for intubation should be low. The use of alkali with the acidemia as a means of delaying intubation is never appropriate.

REFERENCES

1. Bennett, W. M., Luft, F., and Porter, W. A. Pathogenesis of renal failure due to aminoglycosides and contrast media used in roentgenography. J. Am. Med., *69:* 767–774, 1980.
2. Berl, T., Anderson, R. J., McDonald, K. M., and Schrier, R. W. Clinical disorders of water metabolism. Kidney Int. *10:* 117–132, 1976.
3. Byrd, L., and Sherman, R. L. Radiocontrast-induced acute renal failure, a clinical and pathophysiologic review. Medicine, *58:* 270–279, 1979.

4. Carpenter, R., and Rault, R. Parenchymal renal disease and renal failure. In: *Disorders of Fluid and Electrolyte Balance Diagnosis and Management*, edited by J. B. Puschett and A. Greenberg, Chap. 7, pp. 161–188. Churchill, Livingstone, New York, Edinburgh, London, and Melbourne, 1985.
5. Cochran, S. T., Wong, W. S., and Roe, D. J. Predicting angiography-induced acute renal function impairment: Clinical risk model. Am. J. Radiol., *141:* 1027–1033, 1983.
6. Davis, A. N., Phar, B., and Dobbing, J. Neural regulation of water and salt metabolism: Physiologic function and disease. In: *Clinical Neuroendocrinology*, edited by J. B. Martin, S. Reichlin, and G. M. Brown, Chap. 4, pp. 63–92. Davis, Philadelphia, 1977.
7. D'Elia, J. A., Gleason, R. E., Alday, M., Malarick, C., Godley, K., Warram, J., Kaldany, A., and Weinrauch, L. A. Nephrotoxicity from angiographic contrast material, a prospective study. Am. J. Med., *72:* 719–725, 1982.
8. Forrest, N. J., Cox, M., Hung, C., Morrison, G., Bia, M., and Singer, I. Superiority of demeclocycline over lithium in the treatment of chronic syndrome of inappropriate secretion of antidiuretic hormone. N. Engl. J. Med., *298:* 173, 1978.
9. Fox, J. L., Falik, J. L., and Shalhoub, R. J. Neurosurgical hyponatremia: The role of inappropriate antidiuresis. J. Neurosurg., *34:* 506–514, 1971.
10. Goldberg, M., Green, S. B., Moss, M. V., Marbach, C. B., and Garfinkel, D. Computer-based instruction and diagnosis of acid-base disorders, a systemic approach. J.A.M.A., *223:* 269–275, 1973.
11. Goldberg, M., and Handler, J. S. Hyponatremia and renal wasting of sodium in patients with malfunction of the central nervous system. N. Engl. J. Med., *263:* 1037, 1960.
12. Greenberg, A. Common emergencies of acid-base balance. Topics Emerg. Med., *5:* 1–16, 1983.
13. Greenberg, A. Disorders of body water metabolism. In: *Disorders of Fluid and Electrolyte Balance Diagnosis and Management*, edited by J. B. Puschett, and A. Greenberg, Chap. 5, pp. 113–136. Churchill, Livingstone, New York, Edinburgh, London, and Melbourne, 1985.
14. Greenberg, A., and Goldfarb, S. Acid-base disturbances in the surgical patient. In: *Medical Care of the Surgical Patient*, edited by F. H. Brown, and D. R. Goldmann. Lippincott, Philadelphia, 1982.
15. Hantman, D., Rossier, B., Zohlman, R., and Schrier, R. Rapid correction hyponatremia in the syndrome of inappropriate secretion of antidiuretic hormone. Ann. Intern. Med., *78:* 870, 1973.
16. Hayes, R. M. Antidiuretic hormone. N. Engl. J. Med. *295:* 659, 1976.
17. Hilberman, M. Renal protection. In: *The Society of Critical Care Medicine, Textbook of Critical Care*, edited by W. C. Shoemaker, W. L. Thompson, and P. R. Holbrook, Chap. 80, pp. 597–604. W. B. Saunders, Philadelphia, London, Toronto, Mexico City, Rio de Janeiro, Sydney, Tokyo, 1984.
18. Howrie, D. L., and Kroboth, P. D. Drug dosing and renal failure. In: *Disorders of Fluid and Electrolyte Balance Diagnosis and Management*, edited by J. B. Puschett and A. Greenberg, Chap. 11, pp. 231–246. Churchill, Livingstone, New York, Edinburgh, London, and Melbourne, 1985.
19. Peitzman, A. Principles of circulatory support and the treatment of hemorrhagic shock. In: *Oxygen Transport in the Critically Ill Patient*, edited by J. V. Snyder, Yearbook Medical Publishers, Chicago, in press, 1985.
20. Peters, J. P., Welt, L. G., Sims, E. A. H., Orloff, J., and Needham, J. W. A salt-wasting syndrome associated with cerebral disease. Trans. Assoc. Am. Physicians, *63:* 57, 1950.
21. Puschett, J. D., and Pirarno, B. Disorders of acid-base balance. In: *Disorders of Fluid and Electrolyte Balance Diagnosis and Management*, edited by J. B. Puschett and A. Greenberg, Chap. 1, 1–38. Churchill, Livingstone, New York, Edinburgh, London, and Melbourne, 1985.
22. Robertson, G. L. Diseases of the posterior pituitary. In: *Endocrinology and Metabolism*, edited by P. Felig, J. D. Baxter, A. E. Broadus, and L. A. Frohman, Chap. 9, pp. 251–277. McGraw-Hill, New York, St. Louis, San Francisco, Auckland, Bogota, Guatemala, Hamburg, Johannesburg, Lisbon, London, Madrid, Mexico, Montreal, New Delhi, Panama, Paris, San Juan, Sao Paulo, Singapore, Sydney, Tokyo, Toronto, 1981.
23. Rosse, E. J., and Christie, S. B. M. Hypernatremia. Medicine, *48:* 441–473, 1969.
24. Roxe, D. M. Toxic nephropathy from diagnostic and therapeutic agents. Am. J. Med., *69:* 759–766, 1980.
25. Schwartz, W. B., Bennett, W., Curelop, S., and Bartter, F. C. A syndrome of renal sodium loss and hyponatremia probably resulting from inappropriate secretion of antidiuretic hormone. Am. J. Med., *23:* 529–542, 1957.
26. Thomas, T. H., Morgan, D. B., Swaminathan, R., Ball, S. G., and Lee, M. R. Severe hyponatremia a study of 17 patients. Lancet, *1:* 621–624, 1978.
27. Shoemaker, W. C. Fluids and electrolytes in the acutely ill adult. In: *The Society of Critical Care Medicine, Textbook of Critical Care*, edited by W. C. Shoemaker, W. L. Thompson, and P. R. Holbrook, Chap. 82, pp. 614–640. W. B. Saunders, Philadelphia, London, Toronto, Mexico City, Rio de Janeiro, Sydney, Tokyo, 1984.
28. Shoemaker, W. C. Pathophysiology and therapy of shock syndromes. In: *The Society of Critical Care Medicine, Textbook of Critical Care*, edited by W. C. Shoemaker, W. L. Thompson, and P. R. Holbrook, Chap. 11, pp. 52–72. W. B. Saunders, Philadelphia, London, Toronto, Mexico City, Rio de Janeiro, Sydney, Tokyo, 1984.

CHAPTER 4

Metabolic Physiology, Pathophysiology, and Management

BRIAN J. ROWLANDS, M.D., F.R.C.S., F.A.C.S.,
N. SCOTT LITOFSKY, M.D., and
HOWARD H. KAUFMAN, M.D., F.A.C.S

INTRODUCTION

Following neurosurgical procedures or injury to the nervous system, a series of changes in metabolism and hormone secretion occur which constitute an important biologic defense mechanism. There is a complex inter-relationship between energy production, fluid and electrolyte balance, and endocrine activity which is directed toward survival and recovery. The metabolic response to injury is dependent upon a variety of factors, the most important of which is the severity of injury, but the age and gender of the patient, body size, and previous nutritional status also make important contributions to this response. Surgical stress is usually associated with a period of food deprivation and is accompanied by an increase in resting metabolic expenditure which is proportional to the magnitude of the injury. Under these circumstances energy is derived from endogenous tissue stores and there are increased rates of gluconeogenesis, glycogenolysis, and proteolysis associated with an increased mobilization of body stores of protein and fat. These metabolic changes are regulated by alterations in neuroendocrine activity and are reflected in increased urinary nitrogen excretion and changes in plasma substrate and hormone concentrations. These changes will be discussed in detail in this chapter together with consideration of the unique characteristics of the metabolic response in the patient with brain injury.

The outcome of trauma depends on the ability of the protective physiologic responses to preserve optimum cellular metabolism and function throughout the body. In addition to local effects produced at the site of injury, there may be a general disturbance of the metabolism and function of other organs. These metabolic changes are manifested as alterations in protein synthesis and energy metabolism, and an understanding of changes in body homeostasis has led to the evolution of effective preventive and supportive therapy. The rational use of metabolic and nutritional support techniques has had a dramatic impact on patient management by improving the morbidity and survival of hospitalized patients. These regimens have now been extended to the management of neurosurgical patients, especially following head injury, and the importance of the provision of adequate protein, calories, vitamins, and minerals for *all* patients under *all* conditions has been recognized.

Provision of nutritional support by the oral, enteral, or parenteral route has become part of the standard therapeutic regimen of many neurosurgical patients, but is especially important in those patients whose metabolic requirements are increased secondary to major injury and its complications. Accidental head injury is the most frequent cause of death between the ages of 2 and 42 years, has a mortality rate between 5% and 50%, and is associated in 50% of patients with multiple system injury (20). Approximately 60% of deaths from head injury occur within 24 hours of injury (5), but in those patients who survive beyond this time, the quality and morbidity of survival has been improved by advances in intensive care unit monitoring and management, and a better understanding of the secondary effects of head injury such as hypotension, hypoxia, hypovolemia, increased intracranial pressure, and infectious complications. An important component of this improvement in metabolic management is a recognition that there is a high incidence of clinical and subclinical malnutrition in hospitalized patients (24) and that preoperative malnutrition is one of the most important determinants of the development of surgical sepsis (35). Many conditions associated with an increased incidence of infection have accompanying abnormalities of normal host defense mechanisms that manifest themselves as neutropenia and abnormalities of the antibacterial functions of neutrophils, T lymphocytes and B lymphocytes, and as depression of the reticuloendothelial, opsonic, and complement systems. Anergy in surgical patients is associated with an increased risk of infection and death and is closely associated with erosion of body cell mass. Increased metabolic expenditure and depleted nutritional reserve may precipitate acute malnutrition, severely compromising the body's protein and energy stores and giving rise to impairment of humoral and cell-mediated immunity. Improvement of the immune mechanisms may be achieved by aggressive nutritional therapy with consequent reduction of morbidity and mortality. To avoid a vicious cycle of malnutrition and infection, it is important to identify "at risk" patients early in their hospital course and to provide adequate protein and energy substrates to replete and maintain adequate nutrition and to match the increased metabolic demands of illness, injury, and infection (52). Thus, the neurosurgical patient who survives a surgical procedure or neurologic injury may require prolonged metabolic support to achieve optimum recovery and function.

ENERGY REQUIREMENTS OF THE NEUROSURGICAL PATIENT

Normal Metabolic Homeostasis

When oral intake of nutrients is restricted or energy expenditure is increased, energy substrates are mobilized from endogenous sources to satisfy the requirements for vital functions. Fuel is stored in three forms—carbohydrate, protein, and fat. Carbohydrate is stored as glycogen in muscle or liver and yields about half of its theoretical 4 kcal/gm of dry carbohydrate. The main function of protein is not to serve as an energy substrate but to function as an enzyme, contractile or structural protein. When extra protein is eaten and metabolized, the nitrogen is excreted as urea and the calories, if they are in excess of those expended, are stored as adipose tissue. Proteins, like glycogen, are mainly in solution and account for only one fifth of the total tissue weight. As conversion of protein is an energy-consuming process, this is also an inefficient form of tissue fuel. Fat is stored in cells in an extra-aqueous environment and has an energy yield of close to the theoretical 9.4 kcal/gm of pure triglyceride.

A normal fasting man with a resting metabolic expenditure of 1800 kcals/day burns about 75 gm of protein, primarily derived from muscle and 160 gm of adipose tissue triglyceride (10). Liver and muscle glycogen stores are small and are soon utilized and, therefore, the two major fuel depots are muscle protein and adipose triglyceride. Some tissues, e.g. brain, peripheral nerves, and erythrocytes, rely on glucose as an energy source and this is provided by hepatic gluconeogenesis from amino acids, lactate, pyruvate, and glycerol. The splanchnic glucose output is about 180 gm per day of which about 140 gm is used by nervous tissue, mainly the brain (10). The remaining tissues, e.g. heart, kidney, skeletal muscle, use either nonesterified fatty acids released directly into the circulation, or nonesterified fatty acids partially oxidized to acetoacetate or β-hydroxybutyrate (ketone bodies) by the liver. The exclusion of glucose metabolism by these tissues spares the need for *de novo* glucose synthesis and thereby conserves protein. The liver is the most important single organ in any adaptation to endogenous fuel utilization as it synthesizes glucose from its precursors and oxidizes nonesterified fatty acids to ketone bodies. This latter process also provides the energy required for hepatic gluconeogenesis and ketogenesis.

All cellular functions such as ion transport, maintenance of osmolality, and synthesis are dependent on the conversion of energy derived from food substrates to adenosine triphosphate (ATP) and other high energy phosphate bonds.

Oxygen is the hydrogen acceptor required for complete oxidation to carbon dioxide and water. In the absence of oxygen, energy metabolism is dependent on the inefficient degradation of carbohydrate to lactate. The metabolic pathways of glucose and fat indicate that the maximum amount of energy that they contain which can be converted to ATP is about 40%, the remainder being converted to heat which is wasted apart from supporting body temperature. The maximum yield for protein is about 33% depending on the amino acid composition of the protein.

Metabolic Homeostasis in Disease

The resting energy expenditure of a normal 70-kg man is about 1,800 kcal per day. Decreased food intake is accompanied by weight loss and a reduction in resting energy expenditure. Surgical stress, injury, and infection are characterized by an increase in resting energy expenditure. In ambulatory hospitalized surgical patients, daily energy expenditure may be increased by 20% above basal level as a result of physical activity and food consumption. Following elective surgical operation, the postoperative energy expenditure will not differ by more than 10% from preoperative values in the absence of significant complications. Fever increases the resting energy expenditure by 13% for each degree Celsius of fever. Previously well-nourished patients with multiple fractures may have an increase of resting metabolic expenditure of 10% to 25% and major infection such as peritonitis may cause increases up to 50% above predicted normal levels. Sustained higher levels of energy expenditure up to 125% above predicted normal levels may occur with major thermal burns. The increase in daily resting metabolic expenditure in neurosurgical patients will vary according to the extent of local and associated injuries and the presence of complications such as coma, posturing, and infection, but has been reported between 25% and 120% above basal energy expenditure. In addition, the period of hypermetabolism which peaks 5 to 10 days after systemic injury appears to persist throughout the duration of coma.

The increase in resting metabolic expenditure following injury may represent an increase in tissue and organ work, or an increase in neuroendocrine stimuli for heat production, or an increase in obligatory heat loss which demands an increase in heat production to maintain body temperature (33). Alterations in thermoregulation, increases in heat production, and changes in substrate and hormone flow are related to the stress and severity of illness, and return to normal during recovery.

Resting metabolic expenditure and endogenous urinary nitrogen excretion change in parallel following injury (38). It has been suggested that the increased heat production represents an increase in protein oxidation and that in the absence of adequate calorie intake, dietary protein can be utilized for general energy needs. However, in cases with sepsis and burns, calculations suggest that the increased protein oxidation is not sufficient to account for measured increases in energy expenditure (33). In mammals, the main energy requirements are met by the oxidation of two carbon fragments (acetyl CoA) in the tricarboxylic acid (Krebs) cycle and nonesterified fatty acids mobilized from adipose tissue cannot be converted to glucose, glycogen, or carbohydrate intermediaries. Thus, in clinical conditions associated with increased energy expenditure, the nitrogen excretion represents accelerated gluconeogenesis to supply energy for glucose-dependent tissues, rather than a need to supply additional two carbon fragments for general fuel at the expense of body protein (34).

Metabolic Response to Starvation, Stress, and Infection

The metabolic response to injury is classically described as being separated into an acute phase in which there is mobilization of endogenous substrates to provide energy, and an adaptive phase in which metabolism is dependent on the availability of nutrient substrates. These phases correspond to the "ebb" and "flow" phases of the metabolic response to trauma described by Cuthbertson in 1942 (16). The metabolic response to starvation differs from that of stress and infection, and it is important to realize that in an individual patient, varying degrees of starvation and stress from injury and infection may contribute to the overall changes in hormonal and substrate homeostasis. These metabolic changes and their inter-relationships are briefly reviewed here, as an understanding of them is important in assessing and meeting the nutritional requirements of the neurosurgical patient.

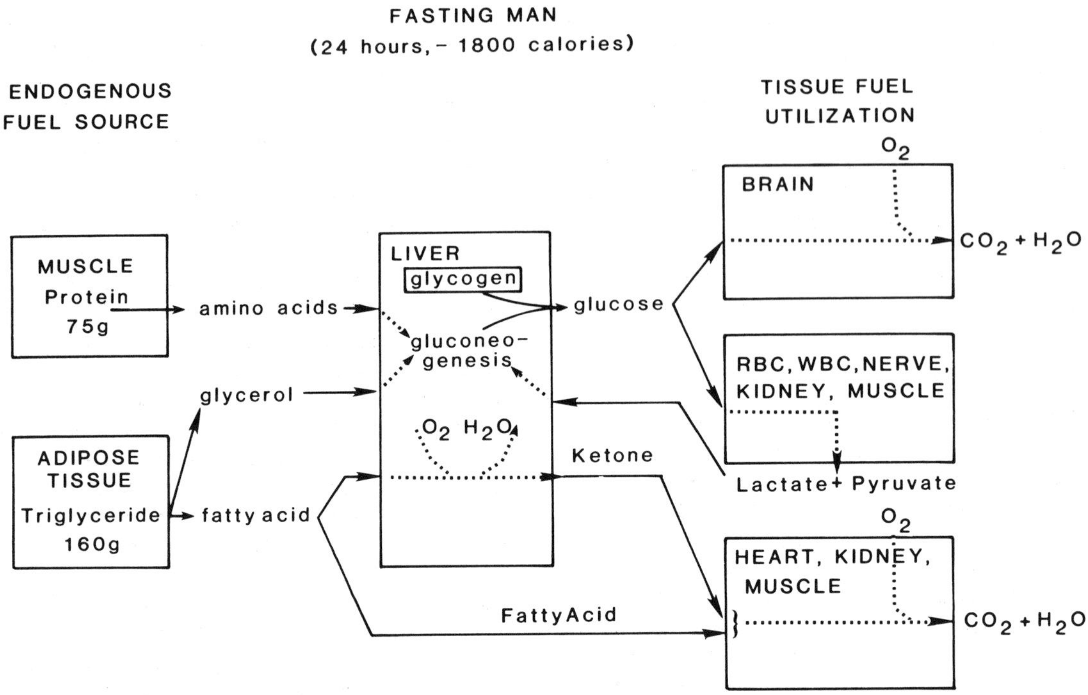

Figure 4.1. The metabolic response to fasting in man is characterized by the rapid consumption within 24 hr of muscle and liver glycogen stores. Energy demands for vital functions are met by mobilization of protein from muscle and triglyceride from adipose tissue stores. Gluconeogenesis in the liver ensures adequate energy provision for glucose-dependent tissues, but the majority of energy needs are satisfied by fat mobilization.

Starvation (Fig. 4.1)

The sequence of events leading to death in starvation is usually decreased food intake, protein wasting, weakness of respiratory muscles, atelectasis, pneumonia, and death. The inability to conserve protein often reflects a failure of normal adaptive mechanisms. The main endogenous fuel in all but the postprandial state is fat and in prolonged fasting up to 90% of daily energy utilization is derived from adipose tissue stores (10). The metabolic response to starvation in man has an initial and a late phase: in the initial phase glucose production is maintained to meet the needs of the brain, nervous tissue, and red cells (gluconeogenic phase) and in the late phase the rate of protein breakdown is minimized (protein conservation phase).

During starvation, in the absence of exogenous carbohydrate supply, glucose homeostasis requires an increase in glucose production and a reduction in extracerebral glucose utilization. Despite this, blood glucose concentration declines and results in a decrease in circulating insulin and glucagon (19). The reduction in circulating insulin stimulates lipolysis, providing nonesterified fatty acids for energy requirements of muscle and liver and hepatic ketogenesis. Early in starvation liver and muscle glycogen stores become depleted rapidly and glucose production depends on hepatic gluconeogenesis from lactate and amino acids, principally alanine and glutamine derived from muscle protein. Glutamine is utilized by the intestine but alanine is used solely for gluconeogenesis by the liver. Alanine is synthesized in muscle tissue by transamination of glucose-derived pyruvate and represents approximately 35% of the total amino acid output from muscle. The main source of amino groups for alanine synthesis are the branched chain amino acids—valine, leucine, and isoleucine. During the initial 72 hours of starvation, alanine output increases and hepatic glucose output is able to keep pace with the rapid rates of glucose utilization in the brain. Pyruvate, lactate, and the glycerol skeleton of triglyceride are also gluconeogenic substrates. The endoglycolytic

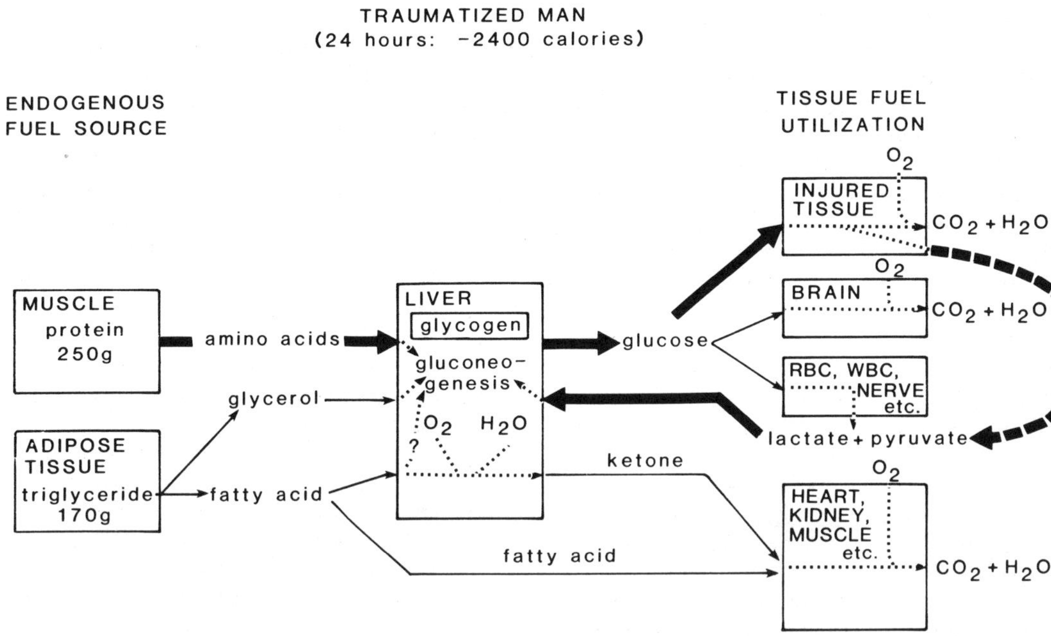

Figure 4.2. The metabolic response to surgical stress trauma and infection differs from that of starvation in that there is a larger and more rapid mobilization of muscle protein to satisfy increased requirement for gluconeogenesis. Energy requirements are increased in all tissues, especially injured tissues, and fat still accounts for the majority of energy expenditure.

product, lactate, may be resynthesized back to glucose in the liver and kidney (Cori cycle). This, however, does not provide net glucose or net energy since the lactate was originally glucose-derived, and the energy required for resynthesizing glucose offsets that derived from glycolysis. The advantages of the Cori cycle are that energy for hepatic glucose synthesis is derived from fatty acid oxidation and recycling the glycolytic product reduces the tissue requirement for protein-derived glucose. Glucose synthesis from the glycerol skeleton of triglyceride becomes a significant contribution to total glucose production as lipolysis increases.

As fasting extends beyond 7 days, loss of nitrogen (particularly urea excretion) progressively declines and there is a reduction of hepatic gluconeogenesis. Blood glucose levels remain unchanged and glucose utilization is reduced. There is an increase in circulating ketone bodies which are formed from fatty acids in the liver, and when prolonged fasting is accompanied by significant ketosis, the brain adapts to the use of ketone bodies for half of its energy requirements. This reduced need for gluconeogenesis is reflected in a decreased flux of alanine from muscle and a fall in plasma alanine concentration due to inhibition of oxidation of branched-chain amino acids in muscle.

Stress and Infection (Fig. 4.2)

Following the stress of injury or infection, the pattern of endogenous fuel substrate utilization differs from that observed in uncomplicated starvation. The most obvious differences are protein wastage, hyperglycemia, and anaerobic glycolysis with lactate production. Injury induces a wide range of integrated changes in hemodynamics, neuroendocrine secretions (in particular, insulin, glucagon, corticosteroids, and catecholamines), and tissue metabolism that are directed initially toward survival and later to healing. Provided that the injury is not fatal, the immediate phase of depressed local metabolism is followed by a period of increased general metabolism due to the increased cellular activity of the repair process, elimination of damaged and devitalized tissue, and increased catabolism of protein.

The immediate local effect of tissue damage is an increase in vascular permeability due to locally released endogenous mediators, e.g. 5-hydroxytryptamine, histamine, bradykinin, and possibly prostaglandins, which give rise to the classical signs of inflammation. This leads to edema and depression of local metabolism and is referred to as the "ebb" phase of injury (16). The effects of the injury then become more widespread and a generalized vasoconstrictive reaction, mediated through catecholamines, occurs in response to fluid loss associated with hemorrhage, burn, crush injury, and infection. Provided the injury is not fatal, a period of increased metabolism ensues due to increased cellular activity, increased oxygen consumption, and increased heat production. The increased rate of nitrogen excretion that characterizes this catabolic response closely parallels the increased energy expenditure. This response is described as the "flow" phase of injury (16).

Of the many metabolic changes that occur following injury, the changes in energy metabolism are the most important. In nonfatal injuries, there is increased sympathetic activity for 48 to 72 hours which ensures an adequate substrate supply by mobilizing carbohydrate and fat stores, resulting in hyperglycemia and increased plasma nonesterified fatty acids. Provided that there is adequate tissue perfusion, the rates of oxidation of both glucose and nonesterified fatty acids are unaltered. Decreased heat production also occurs secondary to a change in the thermoregulatory capacity of the hypothalamus which is related to the severity of injury. Thus, a reduced "steady state" of energy metabolism prevails at a lower level of heat production. In fatal injuries, progressive failure of oxygen supply to the tissue leads to a further fall in heat production, cellular hypoxia, decreased blood glucose and nonesterified fatty acid levels, accumulation of lactate, disruption of acid-base buffering systems, and eventual cellular death.

Following the acute reaction to injury, which may last up to 72 hours, there is an increase in heat production and rise in body temperature associated with an increase in urinary excretion of nitrogen, inorganic sulfate, phosphate, potassium, and creatinine. The excess nitrogen is derived from catabolism of muscle protein and the oxidation of non-nitrogenous residues accounts for some of the extra heat production. The size of the nitrogen loss is related to the severity of injury, the age and gender of the patient, and the patient's previous nutritional status; some of the largest nitrogen losses occur in previously healthy young males with major burns and multisystem trauma. This obligatory protein loss cannot be completely abolished in the immediate post-traumatic period, even with large intakes of protein and calories. Protein catabolism is accelerated to a greater extent than protein synthesis following injury, and the prolonged proteolysis of muscle protein leads to excessive hepatic gluconeogenesis, depletion of muscle protein, weakness, reduction of protein synthesis, diminished enzyme function, and loss of immunocompetence.

Hyperglycemia and a diabetic glucose-tolerance curve are characteristic of the response to injury and infection, despite a normal insulin response to hyperglycemia. However, glucose uptake is unaltered, suggesting insulin resistance in the tissues. Adipose tissue still responds to hyperinsulinemia by suppression of lipolysis. Alanine, lactate, and glycerol all provide an increasing flow of gluconeogenic substrate to the liver which releases more glucose under the influence of alanine-induced hyperglucagonemia. There may be impairment of uptake of other metabolic fuels (nonesterified fatty acids, ketone bodies) leading to the oxidation of locally derived branched-chain amino acids in the muscle to satisfy its energy requirements. Thus, hyperglycemia reflects an augmentation of the glucose pool to maintain glucose oxidation rates rather than a need for overall energy provision from proteolysis. Although the nitrogen excretion following injury parallels the increased resting metabolic expenditure and weight loss, the calorie contribution of protein is only about 20% of daily expenditure, the residual energy requirement being met by mobilization of fat stores.

Several features of neurosurgical injury may contribute to the increase in body metabolism. Fever is often a major stimulus to initiating catabolic losses. Changes in cardiac output, peripheral resistance and tissue oxygenation may exaggerate local fuel deficits. Circulating insulin antagonists such as catecholamines, cortisol, and other "active agents" in the blood may alter peripheral tissue metabolism. The "agents" may be released from damaged tissue (lysosomal enzymes), may be associated with the release of bacteria and toxins into the bloodstream, or may represent circulating denatured proteins and peptides. The liver plays a central role in all metabolism, and damage to its ultrastructure secondary to infection, endotoxemia, hemorrhage, and hypoxia will inevitably adversely affect substrate homeostasis. Damage to the brain and nervous system may influence or modify the neuroendocrine responses to injury and infection.

Neuroendocrine Response to Starvation, Stress, and Infection

The complex inter-relationship between energy production, fluid and electrolyte balance, and endocrine activity following elective surgery and trauma is important for normal recovery, repair, and convalescence. The endocrine response is characterized by an increased secretion rate of many glands and an altered tissue utilization of most hormones. This is reflected in altered concentrations of these hormones in blood and urine. The response to injury is the result of factors such as fear, peripheral, and central nervous system stimulation, temperature changes, anesthetic agents, endotoxins, and blood volume changes, which activate the neuroendocrine and metabolic responses. The exact sequence of events that initiates these changes is not fully defined.

There are three main components to the neuroendocrine response to injury: the afferent impulses that activate the pituitary adrenal axis, the neurohumoral control of the pituitary-adrenal axis including adrenal cortex and medulla, and factors affecting the balance between insulin and glucagon as regulators of the body fuel economy.

Afferent Pathways

The wound directly or indirectly initiates the metabolic and physiologic alterations that occur following injury. Local circulatory changes and the inflammatory response give rise to nervous signals to the central nervous system, and both animal and human studies have demonstrated the importance of afferent nerve impulses in the endocrine response. Direct stimulation of the peripheral nerve produces increased adrenocortical activity but this activity is diminished or absent if the limb is denervated. In animals the adrenocortical response to injury does not occur after transection of the spinal cord above the level of injury, or section through the medulla oblongata, and the brain plays a central role in the control of adrenal and other hormone activity (25). The initial response of adrenalin and noradrenalin, vasopressin, and antidiuretic hormone is also dependent on nervous signals from the injured area.

Similar responses have also been demonstrated in man. Growth hormone and adrenocorticotrophic hormone (ACTH) concentrations rise within 1 hour of cholecystectomy or inguinal herniorrhaphy under general anesthesia, but not with spinal anesthesia. The hyperglycemic response is abolished in patients undergoing abdominal and thoracic surgery when epidural anesthesia is used to the level of the fourth thoracic dermatome but increases of cortisol do occur suggesting that there are also efferent vagal pathways. In paraplegic patients, the sympathetic nervous system response is diminished when operation is performed in a denervated area.

Circulating factors interacting with or arising from the area of injury influence the post-traumatic endocrine response, but the role of amino acids and peptides in initiating hormone responses is not yet well-defined. Substances such as histamine, 5-hydroxytryptamine, and acetylcholine, which are released by damaged tissue, can stimulate the adrenal gland when injected directly into the adrenal blood supply. A variety of homeostatic responses also occur locally due to alterations in blood volume, tissue nutrients, pH, and serum osmolality. Acute hypovolemia and dehydration stimulate sympathetic activity which returns to normal after transfusion and rehydration (57). Hypoxia and hypoglycemia also stimulate the autonomic nervous system to produce changes in respiratory rate and substrate flow (48). Anxiety and fear may also increase cortisol and catecholamine secretion which augments or exceeds the physiologic response to the injury. Total or partial starvation, which is a feature of many injuries, also influences the central nervous and hormone regulators and disturbances of circadian rhythms will add to the stress of illness and alter the normal restorative process of the body.

In 1877, Claude Bernard was the first to demonstrate the role of the central nervous system in the response to trauma when he reported glycosuria following puncture of the fourth ventricle in dogs. The final common pathway for all the afferent impulses that activate the pituitary-adrenal axis is the hypothalamus. Animal experiments show that removal of the brain above the hypothalamus does not affect the increase in pituitary-adrenal secretions following injury but that removal of the hypothalamus obliterates the response (25). It is now generally agreed that the adrenocortical response is initiated by the production of corticotrophin-releasing factor by the hypothalamus which then stimulates the anterior pituitary via the hypophyseal portal vessels. Substrate and energy metabolism is subsequently controlled through the sympathetic and parasympathetic nervous systems and their effects on adrenal and pancreatic secretions.

Catecholamines—Hormones of Stress

Catecholamines are released by the adrenal gland in response to a variety of stimuli. The response to sudden sympathoadrenal discharge, which is necessary for survival, is characterized by tachycardia, papillary dilation, piloerector activity of the skin, alterations of skin and muscle blood flow, and an increased respiratory rate associated with bronchial dilation. This response is accompanied by mobilization of glucose and fatty acids together with salt and water retention. There are several factors that contribute to the resultant hyperglycemia. There is a direct effect on the liver with an increased conversion of liver glycogen and three-carbon precursors to glucose. In skeletal muscle, muscle glycogen is converted to lactic acid and transported to the liver for gluconeogenesis (Cori cycle). There is also suppression of insulin release by the pancreas in response to hyperglycemia and pancreatic glucagon release. Nonesterified fatty acids are mobilized as a result of direct stimulation of fat cells and the response is potentiated by suppression of insulin release. Catecholamines also facilitate neuromuscular transmission and increase the basal metabolic rate in both man and animals.

Insulin—The Storage Hormone

Insulin promotes the storage of metabolic fuels. It normally facilitates the entry of glucose into cells in response to changes in blood sugar and promotes the synthesis of liver and muscle glycogen. When insulin values are low, the rate of triglyceride breakdown is increased and hyperketonemia and hypoaminoacidemia often occur. Insulin also facilitates transport of potassium and phosphorus into cells. Following stress, hyperglycemia and glycosuria occur and may persist for several days. Glycogenolysis and gluconeogenesis are both increased. In the "ebb" phase of injury, the insulin inhibitory effect of the sympathetic nervous system (alpha-receptor effect) predominates, resulting in glucose intolerance. In the "flow" phase, which is characterized by an increased heat production (beta-receptor effect), there is an increased mass flow of glucose from the liver to the peripheral tissues. Beta-adrenergic receptors may augment insulin elaboration during the flow phase of injury. Other feedback mechanisms which may aid in glucose homeostasis following stress are the suppression of insulin by lactic acid, its stimulation by high levels of glucagon, and alterations in blood flow to the endocrine pancreas. The insulin response to stress is nonspecific and the initial suppression of insulin secretion is followed in the flow phase by hyperglycemia associated with hyperinsulinemia which persists for several days (21, 22).

Glucocorticoids, Glucagon, and Growth Hormone—The Permissive Hormones

The glucocorticoid hormones are permissive, augmenting and amplifying specific metabolic responses to stress. They augment hepatic gluconeogenesis by stimulating enzymes that direct the conversion of three carbon fragments into the synthesis of new glucose, and augment lipolysis and glycogen oxidation in skeletal muscle.

Glucagon has opposite effects to insulin and anabolism and protein conservation occur when insulin is increased relative to glucagon. This environment favors the storage of energy, limits gluconeogenesis, and causes increased protein biosynthesis and decreased urea nitrogen excretion. An increase in glucagon relative to insulin is associated with increased glycogenolysis, gluconeogenesis, and ureagenesis at the expense of protein biosynthesis. Glucagon is released in response to hypoglycemia, increased sympathetic activity, and certain amino acids and there seems to be a close correlation between catecholamine activity and glucagon activity. Following injury, glucagon levels are elevated even when hyperglycemia is present.

Growth hormone is stimulated during stress and resets the insulin response to glucose. It also stimulates release of nonesterified fatty acids allowing fat utilization peripherally and nitrogen retention in "fed" man. Growth hormone administration to critically ill patients improves nitrogen retention during the catabolic phase of injury, the effects being mediated by alterations of carbohydrate metabolism (59).

Summary of Endocrine Responses to Trauma (Table 4.1)

The major hormone changes that occur following injury are directed toward survival and maintenance of energy production. Insulin favors hepatic glucose storage, while catecholamines, augmented by glucagon and glucocorticoids, stimulate hepatic glucose production. Increased sympathetic activity directs the response of the pancreatic hormones which then regulate the disposition of key substrates under their control. Peripheral mobilization of substrates is stimulated by catecholamines and augmented by insulin deficiency. Increased adrenergic activity is the initiator of the metabolic responses following injury, stimulating calorigenesis, regulating substrate mobilization through the Cori and alanine cycles, and controlling hepatic gluconeogenesis.

METABOLIC AND NUTRITIONAL MANAGEMENT OF THE NEUROSURGICAL INTENSIVE CARE UNIT PATIENT

The changes in substrate and hormone flux that accompany injury, neurosurgical stress, starvation, and infection are designed initially to ensure survival and subsequently to initiate the repair process. The consumption of endogenous tissue stores as a result of catabolism of lean body mass and reduction of synthetic processes further compromises host metabolism. Unique problems associated with neurosurgical patients, e.g. raised intracranial pressure, diabetes insipidus, and gastrointestinal dysfunction, further complicate the delivery of appropriate metabolic and nutritional support. Optimum metabolic support is usually regulated by monitoring several metabolic parameters, e.g. arterial blood gases, intracranial pressure, and making appropriate therapeutic decisions based on these observations. The nutritional support plan should be designed to replenish existing deficiencies effectively, to minimize further tissue losses, and to provide sufficient energy and protein substrate to support vital functions and to stimulate and maintain anabolism and repair.

Every disease, injury, or surgical procedure can induce or intensify a state of clinical or subclinical malnutrition by altering nutrient requirements, ingestion, absorption, and metabolism. These deficiencies must be recognized and treated to provide optimum conditions for recovery of the patient. Many clinicians recognize and acknowledge only the most extreme nutritional deficiencies. The history and physical examination which documents marked weight loss or obesity, pitting edema, the presence of massive ascites, or a scaphoid abdomen provide a rough assessment of the more extreme nutritional aberrations. More subtle forms of depletion, however, may escape attention. A multidisciplinary nutritional assessment program can provide nutritional data throughout the patient's full clinical course—from admission through diagnosis, treatment, convalescence, and rehabilitation. Thus, the early malnourished state may be identified, guidelines for nutritional support may be provided, and the response to nutritional therapy may be evaluated sequentially.

General Management

Neurosurgical patients admitted to the intensive care unit should be adequately monitored to ensure that changes in the neurologic status and general condition are recognized early and treated promptly. This is particularly important in the comatose patient with increased intracranial pressure. The following invasive monitoring devices are appropriate in such patients: arterial line, intracranial pressure monitor, central venous or pulmonary artery catheter (depending on cardiovascular/hemodynamic status and state of hydration), urinary catheter, nasogastric tube, and jugular bulb catheter. Important therapeutic decisions are based on regular data collection and assessment of improvement or deterioration of neurologic and general condition. Neurologic status is reassessed at frequent intervals by physical examination. Ventilator settings should be adjusted to provide adequate oxygenation and changes should be directed by frequent arterial blood gas analysis. Circulating volume should be maintained with isotonic intravenous solutions to give ad-

TABLE 4.1
Summary of Neuroendocrine Responses to Trauma

	Proteolysis (in muscle)	Gluconeogenesis (in liver)	Glycolysis (in adipose tissue)	Glycogenolysis		Lipolysis (adipose tissue, liver, muscle)	Insulin Antagonism	Insulin Secretion
				Liver	Muscle			
ACTH-cortisol	++	++	−	−	−	+	+	+
Epinephrine, norepinephrine	+	+	+	++	+	++	++	−
Growth hormone	−	+	+	−	−	+	+	++
Glucagon	+	++	−	+	−	++	+	++

equate hydration and urine output and the rate of infusion should be adjusted according to changes in central venous pressure, intracranial pressure, and urinary excretion rate. Adjustments in maintenance intravenous fluid will also take into account fluid content of intravenous and enteral medications and nutritional regimen. Initially intermittent gastric aspiration via nasogastric tube should be used for gastric decompression and therapy with antacids or histamine H_2-antagonists should be instituted if gastric pH measurements indicate high acidity. A detailed description of the management of raised intracranial pressure, hyperventilation, barbiturate coma, abnormal hemodynamic profiles and the nuances of arterial and venous blood gas analysis, gastric hyperacidity, and anticonvulsant therapy are beyond the scope of this chapter and are discussed elsewhere in this volume. However, the principles underlying the use of nutritional assessment, enteral and parenteral nutritional support, and the special considerations that relate to their use in neurosurgical patients will be discussed in detail below.

NUTRITIONAL ASSESSMENT

The protocol for nutritional assessment of the neurosurgical patient utilizes a variety of data to identify and classify subclinical and clinical malnutrition. Commonly used indices to define malnutrition are rapid weight loss of 5 kg or more, a weight of less than 80% of ideal body weight, a serum albumin concentration of less than 3.4 gm%, and a total lymphocyte count of less than 1,500 cells/mm^3. Evidence of protein and/or calorie malnutrition, hypermetabolism associated with multiple trauma and infection, unwillingness or inability to eat due to pathologic process or surgical treatment, and specific illnesses requiring therapeutic use of intravenous or enteral nutrition are all indications for nutritional assessment. The consumption of endogenous tissue stores that accompanies the metabolic and endocrine response to stress, starvation, and infection may be characterized by using a standard battery of anthropometric, biochemical, immunologic, and hematologic tests that evaluate body fat, somatic protein mass, visceral protein status, and immune competence (Fig. 4.3). In addition, calorie and protein expenditure can be either estimated or measured to define more clearly the daily metabolic cost of illness or injury, and provide information on which a logical therapeutic nutritional regimen may be based.

Nutritional Assessment Methods

The protocol for clinical nutritional assessment combines both subjective and objective data to characterize nutritional status. Subjective data is obtained from history and physical examination of the patient or interview with the patient's relatives. The physician records any physical signs and symptoms that may indicate subclinical or clinical malnutrition. The dietitian inquires about changes in appetite or food intake, recent changes in body weight especially marked losses, the presence of pre-existing chronic medical conditions such as diabetes or alcoholism which may affect nutrient intake, absorption and assimilation, and documents any specific dietary restrictions, aversions or allergies. The daily average nutrient intake is assessed. Problems with mastication, swallowing, nausea, vomiting, and disturbances of bowel habit are noted together with occupation, daily activity, past medical history, and current medications. This subjective assessment provides the background for further objective assessment and allows an estimate of protein and calorie needs.

The objective measurements of nutritional status include anthropometric measurements, biochemical and hematologic testing, recall skin antigen testing, estimation or measurement of resting metabolic expenditure, and daily assessment of nutrient intake and body weight (Table 4.2).

Anthropometric Measurements

The patient's height, total body weight, triceps skinfold thickness, and upper arm circumference are measured. The body weight is a simple but gross quantitative measurement of body composition. Ideal body weight is determined from the Metropolitan Life Insurance Standards. The percentage of ideal body weight is calculated, and percentage of usual weight and percent weight change over a defined period are recorded. Caution is essential in interpreting these measurements. Ascites, pleura effusion, and edema may be accompanied by weight gain, and in malnutrition there is simultaneous expansion of the extracellular fluid and depletion of lean body mass. Body weight

Energy stores (kcal)	Test	Protein stores (kg)	% Body weight		
160 000 kcal	Triceps skinfold (mm)				Fat (25%)
30 000 kcal	Arm muscle circumference (cm) Creatinine height index	4.5 kg	Skeletal muscle (30%)	Body cell mass (40%)	Lean body mass (75%)
	Serum albumin, Iron binding capacity (transferrin), skin antigens, delayed hypersensitivity, total lymphocyte count	1.5 kg	Viscera, etc (10%)		
None		0.3 kg	Plasma protein (5%)		
		6.3 kg	Extracellular fluids (20%)		
			Skeleton (10%)		

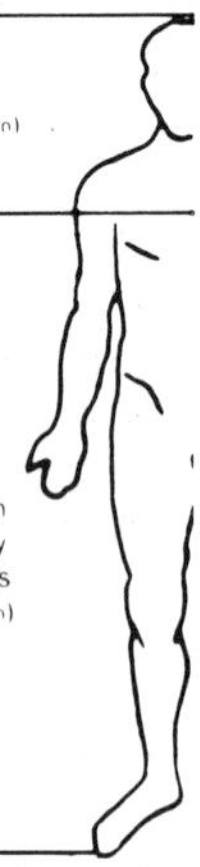

Figure 4.3. The body can be divided into various compartments that represent endogenous stores of energy substrate. In starvation and stress, these stores are mobilized to satisfy energy demands. Nutritional assessment techniques can be utilized to estimate the speed at which substrates derived from the various body compartments are consumed following starvation and injury and to document repletion of these stores during nutritional support.

tends to underestimate the actual nutritional depletion. The percent of usual weight and recent weight change are more accurate indicators of recent or chronic nutritional deprivation.

The thickness of the triceps skinfold is an indirect estimate of body fat stores. Fat is the primary caloric reserve of the body and is readily mobilized to meet the energy requirements of stress, infection, and starvation. A decrease in the triceps skinfold thickness reflects chronic inadequate caloric intake. The arm muscle circumference is a measure of the skeletal muscle mass and is calculated from the midarm circumference and the triceps skinfold thickness; arm muscle circumference (cm) = arm circumference (cm) − (3.14 × triceps skinfold measurement in cm). This figure is then compared with published standards.

Biochemical and Hematologic Measurements

The degree of visceral protein depletion can be estimated from albumin and transferrin serum concentrations. Serum albumin is a gross indicator of visceral protein status because of its long serum half-life (20 days) and its large total body pool. It usually decreases slowly during malnutrition, but serum concentrations fall more rapidly in patients with acute metabolic stress. Interpretation of the serum albumin may be complicated by the state of hydration, edema, recent blood loss, or recent blood product transfusion. Although the plasma albumin is a valid index of severe chronic protein-calorie malnutrition, it responds poorly to short-term changes in protein and energy intake.

Serum transferrin may be a more sensitive indicator of visceral protein status; it falls rapidly during starvation and stress and has a shorter half-life than albumin (8 days). Thyroxin-binding pre-albumin which has an even shorter biological half-life (2 days) and retinol-binding protein (12 hours) respond rapidly to both protein and calorie deprivation and repletion. They may prove to be more sensitive indices of subclinical malnutrition and of early response to enteral and parenteral nutrition.

At the initial screening and at regular intervals throughout hospitalization, hemoglobin, hematocrit, and total white blood cell count and differential should be assessed so that anemia may be corrected and response of the patient to treatment for infection may be followed. SMAC-20 is a good screening test of liver and renal function and of fluid and electrolyte status and should be repeated daily until the patient's condition stabilizes. Twice-weekly estimations are sufficient thereafter. Trace element deficiencies may be detected by measuring serum copper, zinc, magnesium, and manganese, and specific deficiencies should be corrected.

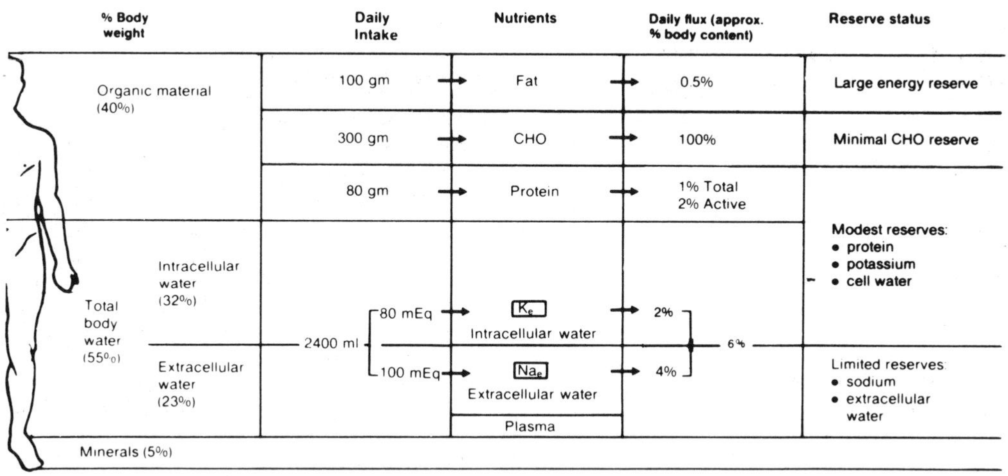

Screening for vitamin deficiencies when available should be part of the initial assessment.

Twenty-four-hour urine samples are collected to measure urinary nitrogen, urea, and creatinine excretion. Nitrogen is the primary component which differentiates protein from other basic nutrients and nitrogen balance measurements present an index of overall protein nutritional status. Urinary nitrogen excretion is either measured directly or estimated from urine urea, and, in estimating daily nitrogen balance, allowance is made for nitrogen losses in the stool and from the skin. The creatinine-height index is an indirect measure of muscle mass and is used to estimate somatic protein mass by calculating the 24-hr urinary creatinine excretion and expressing it as a percentage of the predicted creatinine excretion based on ideal body weight for height.

Skin Antigen Testing

Skin testing with common recall skin test antigens is used to evaluate cellular immune function which may be compromised by moderate to severe protein calorie malnutrition: 0.1 ml. of Dermatophytin, Candida, Varidase, mumps and intermediate-strength purified protein derivative (PPD.) are injected in the dermis of the volar aspect of the forearm, and the reactions are measured 24 and 48 hr following injection. A positive reaction is defined as induration of at least 10 mm in diameter of one or more of the antigens at 48 hr. Patients are defined as being anergic if there is no response to these recall skin test antigens. If there is a measurable area of induration at one or more of the test sites, but there is not one area at least 10 mm in diameter, the patient is considered relatively anergic. Other factors that influence skin test reactivity are age, presence of malignancy or infection, recent surgery or trauma, immunosuppressive therapy, anemia, and diseases affecting the immune system.

Estimating Energy Expenditure

Daily energy requirements are calculated as the sum of the basal energy expenditure (BEE), the calories consumed for physical activity, the specific dynamic action of food, and the increased energy requirements of infection, fever, trauma, disease, and surgery (Table 4.3). BEE is calculated from the Harris-Benedict equation, which is based on the age, gender, height, and weight of the patient (Carnegie Institute of Washington, Publication No. 279, Washington, 1919). Approximate values for the increase in resting metabolic expenditure above BEE in injury, infection, and stress have been established by indirect calorimetry and nitrogen balance techniques in surgical patients and are used to estimate the total daily energy requirements (34, 38). The recommended daily calorie

TABLE 4.2
Components of Initial Nutritional Assessment of the Neurosurgical Patient

Clinical		
Diagnosis		
Complications		
Physical examination		
Weight-actual, % usual, % ideal, % loss		
Dietary history		
Medical history		
Fat		
Triceps skinfold thickness		
Protein, somatic		
Mid-arm muscle circumference		
Creatinine - height index		
Protein, visceral		
Albumin		
Retinol-binding protein		
Thyroxin-binding prealbumin		
Transferrin		
Total lymphocyte count		
Cell-mediated immunity		
Recall skin test antigens		
Hematologic		
Hemoglobin		
Total white cell count		
Prothrombin time		
Hematocrit		
Total lymphocyte count		
SMAC 20 (serum)		
Sodium	Bilirubin	Total protein
Potassium	Glucose	Urea nitrogen
Chloride	LDH	Creatinine
Calcium	SGOT	Uric acid
Phosphate	SGPT	Iron
CO_2	Albumin	Cholesterol
Alkaline phosphatase		Triglycerides
Trace elements		
Copper		
Magnesium		
Zinc		
Manganese		
Urinalysis		
Glycosuria		
Urea nitrogen		
Creatinine		
Nitrogen (N)		
N balance = N intake − (N output urine + N output skin, feces, fistula)		
Calories		
BEE (Harris-Benedict) - See Table 4.3		
Indirect calorimetry		

TABLE 4.3
Estimating Daily Energy Requirements from Harris-Benedict Formula

A. Basal energy expenditure (BEE)
Men BEE = 66 + (13 × wt. in kg) + (5 × ht. in cm) − (6.8 × age)
Women BEE = 655 + (9.6 × wt. in kg) + (1.7 × ht. in cm) − (4.7 × age)
B. Specific dynamic action of food
10% of consumed food calories
C. Activity
10% confined to bed
20% ambulatory
D. Trauma, injury, infection

0–5%,	elective surgery, postoperative
10–15%,	soft tissue trauma
15–20%,	peritonitis
20–25%,	fracture
20–50%,	multisystem trauma
0–20%,	mild infection
20–40%,	moderate infection
40–60%,	severe infection
10–25%,	burn 10%
25–50%,	burn 25%
50–100%,	burn 50%
10–30%,	head injury alone
20–50%,	head injury with posturing

SUMMARY: Daily energy requirements = A + B + C + D

intake during the acute phase of injury should be 30 to 40 kcal/kg per day for adults and 100 to 200 kcal/kg per day for children and infants, with appropriate reductions during convalescence. The requirement for protein in the stressed patient, based on measurements of urinary nitrogen excretion, varies from 1.34 gm/kg per day in patients undergoing elective surgery to 2.30 gm/kg per day in patients with burns and sepsis (38), and the requirements for individual patients can be assessed by measuring 24-hr excretion of nitrogen or urea. The protein requirements can also be estimated by calculating the daily calorie requirement and providing protein on the basis of 150 kcal/gm of nitrogen (37). This ratio is adequate for most catabolic patients but may need to be increased in renal and hepatic dysfunction and decreased in severe infections. The recommended protein intake following injury is 2.0 to 3.0 gm/kg per day for children. The protein intake should at least match measured losses, be increased to match the severity of illness, and be adjusted during the convalescent period (Table 4.4).

TABLE 4.4
Recommended Protein and Calorie Intakes During Surgical Stress*

	Protein	Calories
Adults	1.3–3.0 gm/kg of body wt./day	25–40 kcal/kg of body wt./day
Children†	2.0–3.0 gm/kg of body wt./day	100–150 kcal/kg of body wt./day
Infants†	2.0–3.5 gm/kg of body wt./day	+200 kcal/kg of body wt./day

*1. Protein intake should match measured losses.
2. Protein and calorie intake should increase to match severity of injury and infection.
3. Proportional increase in protein intake should be greater than increase in calorie intake during stress.
4. Calorie:nitrogen ratio should be 150:1 for mild stress.
5. Calorie:nitrogen ratio should decrease to approximately 100:1 for moderate to severe stress.

†For further information on recommended nutrient intakes for injured and infected children and infants, see Rowlands and Dudrick (52).

Measuring Energy Expenditure

Oxidation of organic nutrients to produce energy also produces heat that is lost from the body and has been measured experimentally by direct calorimetry. This technique is expensive and cumbersome and has no application to clinical practice, but has been used to develop standards. Indirect calorimetry uses a microprocessor-controlled system for measurement of respiratory gas exchange in expired air, which in the steady state accurately reflects intracellular oxygen consumption and carbon dioxide production. These measurements together with nitrogen excretion and appropriate adjustments for age, gender, and body weight or surface area are used to calculate resting energy expenditure.

Data Interpretation

The subjective and objective findings are used to generate a metabolic and nutritional profile and several systems have been described for clinical presentation and application of the data (1, 7, 28, 52, 56). The nutritional assessment profile accurately defines any existing nutritional aberration. Protein malnutrition is characterized by depressed serum albumin, serum transferrin and total lymphocyte count, and nonreactive recall skin test antigens. In protein-calorie malnutrition, there is a decrease in anthropometric measurements in the presence of normal serum protein levels. Following severe injury it is common to develop or aggravate protein-calorie malnutrition which is characterized by a combination of these abnormal indices. The initial nutritional assessment is used to determine the daily energy and protein requirements of the patient, and the nutritional support regimen is designed to match these requirements. Subsequent profiles (repeated at 10-day intervals) monitor the patient's clinical course and the effectiveness of the nutritional support techniques that are used to maintain nutritional balance or correct nutritional abnormalities. Several authors have recommended that certain nutritional parameters may be used as a predictive index of eventual outcome in a similar fashion to the use of Injury Severity Score, Glasgow Coma Scale, and Burn size and depth as predictors of outcome following trauma, head injury, and thermal injury respectively (9, 43).

NUTRITIONAL SUPPORT TECHNIQUES

When the nutritional requirements of an individual patient have been determined, the most appropriate route and type of nutritional support regimen must be defined. Nutrition may be delivered to the patient orally, directly into the gastrointestinal tract via gastrostomy or jejunostomy tube, or intravenously.

The major determinant of the need for nutritional support is the ability of the patient to satisfy his caloric and protein requirements by consuming a normal oral diet. The patient's actual oral intake should be measured over a 24-hr period. Neurosurgical injury is often accompanied by inability to consume food by mouth or by anorexia or voluntary withdrawal of solid food and substitution with fluids which are inadequate for maintenance of nutritional balance. Diarrhea and rapid intestinal transit may lead to malabsorption of nutrients as may the use of purgatives and antibiotics or the presence of specific enteric infections. All of these problems and the additional stress of investigations and surgical treatment involving a period of fasting may induce or aggravate a state of malnutrition. Prior to the introduction of nutritional supplements or complete nutritional support, efforts should be made to correct hypovolemia, fluid and electrolyte and acid-base abnormalities, and to ensure that the patient is hemodynamically stable.

ENTERAL NUTRITIONAL SUPPORT

Oral Nutritional Supplements

These may be used to augment the elective intake of conventional foods and beverages, but they do not provide full nutritional support. The supplement is usually provided in the form of a commercially formulated liquid powder containing one or more concentrated nutrients. They should be ordered with a balanced diet and be given between meals in place of noncaloric beverages. Modular supplements provide a source of a single nutrient (carbohydrate, protein, or fat) and can be mixed with food and beverages to increase overall or specific nutrient density.

Nutrient Formulas for Tube or Ostomy Feeding

When nutritional needs cannot be met orally via a normal diet, commercial formulas are available which can provide adequate maintenance nutrition and can be given by mouth, tube, or ostomy. These products require an intact digestive and absorptive process and vary considerably in their nitrogen and caloric composition and in their osmolality, lactose, vitamin, and mineral content. However, if sufficient calories are delivered, recommended daily allowances of all nutrients can be met or exceeded. Tube and ostomy feedings should be introduced in dilute concentrations and small volumes initially and increased over several days to avoid inducing diarrhea by a sudden delivery of a large volume and osmotic load into the gastrointestinal tract.

Defined Formula Diets

These are nutritionally complete, chemically formulated powders which provide an easily digested liquid diet when reconstituted. The ingredients include amino acids, hydrolyzed protein, polysaccharides, oligosaccharides, medium-chain triglycerides, essential fatty acids, vitamins, and minerals. They require little digestion, are readily absorbed, leave minimal residue, and are usually lactose free. Defined formula diets may be useful in patients with gastrointestinal diseases but are also used for early support of the neurosurgical patient via fine bore nasoduodenal or needle catheter jejunostomy tubes. In introducing defined formula diets, similar precautions to those used with nutrient formulas for tube and ostomy feeding should be used.

Enteral Products

A wide range of commercial products is available for nutritional support via the gastrointestinal tract. A comprehensive discussion of their specific indications and properties is beyond the scope of this chapter, but may be found elsewhere (41). Before prescribing an enteral product its protein, fat and carbohydrate content should be ascertained together with its caloric density, osmolality, and electrolyte composition. Ideally, the enteral supplement should contain adequate protein and have a high caloric density at a reasonable osmolality for use in hypermetabolic patients allowing nutrient requirements to be met without precipitating side effects.

Management of Tube and Ostomy Feeding

Fine-bore nasogastric or nasoduodenal tubes can be used to feed patients via the gastrointestinal tract. Several delivery systems are available commercially which have the advantage that full nutritional requirements or supplements can be given by constant infusion, thereby reducing the risk of hyperosmolar diarrhea and making optimal use of absorption capacity. Constant infusion also obviates the problem of formula unpalatability. Provided that there is no impairment of gastric emptying or prolonged ileus, this form of feeding can be introduced early in the postoperative period. The placement of a gastrostomy or jejunostomy tube either at the time of major operation or electively avoids the problems of prolonged nasogastric intubation, but strict attention to the details of surgical technique is important to avoid unnecessary complications, such as intraperitoneal leakage, obstruction, adhesions, and wound sepsis. In addition, the position of any tube should be checked radiologically prior to commencing the feeding regimen.

Diarrhea is the most frequent complication of this technique when tube feedings are introduced too quickly, are too large, or are too hyperosmolar. This may lead to dehydration, fluid, electrolyte and acid-base imbalance, as well as malabsorption of nutrients. Continuous feeding, the use of codeine phosphate, and the elimination of lactose from the formula may prevent this complication. Strict adherence to asepsis in the preparation of feedings and frequent changes of delivery tubing will minimize the complications of contamination. The delivery system should be unique to gastrointestinal feeding and the feedings prepared with brightly colored food dyes to avoid the disastrous complication of accidental intravenous administration. Tube and ostomy feeding should be maintained until the patient is able to take a normal diet, taking several days for the transition from the use of liquid or low-residue feedings to normal diet.

INTRAVENOUS NUTRITIONAL SUPPORT

Management

Intravenous nutrition is indicated when specific metabolic requirements are better met by intravenous techniques rather than orally or enterally, because the latter techniques are impossible, inadvisable or hazardous, or the nutrient requirements are greater than can be achieved via the gastrointestinal tract. Increased metabolic requirements in many conditions may dictate the use of intravenous nutrition either alone or in addition to nutrients via the gastrointestinal tract. Intravenous nutrition should be instituted in any patient who is expected to receive intravenous therapy for longer than 5 days, even if the patient has previously been in good health and is nutritionally normal. Intravenous and oral nutrient supplements are important adjuncts to appropriate surgical treatment and should be introduced early, before significant nutrient deficits occur. Patients with hepatic and renal impairment may need adjustment of their intravenous nutritional regimen to accommodate their unique metabolic derangement, and pediatric patients have relatively greater calorie, protein, mineral, and vitamin requirements than adults. Intravenous nutrition is an important aspect of therapy in many clinical situations, and there is good evidence that appropriate intravenous nutritional support of the hypermetabolic patient restores body cell mass and immunologic competence, and improves morbidity and survival. An important limiting factor of this technique is the ability of the tissue to metabolize the infused nutrients. The injured patient presents a difficult clinical problem in meeting metabolic requirements intravenously for, on the one hand, there is a requirement for larger quantities of exogenous nutrient substrate while, on the other hand, there is less efficient utilization of those substrates by the tissues because of local and general metabolic responses to injury. In order to meet this increased requirement, nutrients are necessarily hyperosmolar and should be delivered into a central vein via a subclavian vein catheter. The subclavian vein catheter should be inserted under aseptic conditions by someone familiar with the technique; thereafter, the catheter should be maintained and solutions infused in accordance with a strict management protocol (55). The position of the subclavian catheter must be checked radiologically immediately after insertion, and if the placement is satisfactory, the nutrient regimen should be introduced slowly over the next 24 to 48 hr until requirements are fully satisfied or maximum tolerance achieved.

Basic guidelines for the management of intravenous nutrition include accurate measurement of temperature, pulse rate, respiratory rate, and blood pressure every 4 hr, urinalysis for glucose and acetone every 6 hr, fluid balance every 8 hr, and body weight at the same time and under the same conditions daily. Biochemical monitoring should include serum electrolytes, urea nitrogen, and glucose on a daily basis until the full nutritional regimen is achieved and the patient is stabilized. Thereafter, liver function tests, serum calcium, phosphorus, magnesium, albumin and globulin, and hematologic indices should be measured at least weekly. Patients with hypoproteinemia or anemia should be given salt-deficient human albumin, whole blood and packed erythrocytes when indicated to restore normal plasma oncotic pressure and oxygen-carrying capacity by

TABLE 4.5
Mechanical, Technical, and Thrombotic Complications of Intravenous Nutrition

At Insertion	During Use
Pneumothorax	Pump malfunction
Hemothorax	Kinking of tubing
Misplaced catheter	Occlusion of catheter
Catheter embolism	Air embolism
Air embolism	Hydrothorax
Subclavian artery laceration	Hydromediastinum
Subclavian vein laceration	Subcutaneous emphysema
Brachial plexus injury	Venous thrombosis
Phrenic nerve injury	Pulmonary embolism
Thoracic duct injury	
Tracheal injury	

maintaining a serum albumin above 3.5 gm% and a hemoglobin greater than 12 gm%. Albumin should not be regarded primarily as a nutrient because its plasma half-life of 20 days is too long for it to be an immediate or efficient source of utilizable nitrogen. Periodic evaluation of arterial and central venous pressure, arterial blood gases, pH, lactate, and ammonia may be necessary or desirable in the management of critically ill patients with significant cardiovascular, respiratory, renal, hepatic, or metabolic derangements. If serious fluid, electrolyte, acid-base, or hyperosmolar problems develop, intravenous nutrition should be reduced or discontinued until the metabolic derangement responds to appropriate therapy.

Complications

Several metabolic, mechanical, infective, or thrombotic complications may be associated with intravenous nutritional support, many of which are more common and more difficult to manage in the intensive care unit patient (Tables 4.5, 4.6, 4.7). One of the most common complications following the initiation of intravenous nutrition in the injured patient is hyperglycemia associated with persistent, excessive glycosuria, osmotic diuresis, increased fluid and electrolyte loss, dehydration, and nonketotic coma. Thus, accurate monitoring of blood glucose and glycosuria is mandatory. Patients with persistent elevations of blood glucose above 250 mg% and glycosuria above 2 gm% manifest impairment of substrate utilization and a significant loss of nutrient in the urine which requires treatment with exogenous insulin. The selection of the appropriate dose of insulin is

TABLE 4.6
Metabolic Complications of Intravenous Nutrition

Glucose metabolism
- Hyperglycemia, glycosuria, osmotic diuresis, hyperosmolar nonketotic dehydration and coma
- Ketoacidosis in diabetes mellitus
- Postinfusion (rebound) hypoglycemia

Amino acid metabolism
- Hyperchloremic metabolic acidosis
- Serum amino acid imbalance
- Hyperammonemia
- Prerenal azotemia

Calcium and phosphorus metabolism
- Hypophosphatemia, decreased, 2,3-diphosphoglycerate, increased hemoglobin affinity for oxygen, erythrocyte metabolic aberrations
- Hypocalcemia
- Hypercalcemia
- Vitamin D deficiency or excess

Essential fatty acid metabolism
- Serum deficiencies of phospholipid linoleic acid and arachidonic acid
- Serum elevations of 5,8,11-eicosatrienoic acid

Miscellaneous
- Hypokalemia
- Hyperkalemia
- Hypomagnesemia
- Hypermagnesemia
- Biochemical liver dysfunction
- Bleeding
- Anemia
- Hypervitaminosis A
- Cholestatic hepatitis

based on frequent measurements of blood and urine glucose concentration which may vary considerably and abruptly as the patient's clinical condition changes. Hypoglycemia must also be avoided. To obtain optimal control of hyperglycemia, insulin should be added to the intravenous regimen and given as a continuous infusion rather than as intermittent doses of subcutaneous or intramuscular insulin, the absorption of which may be unpredictable due to local impairment of tissue perfusion. Insulin is an anabolic hormone which, when given with intravenous nutrients, improves glucose utilization and nitrogen balance and decreases ureagenesis (61).

Metabolic acidosis, which may accompany severe injury and shock, may be further aggravated by the infusion of hypertonic dextrose and amino acid solution (53). This may be due to high concentration of chloride, amino acid imbalances, or the use of carbohydrate substitutes

TABLE 4.7
Septic Complications of Intravenous Nutrition

Catheter sepsis
- Bacteremia
- Septicemia
- Septic thrombophlebitis
- Septic embolism

Catheter misuses
- Frequent disconnection
- In-line filter and stopcocks
- Manometer for CVP measurement
- Piggy-back infusions
- Environmental contamination

Solution contamination
- Poor preparation
- Defective bottles
- Additives
- In-use contamination

Patient's disease
- Any condition causing increased susceptibility to local or disseminated infection, e.g. diabetes, malignancy, chronic malnutrition, burns, tracheostomy, extremes of age.

such as fructose or sorbitol. Steps should be taken to treat the primary cause of acidosis and to adjust the feeding regimen. Hypophosphatemia occurs in patients who are not receiving adequate phosphate supplements, especially if high-calorie feeding is started in the presence of chronic malnutrition (51). This may cause changes in red blood cell metabolism leading to an increased affinity of hemoglobin for oxygen. Changes in calcium, essential fatty acid, potassium, magnesium, and vitamin metabolism may also occur. Liver function is often impaired, especially with infection, and further alterations in liver enzymes are more common if biochemical liver function test abnormalities are present at the start of intravenous nutritional therapy. Cholestasis and periportal inflammation are seen in association with intravenous hyperalimentation in children with immature hepatic function and in the presence of severe sepsis. All of these metabolic complications can be minimized by attention to the amino acid, carbohydrate, fat, mineral, vitamin, and trace element content of the infusion regimen and by careful monitoring of the patient during nutritional therapy.

Infection is a major complication of intravenous hyperalimentation, but strict adherence to protocols for aseptic insertion of the catheter and subsequent dressing changes and catheter maintenance can reduce the overall incidence of infective complications to less than 2%, or fewer than two episodes per 1,000 patient-days of therapy. The chances of catheter contamination can be reduced by using the catheter solely for nutritional solutions—avoid administration of blood or blood products and medications, never use the line to measure central venous pressure or obtain blood samples, and never have Y-connectors or three-way stopcocks in the line. Contamination of the solution can occur during preparation or delivery. A constant-infusion pump equipped with an alarm should be used to deliver solutions and thus avoid unrecognized cessation of infusion and clotting of the line. Although these precautions can decrease the chances of contamination, there is inevitably a higher incidence of catheter-related infections in patients in intensive care units. The major problem in diagnosis is that fever chills, leukocytosis, deteriorating clinical and mental status, failure to gain weight, and unexplained glycosuria may be due to either the patient's disease or catheter sepsis. Clinical and laboratory resources should be used to locate the source of the infection as accurately and as rapidly as possible, and investigation should include blood cultures from the catheter and by venipuncture. If no source is apparent or the patient's condition does not improve after 24 hr, the catheter should be removed and the tip cultured. The catheter should be removed immediately if the patient is in shock. It is customary following removal of a catheter for suspected infection to wait 24 hr before restarting nutritional therapy. Occasionally, in a critically ill patient, it is impossible to maintain one intravenous line exclusively for intravenous nutrition or one part of a multilumen catheter is used. In these circumstances, and in patients with systemic infections, a strong case may be made for electively changing the catheters every 4 days to avoid contamination or hematogenous seeding of microorganisms to the catheter. Fungal infections as well as bacterial infections occur more commonly in this group of patients.

Intravenous Nutritional Regimen

With the information generated from the nutritional assessment profile as a guide to the energy and protein needs of the individual patient, an intravenous nutrition regimen is formulated. This is based on the use of hypertonic dextrose as the calorie source, a crystalline amino acid solution as the nitrogen source, and the addition of minerals, vitamins, and trace elements to satisfy daily requirements (Table 4.8). Adjustments are made to meet the increased demands for all nutrients following injury, stress, and infection, or to cope with the special problems of renal failure or liver dysfunction, or in pediatric patients. In addition, insulin, albumin, and cimetidine may be added as clinically indicated. Several crystalline amino acid solutions which differ slightly in their amino acid composition are available for clinical use, but no single solution appears to have an advantage over the others. The solutions are mixed by the pharmacy under sterile conditions and each bag is labeled to provide information to the physician, nurse, and pharmacist about the contents, rate of infusion, and expiration time. The regimen is delivered continuously over 24 hr in accordance with strict management protocols. Appropriate adjustments to the regimen are made during treatment as the patient's clinical condition either improves or deteriorates, taking into consideration information from serial nutritional assessment.

The nonprotein calorie requirements of an intravenous diet may be supplied by hypertonic carbohydrate solutions or fat emulsions. In all situations, dextrose is the carbohydrate calorie source of choice as it is inexpensive, associated metabolic acidosis is unusual, and hyperglycemia is easily treated with exogenous insulin (22). Fat emulsions may be used as an alternative calorie source. The manufacturers recommend that the daily dose should not exceed 2.5 gm/kg of body weight and that fat should not make up more than 60% of the total calorie intake. In normal and starved patients, isocaloric fat and carbohydrate regimen with similar amino acid intakes produce similar nitrogen balances (27, 69). In hypermetabolic patients carbohydrate appears to have a greater impact on nitrogen retention than does fat. Nitrogen retention improves as carbohydrate intake increases, provided that total calorie intake matches total metabolic expenditure. (39). The nitrogen-sparing effect of carbohydrate appears to be mediated through insulin and additional nitrogen retention may be achieved with exogenous insulin (61). The explanation of this apparent difference between fat and carbohydrate as energy sources in hypermetabolic patients is related to the muscle fuel deficit that exists secondary to a failure of keto-adaptive mechanisms and suppression of hepatic ketone body output by glucose. In addition, inflammatory tissues are glycolytic and have a major capacity for anaerobic metabolism. Endogenous fat is the primary fuel for skeletal muscle and hepatic gluconeogenesis, while glucose and lactate provide energy for the injured tissues. Thus, fat

TABLE 4.8
Composition of Standard Intravenous Nutrition Solution for Adults*

Base Solution
Protein = 10% crystalline amino acid solution, 500 ml
Calories = 50% dextrose solution, 500 ml
Electrolytes
Sodium (chloride and/or acetate, lactate, bicarbonate), 50 mEq
Potassium (chloride/acetate), 20 mEq
Phosphate (potassium acid salt, 1 mM = 1.5 mEq K^+), 10 mM
Calcium gluconate, 4.6 mEq
Magnesium sulphate, 10 mEq
Zinc sulphate (as Zn ion), 4 mg
Copper sulphate (as Cu ion), 0.8 mg
Standard formula† - final volume 1060 ml contains:
50 gm protein (8.3 gm nitrogen) = 200 kcal
250 gm carbohydrate = 850 kcal
Total calories = 1,050 kcal
Total calorie:nitrogen ratio = 127:1
Nonprotein calorie:nitrogen ratio = 102:1
Supplements to daily regimen
Added to standard formula by pharmacy:
Vitamins
Multivitamin injection (MVI 12), 10 ml
Vitamin K‡, folic acid‡, and cynacobalamin‡ (vitamin B_{12})
Miscellaneous‡
Heparin
Albumin
Human insulin
Cimetidine
Iron dextran (25 mg Fe/ml)
As separate infusion:
Fat emulsion 10% or 20% emulsion
Daily dosage should not exceed 2.5 g/kg
Proportion of total daily calorie intake 5–50%

*For more details of recommended daily allowances of intravenous nutrients for adults and children, see Rowlands and Dudrick (52).

†Standard formula (base solution plus electrolytes) is dispensed in bags containing total daily regimen for infusion over 24 hr.

‡As indicated by condition of patient.

emulsions will stabilize body fat and serve as an exogenous fuel, but will not affect nitrogen balance, whereas exogenous glucose stimulates insulin which reduces muscle proteolysis and nitrogen excretion (58). Although fat emulsions appear to have limitations as calorie sources in hypercatabolic, injured, or septic adults, it is important that some fat be given in depleted states to ensure that essential fatty acid deficiency does not occur. Deficiency may be prevented by supplying approximately 4% of total calories as polyunsaturated fat by giving 500 ml of 10% fat emulsion on alternate days, or small amounts of safflower oil by tube if the enteral route is available.

Recently, a study of the relative merits of glucose and fat as calorie sources showed that in two groups of patients requiring intravenous nutrition, marked differences in body composition were noted after a 2-week infusion period (42). The group receiving dextrose as its sole source of calories gained weight due to gain in body fat and water, but in the group receiving 60% of its nonprotein energy as fat, there was a significant gain of protein but not water and fat. The study suggested that the differences in water retention may account for the observations and may be particularly significant in the critically ill patient. The ability to preserve muscle and visceral protein mass and stimulate anabolism was important to the successful outcome of hypermetabolic illness. The septic and injured patient seems to utilize endogenous fat preferentially as an energy source even when dextrose is administered in quantities above energy expenditure. Administration of a large dextrose load to hypermetabolic patients does not suppress net fat oxidation as it does in the depleted patient, but there is an increase in oxygen consumption, continued oxidation of fat, and an increase in the conversion of glucose to glycogen (4). This is associated with an increase in CO_2 production which is not seen when fat emulsions are used. The excess CO_2 has to be excreted by the lungs, and in patients with respiratory infection and compromised pulmonary function, respiratory distress may be precipitated. In this situation, a large dextrose intake may represent an additional physiologic stress. However, it must be remembered that fat emulsions must be used with caution in a patient with respiratory distress or "shocked lung," as fat emboli may occur, further compromising respiratory performance.

The protein content of the standard intravenous regimen is supplied as a crystalline, amino acid solution containing a balanced formulation of both essential and nonessential amino acids which provide an available source of nitrogen for tissue synthesis. A variety of commercial formulas are available in a range of concentrations from 3% to approximately 12% and their nitrogen content may be calculated by the formula 1 gm of nitrogen = 6.25 gm of amino acid. Amino acid solutions should always be infused with an appropriate and adequate calorie source for optimum utilization (54). Recently special amino acid formulas have been developed for renal failure, hepatic failure and encephalopathy, sepsis, and hypermetabolism. The renal failure solution contains only essential amino acids and, therefore, is nutritionally incomplete. Its use should be reserved for a small cadre of chronic renal failure patients to supplement inadequate oral protein intake or to obviate the need for regular peritoneal or hemodialysis. In the stressed patient with acute renal failure, it is better to provide a standard intravenous nutritional regimen and dialyse at regular intervals. In hepatic failure and encephalopathy, a formula rich in branched-chain amino acids and low in aromatic amino acids may enable the patient to receive an adequate protein intake without precipatating acute encephalopathy, although so far only one controlled clinical trial has documented the efficacy of this therapy (11). Experience has also been reported of a controlled clinical trial of a high branched-chain amino acid formula in hypermetabolic intensive care unit patients (12). The experimental high branched-chain formula was shown to be superior to a standard formula during the acute catabolic phase following injury, but further studies are required to accurately define the place of this formula in clinical practice. Special amino acid solutions are expensive when compared to standard formulas and whether their impact on mortality and morbidity and the prevention of multisystem organ failure will be sufficient to justify the additional cost of therapy awaits further study. When a standard amino acid formula is used, the protein content of the regimen should be increased to match the increased protein requirements of injury and infection, and decreased subsequently during convalescence.

In children, there is normally a greater requirement for protein, calories, minerals, and vitamins than in adults and there is only limited availability of endogenous energy stores. The requirements for nutrients vary according to weight and maturity and are increased during acute illness. Essential fatty acid deficiency occurs more commonly in infants and children and fat emulsions should be given routinely. The daily fat intake should not exceed 4 gm/kg of body weight and should not make up more than 60% of total calories. The solutions may be administered by peripheral vein or via a central venous catheter which should be inserted under sterile conditions in the operating room. Infusion via a central vein provides a route which is optimum for the provision of higher quantities of protein and energy. Appropriate adjustments are made to the calorie and protein content of the intravenous regimen to satisfy the requirement for energy substrate, tissue repair, and growth (52).

Intakes of sodium, potassium, chloride, magnesium, calcium, and phosphorus may be determined easily by clinical evaluation and laboratory analysis. The requirements for trace elements and vitamins during intravenous nutrition are not well known. Oral daily allowances may provide guidelines, but blood levels provide little information about their distribution in the body, balance state, biologic activity, or metabolism in tissues under various clinical conditions. The requirement for most minerals, trace elements, and vitamins increases with injury and infection, and adequate amounts must be provided for optimum cellular metabolism and tissue repair (52).

Specific Considerations in Metabolic and Nutritional Management of the Neurosurgical Patient

The metabolic response to injury and infection in the neurosurgical patient is similar in many respects to that seen in the general surgical patient. Changes in tissue fuel homeostasis lead to consumption of endogenous energy stores and if allowed to proceed unhindered may place the patient at increased risk from complications of their injury or disease. Most metabolic studies of the neurologically impaired patient have focused on the acute metabolic response to head injury and have demonstrated that several unique factors may influence both the magnitude and duration of the response. A number of general features of head injury including hyperventilation, changes in cardiac output, fever, posturing, restlessness, and seizures are all known to increase metabolism whereas sedation, paralysis, and mechanical ventilation may decrease energy needs. The use of steroids and inappropriate nutritional regimen may give rise to additional metabolic stresses. The goal of nutritional and metabolic support in neurosurgical patients should, therefore, be to minimize catabolism and optimize repair and recovery by considering those unique metabolic derangements that characterize neurologic impairment. Treatment should therefore include an assessment of the needs of the brain itself as well as the need to support general metabolism.

The brain under normal circumstances is extremely active metabolically. It receives 15% of cardiac output and accounts for a quarter of the energy of basal metabolism by using glucose exclusively as an energy source (3). Most of the energy is used for functions such as the conduction of action potentials, neurotransmission, and the maintenance of the blood-brain barrier. During starvation, the energy needs of the brain decrease and adaptation to the use of ketone bodies—acetoacetate and hydroxybutyrate—derived from triglycerides diminishes the need for gluconeogenesis from muscle protein (45). Following injury to the brain, energy needs probably increase and additional substrate flow is required for inflammatory and reparative processes. Head injury also stimulates the endocrine and anatomic nervous systems which are the major regulators of the general metabolic response to injury.

Several studies have demonstrated increases in resting metabolic expenditure, ranging from 120% to 200% of normal, and oxygen consumption to twice the normal value in head-injured patients (14, 23, 50). The magnitude of the increase is influenced by the level of unconsciousness as measured by the Glasgow Coma Score and the presence of decerebration or posturing, and temperature elevation (14, 40, 50). The use of sedation, barbiturate coma, and propranolol ameliorated this response. Persistence of the vegetative state following head injury is known to be associated with persistence of increased metabolism over a longer period than is seen in general surgical patients.

The changes in brain and general metabolism are influenced by changes in endocrine secretions. Several studies have documented elevations of catecholamines which rise in proportion to the magnitude of injury and correlate with the increase in resting energy expenditure and oxygen consumption (14, 44). Cortisol also rises in proportion to the degree of injury and diurnal variations are eliminated (32). A decreasing level of consciousness corresponds with an increased cortisol level in patients who die within 2 weeks of injury, peak elevations of plasma cortisol occur shortly before death (47). Changes in serum insulin concentrations vary according to severity of the injury and the time interval between injury and measurement. During the catabolic phase there may be suppression of insulin release due to elevated catecholamines but subsequently basal and stimulated insulin levels may be elevated due to relative peripheral insulin resistance (29, 30). The other catabolic hormones, growth hormone, and glucagon also rise following head injury (46). These elevations of growth hormone may be sustained over a 2-week period following injury and are enhanced by glucose administration (31). These endocrine changes affect glucose tolerance, hyperglycemia being common and impaired glucose disappearance being greatest in deep coma. Fasting blood sugar is usually persistently elevated in those patients who die within 2 weeks and in those patients who recover progressive decrease in fasting blood sugar accompanies improvement in level of consciousness. Persistent elevation of blood sugar above 300 mg% is associated with an increased mortality (17). These interactions between the endocrine and autonomic nervous system are regulated by the hypothalamus and head injury may disrupt many of the stimulatory and inhibitory activities of the hypothalamus. The important role of cerebral blood in maintaining brain metabolism and influencing the generalized metabolic response has recently been recognized. In the past, fluid restriction and the liberal use of diuretics have been standard therapy for reducing and preventing cerebral edema. However, Clifton and his colleagues (15) have pointed out that maintenance of normovolemia reduces morbidity and is not associated with increased incidence of elevated intracranial pressure. Fluid restriction has the undesirable effect of causing dehydration, hypotension, and hypovolemia, which decreases oxygen delivery to the brain and causes additional sympathetic stimulation. Cardiac output increases to meet the need for increased energy substrate delivery and the highest cardiac outputs are seen in those patients with the greatest oxygen consumption and highest resting metabolic expenditure (15, 50). Finally, two other factors will affect the generalized metabolic response. Decreased spontaneous movement and immobilization leads to reduced synthesis and increased breakdown of muscle protein and may contribute to the negative nitrogen balance. The use of steroids in the management of cerebral edema may also enhance the generalized catabolic response.

All these factors impact on the assessment of nutritional status and the delivery of nutritional support to the neurosurgical patient. Several studies have alluded to the beneficial effects of nutritional support although it is difficult to clearly define the goals of nutritional therapy at this time. Nutritional support has been shown to prevent weight loss and hypoalbuminemia, improve speed and quality of rehabilitation, and may reduce overall incidence of death, infection, and the development of decubiti (6, 8, 18). Although theoretical considerations would dictate that some form of nutritional support was appropriate for most neurosurgical patients, the practical aspects of managing nutritional regimen may appear insurmountable. Nutritional assessment, using a protocol such as the one described above to assess nutritional status within the first 72 hr of hospitalization, and subsequently at 10-day intervals, is labor intensive, may not be practical for all patients on a busy neurosurgical unit, and care must be taken in interpretation of the data obtained. Dietary history and subjective information may be difficult to obtain and anthropometric measurements may be difficult to interpret as the standards are derived from relaxed, cooperative subjects rather than the posturing or unconscious patient. Anthropometric measurements respond slowly to changes in nutritional status and therefore do not reflect accurately acute nutritional compromise and are more useful for epidemiologic surveys of patient populations. Biochemical parameters should also be interpreted with caution especially those reflecting changes in visceral protein status. Albumin responds slowly to changes in nutritional status and the shorter half-life protein, e.g. retinol-binding protein, thyroxin-binding prealbumin, although more sensitive are not available routinely for clinically use. Estimation of daily calorie and protein requirements are hampered by indefinite information concerning the impact of each injury and therapy on resting metabolic expenditure. Indirect measurement of energy expenditure from nitrogen excretion, oxygen consumption, and carbon dioxide production relies on the extrapolation of data obtained over a short period of observation (30 min) to calculate daily energy expenditure. The use of delayed hypersensitivity skin antigen testing may also be difficult to interpret following injury and the use of steroids and in the face of septic complications. These limitations should not condemn the use of nutritional assessment techniques, but their application will more clearly define the neurosurgical patients who are most likely to benefit from nutritional support. At present, the most useful assessment of the level of nutritional support required for a given patient is to accurately measure daily urinary urea nitrogen, or total nitrogen excretion, and add 4 gm of nitrogen for insensible losses through skin, lungs, and feces. The nitrogen intake should match nitrogen output and it should be remembered that in the catabolic phase, which may last up to 2 weeks in uncomplicated head injury, that increasing nitrogen intake will automatically increase urinary nitrogen excretion. No attempt should be made to escalate protein intake to meet this increasing output. However, calorie intake should be given in sufficient quantities to obtain efficient utilization of the protein. The calorie intake should match daily metabolic expenditure and should be either calculated or measured by indirect calorimetry. Appropriate adjustments in calorie and protein intake are made if complications ensue or during convalescence. An alternative method of calculating calorie requirements is to provide them in a fixed ratio to protein intake by using a calorie:nitrogen ratio of approximately 150:1 in uncomplicated injury and of approximately 100:1 when infection increases metabolic requirements. With these practical guidelines the objective of the nutritional regimen should be to provide nutrients in sufficient quantities to minimize losses rather than to achieve positive nitrogen balance, for in the acute phase following injury this may be neither possible nor desirable.

Several factors may limit the provision of nutrients to neurosurgical patients which do not impact on the management of general surgical patients. Large volumes of hypertonic fluid may elevate intracranial pressure, hyperglycemia may worsen outcome of cerebral ischemia, and increased carbon dioxide production due to carbohydrate metabolism may also increase intracranial pressure. When the enteral route is used, there is a danger of aspiration, gastric distention, and atony, acute erosive gastritis and diarrhea (2, 13, 36). The uncooperative patient may remove tubes placed into the stomach, duodenum, or jejunum; or the tubes may become dislodged or blocked during administration of the enteral feeding regimen. Additional surgical procedures such as tracheostomy, ventriculostomy, or orthopaedic procedures may require cessation of the regimen during the perioperative period. These factors may lead to significant problems in the delivery of enteral nutrition during the early post-injury period, but whether adequate nutritional intake can be maintained in most patients is still a topic for debate (13, 26). In the absence of other information, the guidelines for enteral nutrition suggested by Clifton *et al.* (13) seem adequate goals for most patients, but Hunt *et al.* (26) believe that optimum nutritional support following moderate to severe head injury should include a period of intravenous nutrition during the immediate post-injury period, and until gastrointestinal tolerance of enteral feeding is well established.

Intravenous nutrition can be managed safely by using strict management protocols to avoid the technical, metabolic, and infective complications. Following head injury, particular care should be taken to avoid overhydration and catheter sepsis. The regimen should be designed to meet metabolic needs and should be used in the early postinjury period for patients with head injury complicated by multisystem injury or intolerance to enteral feedings and for patients sedated with morphine or in barbituate coma (26, 49, 50). Although intravenous nutrition is more expensive than enteral nutrition, its use under these circumstances is justified due to its beneficial support of host metabolism in comparison with inadequate or minimal nutrition.

SUMMARY

The neurosurgical patient presents a unique problem in metabolic and nutritional management. Neurologic injury produces a generalized metabolic response which is designed to mobilize substrates from endogenous tissue stores to provide energy for vital functions and substrates for tissue repair. The autonomic and endocrine regulation of this response may be modified and the high metabolic demands of the brain and nervous tissue may be increased. The additional problem of abnormal neuromuscular activity, such as posturing or seizure, contributes to a metabolic response, the magnitude of which is out of proportion to the degree of injury and has not yet been clearly defined. The catabolism of lean tissue and reduced synthesis of visceral proteins rapidly leads to impairment of host defense mechanisms and exposes the patient to increased morbidity and mortality. Initially, metabolic and nutritional support should be capable of attenuating this problem so that the erosion of body cell mass is minimized, neurologic metabolism and function is preserved, and optimum conditions are provided for repair and recovery of the neurologic injury. Although studies are available that attest to the beneficial effects of nutrition in supporting general metabolism following head injury, future studies will be needed to define the optimum protein and calorie needs for these patients and the precise relationship between the metabolic needs of the injured brain and the maintenance of body homeostasis.

REFERENCES

1. Agarwal, N. R., Savino, J. A., Feldman, M., Dawson, J., Gupte, P., and DelGuercio, L. R. M. The automated metabolic profile. Crit. Care Med., *11:* 546-550, 1983.
2. Anderson, B. J. A theoretical protocol for nutritional maintenance in head injured patients. J. Neurosurg. Nurs., *16:* 50-53, 1984.
3. Anderson, G. H. Diet, neurotransmitters, and brain function. Br. Med. Bull., *37:* 95-100, 1981.
4. Askanazi, J., Carpentier, Y. A., Elwyn, D. H., Nordenstrom, J., Jeevanandam, M., Rosenbaum, S. H., Gump, F. E., and Kinney, J. M. Influence of total parenteral nutrition on fuel utilization in injury and sepsis. Ann. Surg., *191:* 40-46, 1980.
5. Becker, D. P., Miller, J. D., Ward, J. D., Greenberger, R. P., Young, H. F., and Sakalas, R.: The outcome from severe head injury with early diagnosis and intensive management. J. Neurosurg., *47:* 491-502, 1977.
6. Bildsten, C., and Lamid, S. Nutritional management of a patient with brain damage and spinal cord injury. Arch. Phys. Med. Rehab., *64:* 382-383, 1983.
7. Blackburn, G. L., Bistrian, B. R., Maini, B. S., Schlamm, H. T., and Smith, M. F. Nutritional and metabolic assessment of the hospitalized patient. J.P.E.N., *1:* 11-22, 1977.
8. Bryan-Brown, C. W., Savitz, M. H., Elwyn, D. H., *et al.* Cerebral edema unresponsive to conventional therapy in neurosurgical patients with unsuspected nutritional failure. Crit. Care Med., *1:* 125-129, 1973.
9. Buzby, G. P., and Mullen, J. L.: Nutritional assessment. In: *Enteral and Tube Feeding*, edited by J. L. Rombeau and M. D. Caldwell, pp. 127-147, W. B. Saunders, Philadelphia, 1984.
10. Cahill, G. D. Starvation in man. N. Engl. J. Med., *282:* 668-675, 1970.
11. Cerra, F. B., Cheung, N. K., Fischer, J. E., Kaplowitz, N., Schiff, E. R., Dienstag, J. L., Bower, R. H., Mabry, C. D., Leevy, C. M., and Kiernan, T. Disease specific amino acid infusion (F080) in hepatic encephalopathy: A prospective randomized double blind controlled trial. J.P.E.N., *9:* 288-295, 1985.
12. Cerra, F. B., Mazuski, J. E., Chute, E. M., Nuwer, M., Teasley, K., Lysne, J., Shronts, E. P., and Konstantinides, F. M. Branched chain metabolic support: A prospective randomized, double blind trial in surgical stress. Ann. Surg., *199:* 286-291, 1984.
13. Clifton, G. L., Robertson, C. S., and Contant, C. F. Enteral hyperalimentation in head injury. J. Neurosurg., *62:* 186-193, 1985.
14. Clifton, G. L., Robertson, C. S., Grossman, R. G., *et al.* The metabolic response to severe head injury. Neurosurgy, *60:* 687-696, 1984.
15. Clifton, G. L., Robertson, C. S., Kyper, K., Taylor, A. A., Dhekne, R. D., and Grossman, R. G. Cardiovascular response to severe head injury. Neurosurgery, *59:* 447-454, 1983.
16. Cuthbertson, D. P.: Post-shock metabolic response. Lancet, *1:* 433-436, 1942.
17. Deloof, T. H., Berre, J., Genette, F., *et al.* Disturbances of the carbohydrate metabolism in acute head trauma. Acta Neurochir. Suppl., *28:* 113-114, 1979.
18. Ensin, J. Nutritional assessment of a severely head-injured, multi-trauma patient. J. Neurosurg. Nurs., *14:* 262-267, 1982.
19. Felig, P. Starvation. In: *Endocrinology*, edited by L. J. DeGroot *et al.*, pp. 1927-1940, Grune & Stratton, New York, 1979.
20. Gamache, F. W. Evaluation of nervous system trauma. Infect. Surg., *3:* 485-488, 1984.
21. Giddings, A. E. B. The control of plasma glucose in the surgical patient. Br. J. Surg., *61:* 787-792, 1974.
22. Giddings, A. E. B., Rowlands, B. J., Mangnall, D., and Clark, R. G. Plasma insulin and surgery. II. Later changes and the effect on intravenous carbohydrates. Ann. Surg., *186:* 687-693, 1977.
23. Haider, W., Lackner, F., Schlick, W., Benzer, F., Gerstenbrand, F., Irsigler, K., Korn, A., Krystof,

G., and Mayrhofer, O. Metabolic changes in the course of severe acute brain damage. Eur. J. Intensive Care Med., *1:* 19-26, 1975.

24. Hill, G. L., Blackett, R. L., Pickford, I., Burkinshaw, L., Young, G. A., Warren, J. V., Schorah, C. J., and Morgan, D. B. Malnutrition in surgical patients: An unrecognized problem. Lancet, *1:* 689-692, 1977.
25. Hume, D. M., and Egdahl, R. H. The importance of the brain in the endocrine response to injury. Ann. Surg., *150:* 697-712, 1959.
26. Hunt, D., Rowlands, B., Allen, S., Stein, D., Hedberg, A., Vizuete, S., and Hickson, J. The inadequacy of enteral nutritional support in head injury patients during the early post-injury period. J.P.E.N., *9:* 121, 1985.
27. Jeejeebhoy, K. N., Anderson, G. H., Nakhooda, A. F., Greenberg, G. R., Sanderson, I., and Marlis, E. B. Metabolic studies in total parenteral nutrition with lipid in man. J. Clin. Invest., *57:* 125-136, 1976.
28. Kelts, D. G., Davidson, F. A., and Jong, M. R. Computerized metabolic assessment and total parenteral nutrition formulation. Update Comput. Med., *2:* 25-32, 1984.
29. Keymolen-Jardini, V., Movawad, E., Claeys-de Clercq, P., *et al.* Glucose metabolism in traumatic brain injury. Acta Endocrinol., *77:* 103-110, 1974.
30. King, L. R., Knowles, H. C., McLaurin, R. L., *et al.* Glucose tolerance and plasma insulin in cranial trauma. Ann. Surg., *173:* 337-343, 1971.
31. King, L. R., Knowles, H. C., McLaurin, R. L., *et al.* Pituitary hormone response to head injury. Neurosurgery, *9:* 229-235, 1981.
32. King, L. R., McLaurin, R. L., Lewis, H. P., *et al.* Plasma cortison levels after head injury. Ann. Surg., *172:* 975-984, 1970.
33. Kinney, J. M. Energy requirements of the surgical patient. In: *Manual of Surgical Nutrition: American College of Surgeons*, edited by W. F. Ballinger, pp. 223-235, W. B. Saunders, Philadelphia, 1975.
34. Kinney, J. M., Duke, J. H., Long, C. L., and Gump, F. E. Tissue fuel and weight loss after injury. J. Clin. Pathol., *23* (Suppl. 4)*:* 65-72, 1970.
35. Kune, G. A. Life threatening surgical infection: Its development and prediction. Ann. R. Coll. Surg. Engl., *60:* 92-98, 1978.
36. Larson, G., Koch, S., O'Dorisio, T. M., Osadchey, B., McGraw, P., and Richardson, J. D. Gastric response to severe head injury. Am. J. Surg., *147:* 97-105, 1984.
37. Long, C. L., Crosby, F., Geiger, J. W., Kinney, J. M. Parenteral nutrition in the septic patient, nitrogen balance, limiting plasma amino acids and calorie to nitrogen ratios. Am. J. Clin. Nutr., *29:* 380-391, 1976.
38. Long, C. L., Schaffel, N., Geiger, J. W., Schiller, W. R., and Blakemore, W. S. Metabolic response to injury and illness: Estimation of energy and protein needs from indirect calorimetry and nitrogen balance. J.P.E.N., *3:* 452-456, 1979.
39. Long, J. M., Wilmore, D. W., Mason, A. D., Pruitt, B. A. Effect of carbohydrate and fat intake on nitrogen excretion during total intravenous feeding. Ann. Surg., *185:* 417-422, 1977.
40. Lutz, H., Peter, K., Van Ackern, K. Total parenteral alimentation in neurosurgical and neurological patients. In: *Total Parenteral Alimentation*, edited by C. Mann, S. I. Magalini, and E. Scrascia, pp. 215-217, Excerpta Medica, Amsterdam, 1976.
41. MacBurney, M. M., and Young, L. S. Formulas. In: *Enteral and Tube Feeding*, edited by J. L. Rombeau and M. D. Caldwell, pp. 171-198, W. B. Saunders, Philadelphia, 1984.
42. Macfie, J., Smith, R. C., and Hill, G. L. Glucose or fat as a non-protein energy source: A controlled clinical trial in gastroenterological patients requiring intravenous nutrition. Gastroenterology, *80:* 103-107, 1981.
43. Meakins, J. L., Pietsch, J. B., Bubenick, O., Kelly, R., Rode, H., Gordon, J., and MacLean, L. D. Delayed hypersensitivity: Indicator of acquired failure of host defenses in sepsis and trauma. Ann. Surg., *186:* 242-250, 1977.
44. Nayak, A. K., Mohanty, S., Nimai Singh, R. K., *et al.* Plasma biogenic amines in head injury. J. Neurol. Sci., *47:* 211-219, 1980.
45. Owen, O. E., Morgan, A. P., Kemp, H. G., Sullivan, J. M., Herrera, M. G., and Cahill, G. F. Brain metabolism during prolonged starvation. J. Clin. Invest., *46:* 1589-1595, 1967.
46. Pentelenyi, T., and Kammerer, L. Changes in blood glucose after head injury and its prognostic significance. Injury, *8:* 264-268, 1977.
47. Pentelenyi, T., and Kammerer, L. Alterations of the serum cortisol and blood glucose in brain-injured patients. Injury, *15:* 397-402, 1984.
48. Porte, D., and Robertson, R. P. Control of insulin secretion by catecholamines, stress and the sympathetic nervous system. Fed. Proc., *32:* 1792-1796, 1973.
49. Rapp, R. P., Young, B., Twyman, D., Bivens, B., Haack, D., Tibbs, P., and Bean, J. R. The favorable effect of early parenteral feeding on survival in head-injured patients. J. Neurosurg., *58:* 906-912, 1983.
50. Robertson, C. S., Clifton, G. L., and Grossman, R. L. Oxygen utilization and cardiovascular function in head-injured patients. Neurosurgery, *15:* 307-314, 1984.
51. Rowlands, B. J. Postoperative hypophosphataemia. J.P.E.N., *2:* 108-11, 1978.
52. Rowlands, B. J., and Dudrick, S. J. Nutritional support of the infected patient. In: *The Physiologic and Metabolic Responses of the Host*, edited by M. C. Powanda and P. G. Canonico, pp. 359-397, Elsevier/North Holland, Biomedical Press, 1981.
53. Rowlands, B. J., Giddings, A. E. B., Clark, R. G. Changes in plasma lactate, phosphate, and uric acid during postoperative carbohydrate infusion. Br. J. Surg., *64:* 424-427, 1977.
54. Rowlands, B. J., Giddings, A. E. B., Johnson, A. O. B., Hindmarsh, J. T., and Clark, R. G. Nitrogen sparing effect of different feeding regimens in the postoperative patient. Br. J. Anaesth., *49:* 781-787, 1977.
55. Rowlands, B. J., Hoelzer, D. J., and Flynn, T. C.

Vascular access for total parenteral nutrition in adults and children. In: *Access Surgery*, edited by G. Koostra and P. J. G. Jorning, pp. 235–241, M.T.P. Press, Lancaster, 1983.
56. Schloerb, P. R. Computer-assisted nutritional support in surgery. Contemp. Surg., *25:* 53–57, 1984.
57. von Euler, U. S. Noradrenalin in hypotensive states and shock-physiological aspects. Lancet, *2:* 151–154, 1955.
58. Wilmore, D. W. Role of lipid as a source of nonprotein calories. In: *Advances in Parenteral Nutrition*, edited by I. D. A. Johnston, pp. 195–207, MTP Press, Lancaster, 1978.
59. Wilmore, D. W., Moylan, J. A., Bristow, B. F., Mason, A. D., and Pruitt, B. A. Anabolic effects of growth hormone and high calorie feedings following thermal injury. Surg. Gynecol. Obstet., *138:* 875–884, 1974.
60. Wolfe, B. M., Culebras, J. M., Sim, A. J. W., Ball, M. R., and Moore, F. D. Substrate interaction in intravenous feeding: Comparative effects of carbohydrate and fat on amino acid utilization in fasting man. Ann. Surg., *186:* 518–540, 1977.
61. Woolfson, A. M. J., Heatley, R. V., and Allison, S. P. Insulin to inhibit protein catabolism after injury. N. Engl. J. Med., *300:* 14–17, 1979.

CHAPTER 5

Neuroendocrine Physiology, Pathophysiology, and Management

DANIEL L. BARROW, M.D., and
GEORGE T. TINDALL, M.D.

INTRODUCTION

Rapid advances in neuroendocrinology have added significantly to our understanding of hypothalamic-pituitary physiology and pathophysiology. Additionally, these advances have made us aware of the incredible complexity of hypothalamic pituitary control and the widespread effects this small anatomic area has on the homeostasis of the entire organism. The isolation of hypothalamic hypophysiotropic hormones, development of accurate hormone assays, and the application of molecular biology to understand gene organization and expression are among the more important achievements.

The concept of neurosecretion, the secretion of hormones into the circulation by nerve cells, was crucial to the development of neuroendocrinology. Secretory cells can be classified into three types. The first type are *exocrine* cells, such as sweat and salivary glands, which secrete into a lumen that communicates with the external environment. These are regulated by secretomotor nerve fibers through the release of a neurotransmitter at a receptor site. The second type of secretory cells are *endocrine*, such as the adrenal and thyroid glands, that secrete into the circulation. These are regulated by the pituitary gland, which is, in turn, regulated by the third type of secretory cell, the *neurosecretory* cells of the hypothalamus. All neurosecretory cells retain the physiologic and morphologic properties of neurons. They are neurons that possess both neural and glandular properties and are therefore capable of translating neural information into chemical output (76).

Anatomy and Physiology of the Hypothalamic-Pituitary Unit

A knowledge of the anatomy of the pituitary gland, pituitary stalk, and hypothalamus is a prerequisite to understanding the physiologic functions of these structures (Fig. 5.1). The pituitary gland, or hypophysis, is anatomically connected to the medial basal hypothalamus by the highly vascular pituitary stalk. The human pituitary is divided into two lobes, the anterior, or *adenohypophysis*, and the posterior, or *neurohypophysis*. Although these two lobes have different embryologic origins, they become intimately related during embryonic life and remain that way.

Adenohypophysis

The adenohypophysis is composed of three parts. The *pars distalis* is the primary site of production and release of the classical anterior pituitary hormones, thyrotropin (thyroid-stimulating hormone, TSH), adrenocorticotropin (ACTH), growth hormone (somatotropin, GH), prolactin (luteotropic hormone, PRL), luteinizing hormone (interstitial cell-stimulating hormone, LH), and follicle-stimulating hormone (FSH). The *pars intermedia* or intermediate lobe is vestigial in man and its relatively few cells are spread diffusely throughout the anterior lobe. The *pars tuberalis* is that small portion of the adenohypophysis that extends upward to surround the pituitary stalk and in-

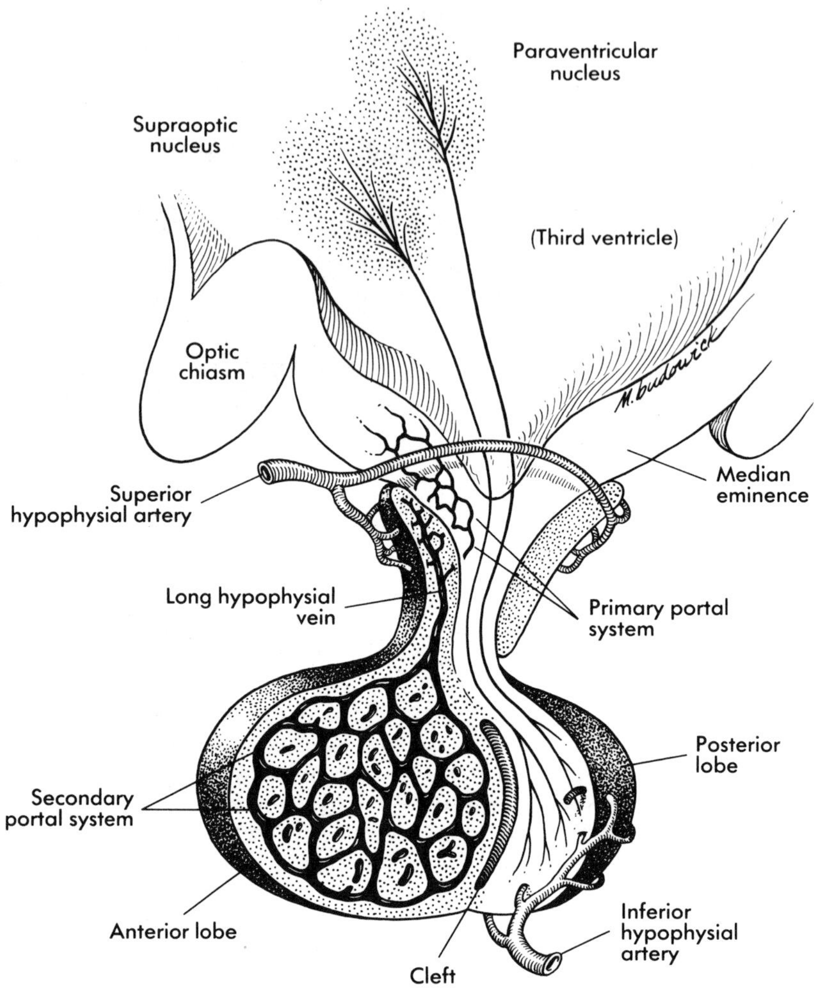

Figure 5.1. Sagittal diagram of pituitary and some of its important anatomic features. (Reprinted with permission from G. T. Tindall and D. L. Barrow, *Disorders of the Pituitary*, C. V. Mosby Co., St. Louis, 1986.)

ferior surface of the hypothalamus. The pars tuberalis consists of cells identical to those in the pars distalis.

Neurohypophysis

The neurohypophysis or posterior lobe of the pituitary develops embryologically as a downgrowth from the ventral diencephalon, and retains its neural connections in adult life. The supraopticohypophysial and paraventriculohypophysial nerve tracts originate in the hypothalamus, descend through the infundibulum and neural stalk, and terminate in the posterior lobe of the pituitary (66, 67, 107). The hormones vasopressin (antidiuretic hormone, ADH) and oxytocin are released from the nerve terminals into fenestrated capillaries of the neurohypophysis.

Cells of origin of these tracts are relatively large and are consolidated into distinctive groups situated in the paired nuclei, the supraoptic and paraventricular nuclei. Cells in these nuclei contain only one peptide, either vasopressin or oxytocin.

The chemical structure of vasopressin and oxytocin is similar, and each hormone is associated with a distinct neurophysin now recognized to be part of their prohormones, termed propressophysin and prooxyphysin, respectively (19, 41, 68). The neurophysins are released simultaneously with their respective neurohypophysial peptide (101, 102).

Pituitary Stalk

The pituitary and hypothalamus are connected by a stalk composed of glandular, vascular, and neural elements. The glandular portion of the stalk is made up of the pars tuberalis. The vascular component consists of nutrient arteries, the portal venous system, and a capillary network. The arterial supply to the median eminence, pituitary gland, and stalk derives from paired superior hypophysial arteries that originate from the cavernous carotid arteries. The portal vessels are formed by the confluence of capillary loops of the median eminence into veins on the anterior surface of the pituitary stalk. Portal vessels also anastomose with capillaries of the neurohypophysis which receives a direct arterial supply from the inferior hypophysial arteries (12, 13, 86). The arteries divide into capillary tufts that come into contact with nerve endings of the hypothalamic peptidergic neurons that synthesize the releasing hormones. The capillary tufts are drained by portal veins and distributed to the sinusoids of the adenohypophysis. This vascular component is thus crucial for the transport of hypothalamic hormones to the adenohypophysis. The neural portion of the pituitary stalk is composed of the unmyelinated supraopticohypophysial and paraventriculohypophysial nerve tracts that originate in the hypothalamic nuclei and terminate in the neurohypophysis. The neural portion of the stalk is essential for the transport of neurohypophysial hormones, vasopressin and oxytocin, to the posterior lobe.

Hypothalamus

The hypothalamus and pituitary gland function as a unit that can be considered as two systems, the hypothalamic-adenohypophysial system and the hypothalamic-neurohypophysial system (Fig. 5.2).

The hypothalamic-adenohypophysial system includes the tuberoinfundibular neurons in the hypothalamus, believed to be the source of the hypophysiotropic hormones. Their axons terminate on the capillary plexus of the hypophysial portal blood vessels. The crucial role of these blood vessels as a conduit for hypothalamic hypophysiotropic hormones from the tuberoinfundibular neurons to the adenohypophysis via the stalk is now well established. Most of the cell bodies of the tuberoinfundibular neurons are located in the medial basal hypothalamus in the arcuate nucleus, the anterior periventricular area, and the medial preoptic area (70, 120).

The tuber cinereum is a convex bulge on the ventral surface of the hypothalamus. Arising from it in the midline is the median eminence, or infundibulum, a specialized region of the third ventricle which gives rise to the pituitary stalk. This median eminence contains the primary plexus of the hypophysial-portal blood vessels which forms a contact zone between the terminals of the tuberoinfundibular (releasing factor) neurosecretory neurons and the capillaries of the hypophysial portal circulation (76). The median eminence contains capillaries with fenestrated endothelium (usually characteristic of glandular-type capillaries in endocrine secretory tissue). Situated within the inferior walls of the third ventricle are specialized ependymal cells known as tanycytes. These cells send processes that terminate in the area of the median eminence, thus establishing a link between the cerebrospinal fluid (CSF) and the median eminence. The function of the tanycytes has been a matter of speculation. Their unusual morphology and anatomical position has led to the suggestion that they may function as conduits for the transfer of hypothalamic hormones from CSF in the third ventricle to capillaries of the median eminence and vice versa (10).

The hypothalamic-neurohypophysial system includes the paired supraoptic and paraventricular nuclei in the hypothalamus, whose axons terminate on blood vessels in the posterior pituitary. These nuclei produce vasopressin and oxytocin which are transported in granules in association with their respective neurophysins to the posterior lobe of the pituitary. There they remain in storage until released by an action potential arising in the cell body.

Hypophysiotropic Hormones

Efforts to identify the hypophysiotropic hormones that stimulate or inhibit the release of each of the known pituitary hormones began in the mid-1950s. Five such peptide hormones have since been isolated. The first releasing factor to be identified was thyrotropin-releasing hormone (TRH), whose structure was elucidated in 1969. In 1971, luteinizing hormone-releasing hormone (LHRH, more recently referred to as gonadotropin-releasing hormone, GnRH) was characterized and in 1973 somato-

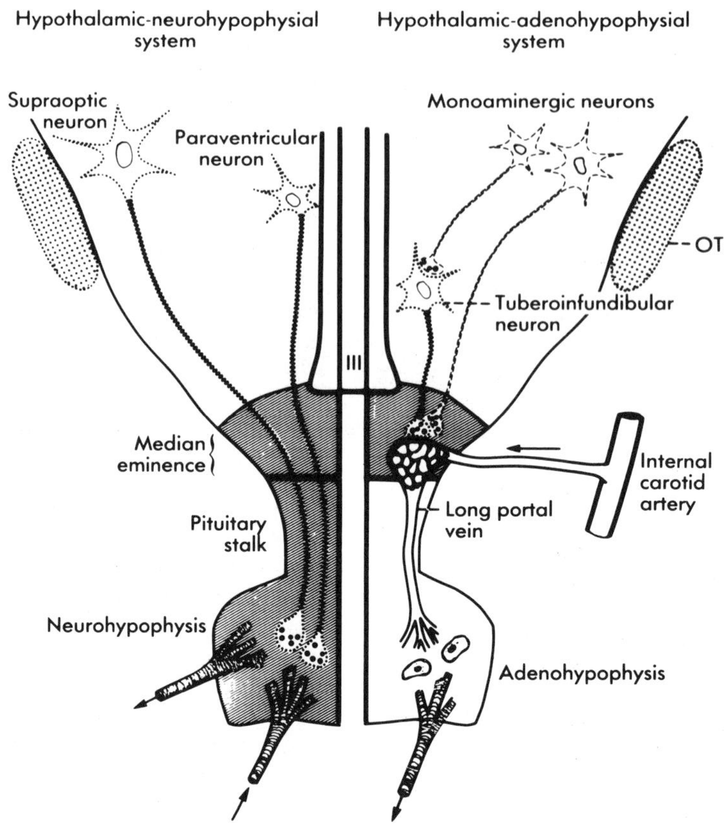

Figure 5.2. Coronal diagram of hypothalamic-pituitary axis. *Left*, Hypothalamic-neurohypophysial system. Supraoptic and paraventricular axons terminate on blood vessels in neurohypophysis. *Right*, Hypothalamic-adenohypophysial system. Tuberoinfundibular neurons, believed to be the source of hypothalamic regulatory hormones, terminate on capillary plexus in median eminence. Pituitary portal system is derived from branches of internal carotid artery, which forms primary capillary bed in median eminence. Portal veins drain capillary plexus into sinusoids of anterior pituitary. (Adapted and reprinted with permission from J. B. Martin, S. Reichlin, and G. M. Brown. *Clinical Neuroendocrinology*. F. A. Davis Co., Philadelphia, 1977; and G. T. Tindall and D. L. Barrow, *Disorders of the Pituitary*, C. V. Mosby Co., St. Louis, 1986.)

statin (somatotropin release-inhibiting factor, SRIF), which inhibits GH release (18), was identified. Corticotropin-releasing hormone (CRF) that stimulates ACTH and beta-endorphin release was sequenced from sheep hypothalami (114) and more recently rat CRF has been characterized and is known to be identical to human CRF (40). Growth hormone-releasing hormone (GHRH) was first identified in 1982 as an ectopic secretion of a pancreatic adenoma that caused acromegaly (47, 99), but an identical factor was demonstrated in the human hypothalamus in 1984 (72). Pituitary prolactin is under a tonic inhibitory influence by the hypothalamus and it appears that dopamine serves as the principal prolactin inhibitory factor (PIF). Possible candidates for prolactin-releasing factor(s) are vasoactive intestinal polypeptide (VIP), peptide histadine isoleucine (PHI), and TRH (57, 115, 119).

It was initially thought that each of the releasing factors were entirely specific in their function. This simplistic view has been altered by the realization that individual hypothalamic hormones have several crossover effects and some affect hormone-secreting tissues other than the pituitary. As examples, TRH stimulates the release of prolactin as well as TSH and somatostatin inhibits TSH as well as GH and further inhibits the release of insulin, glucagon, and gastrin secretion by the gut and pancreas.

The anterior pituitary produces and secretes at least six well-characterized trophic hormones: ACTH, TSH, LH, FSH, GH, and prolactin. Several other pituitary hormones have also been described. The first four hormones mentioned trigger the synthesis and release of families of hormones by the so-called "target organs", the adrenal cortex, thyroid, ovary, and testis. Growth hormone and prolactin appear to act on peripheral tissues without the mediation of another endocrine gland. Immunocytochemical studies have demonstrated that each of the anterior pituitary hormones is produced by a separate set of cells (55, 64, 65). The exceptions are some cells which contain both LH and FSH and cells which produce ACTH also produce other peptides of the opiomelanocortin family. Each cell type has a distinctive morphologic appearance by electron microscopic features including size, shape, and electron density of the secretory granules. The release of anterior pituitary hormones is regulated by the corresponding hypophysiotropic hormones which are under the influence of various hypothalamic and extrahypothalamic factors. In reviewing the physiology of the hypothalamic-pituitary-end organ axes, we will limit the discussion to those systems that are most relevant to the critical care patient, namely the adrenal and thyroidal axes.

Stress, such as that seen in the critically ill patient, evokes changes in the pituitary-adrenal and pituitary-thyroid axes but additionally, there are several other hormones that characteristically respond to a variety of stressful stimuli. For instance, in man, GH and prolactin are commonly released in response to "nonspecific" stress. In addition, a single stimulus may give rise to a multihormonal response that at least in some instances is specific to the stimulus in question; e.g., during exposure to heat, GH elevation is observed in the absence of a cortisol rise. Also, it is well known that pain and emotional stress bring about a rapid release of ADH accompanied by antidiuresis.

Pituitary Thyroidal Axis

The secretion of TSH is regulated by a negative feedback loop from the thyroid hormones, triiodothyronine (T_3) and thyroxine (T_4), and a positive influence mediated by hypothalamic TRH (Fig. 5.3). TRH probably stimulates release of TSH by increasing the intracellular calcium of the thyrotroph cells (28). Both circulating T_4, by its intrapituitary conversion to T_3, and plasma T_3 per se inhibit TSH secretion either directly or by altering the sensitivity of the thyrotroph to TRH.

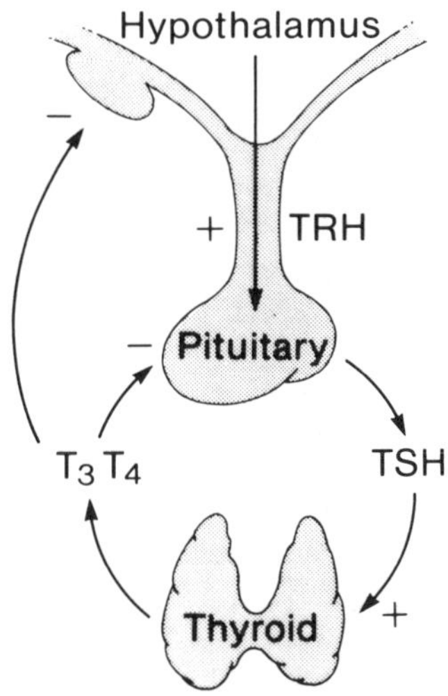

Figure 5.3. Hypothalamic-pituitary-thyroidal axis. Secretion of thyroid-stimulating hormone (TSH) by the anterior pituitary is inhibited by the negative feedback effects of thyroid gland secretions T_3 and T_4, which have a direct effect on the pituitary. The secretion of TSH is stimulated by the hypothalamic tripeptide, TRH.

The factors that control thyrotroph response to TRH secretion are still under investigation but are believed to be integrated into other visceral controls of body temperature, stress, and food intake. The function of the hypothalamus in pituitary-thyroid interactions is to determine the "set point" of feedback control around which the usual feedback regulatory responses are elicited (95).

Although TRH is the major hypothalamic hormone stimulating TSH release, other hypothalamic hormones influence its secretion. Somatostatin release-inhibiting factor (SRIF) and dopamine both appear to inhibit TSH secretion through a direct action on the pituitary. TSH secretion is acutely suppressed by pharmacologic doses of glucocorticoids and estrogens. A circadian variation in TSH secretion is present, with peak values observed between 11:00 PM and 2:00 AM and a nadir in early afternoon (28, 117). The magnitude of this difference, unlike cortisol secretion, is clinically insignificant.

The overall secretion of TSH is ultimately determined by the need to maintain an adequate level of thyroid hormone. The measurement of TSH levels in plasma is an accurate indicator of the condition of the thyroid gland. Hypersecretion of the thyroid or administration of exogeneous thyroid hormone suppresses TSH. Damage to the thyroid, drug effects on the thyroid, or thyroidectomy result in elevated plasma TSH concentrations.

Actions of TSH

TSH is bound by receptors on the surface of thyroid cells and exerts its effects by increasing the cellular content of cyclic AMP (cAMP). TSH exerts profound effects on many aspects of thyroid function including an increase in thyroid size and vascularity. TSH increases iodide uptake, thyroglobulin synthesis, iodotyrosine and iodothyronine formation, thyroglobulin proteolysis, and thyroxine (T_4) release from the thyroid gland (27).

Actions of Thyroid Hormones

The thyroid hormones exert significant influence on various metabolic processes (56). They affect the activity of many enzymes and the metabolism of substrates, vitamins, and minerals. The secretion and degradation rates of virtually all other hormones and the response of their respective target tissues are affected by thyroid hormones.

Calorigenesis. Thyroid hormones have a stimulating effect on calorigenesis reflected by increased oxygen consumption in the animal, increased heart rate, decreased cardiac glycogen content, and increased sensitivity to the lipolytic effect of epinephrine. The precise mechanism of the thermogenic effect of thyroid hormone remains unknown (14, 106, 112).

Protein Metabolism. Protein synthesis is stimulated by thyroid hormones, a process that may be partly responsible for a portion of their calorigenic effect. The effects of thyroid hormones on protein metabolism and overall growth rate are dependent upon the metabolic state of the organism and the dosage of hormone. Moderate doses of T_4 increase protein synthesis and decrease nitrogen excretion in thyroidectomized rats, whereas larger doses inhibit protein synthesis and increase the concentration of free amino acids in plasma, liver, and muscle (56). Likewise, growth is retarded in young patients by hypothyroidism, is restored by replacement doses of thyroid hormone, and is inhibited by excessive doses.

Carbohydrate Metabolism. Almost all aspects of carbohydrate metabolism are affected by thyroid hormones, many being modified by other hormones such as insulin and catecholamines. Thyroid hormones enhance the rate of intestinal absorption of glucose and galactose, increase the rate of uptake of glucose by adipose tissue and muscle, and increase the rate of insulin degradation. The latter fact may be responsible for the decreased sensitivity to exogenous insulin often seen in thyrotoxicosis and increased sensitivity that may occur in hypothyroidism (56).

Lipid Metabolism. Although thyroid hormones appear to stimulate all aspects of lipid metabolism including synthesis, mobilization, and degradation, degradation is affected more than synthesis. The net effect of hormone excess is to decrease the stores and plasma concentration of most lipids (56).

Effects of Stress on Thyroid Function.

Studies of the effects of various stressful situations on thyroid hormone function in man have been sparse and have often resulted in equivocal results (75). Stressful factors may alter hypothalamic-pituitary-thyroid function at many levels of control and include altered TRH secretion, altered metabolism of the thyroid hormones in peripheral tissue, and alterations in the physical state of thyroid hormone-binding proteins in blood. Additionally, other hormones, especially those of the adrenal gland may influence TSH secretion. Nervous stress has been reported to result in an increased protein-bound iodine (PBI) in some studies but not in others. Exercise stress produces no significant changes in serum T_4 or TSH concentration but leads to an increase in the total daily disposal of T_4. In man, acute bacterial sepsis is accompanied by an acceleration of T_3 and T_4 turnover. Surgery has been a means to study the effect of stress on thyroid physiology in animals and man (28, 50). Studies of the effects of surgical stress are complicated by the fact that the effects of anesthesia and of surgery per se have yet to be clearly identified. The most striking change is thyroid function is a decrease in the serum total T_3 (TT_3) and free T_3 (FT_3) concentrations shortly after surgery. The reduction in the concentration of the active forms of thyroid hormone during the postoperative pe-

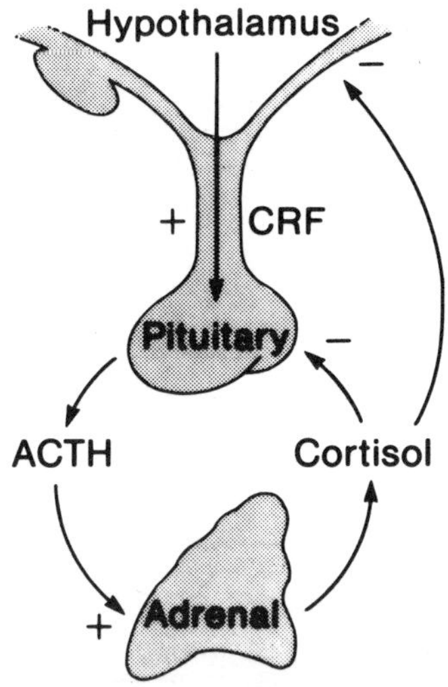

Figure 5.4. Hypothalamic-pituitary-adrenal axis. Secretion of adrenocorticotropin (ACTH) by the anterior pituitary is inhibited by the negative feedback effects of circulating cortisol. The hypothalamic stimulation of ACTH secretion is mediated by corticotropin-releasing factor (CRF). In addition to inhibiting the pituitary response to CRF, cortisol may also inhibit the secretion of CRF itself.

riod is preceded by a small, short-term increase in free T_4 (FT_4) and FT_3 concentrations during surgery (21, 49). The subsequent reduction in T_3 levels correlates with the severity of the trauma and morbidity during the postoperative period (49). The serum TSH levels also tend to diminish (21), except during surgery performed in children under hypothermic conditions (121). The effect of surgery on thyroid function cannot be fully explained on the basis of increased adrenocorticoid activity or caloric deprivation (17).

In animals, exposure to cold causes a prompt increase in TSH secretion giving rise to thyroid hormone release. In humans, although hypothermia causes a dramatic TSH secretion in the newborn, this response is almost totally lost after the first few years of life.

Starvation causes a profound decrease in serum T_3 concentration. Reduction in carbohydrate intake rather than total calorie deprivation seems to be the major factor (20).

In general, TSH secretion is inhibited during severe stress (33). Thyroid hormone may be increased after acute stress and a few reports have claimed that emotional stress in man is followed by increased pituitary-thyroid function. Insulin-induced hypoglycemia also has been reported to cause release of TSH in man.

Pituitary-Adrenal Axis

The secretion of ACTH is regulated by two interacting factors as outlined in Figure 5.4. Hypothalamic CRF stimulates the production and secretion of ACTH and circulating cortisol inhibits its release. Glucocorticoids may also act directly on the brain to inhibit CRF release. The regulation of ACTH secretion by CRF is involved in a number of neurogenic stimuli for ACTH release including circadian rhythm, pulsatile secretion, response to pain, anxiety, pyrogens, hypoglycemia, and vasopressin.

CRF levels fluctuate in relationship to a circadian rhythm linked to the light-dark cycle in which ACTH concentrations are highest in the early morning hours, gradually fall during the day, and reach their lowest levels late in the evening.

Actions of ACTH

Specific receptors exist on the surface of adrenal cortical cells that bind ACTH with a high affinity. In the presence of calcium, the ACTH-receptor complex increases the concentration of cAMP in the adrenal cell through the activation of adenyl cyclase. The elevated concentration of intracellular cAMP results in the phosphorylation of certain enzymes and histones that lead to the biologic action of the hormone (27). The rate-limiting step in the biosynthesis of steroids, the conversion of cholesterol to pregnenolone, is stimulated by ACTH. Furthermore, ACTH maintains adrenal size, stimulates the accumulation of cholesterol within the adrenals, and maintains enzymes active in the conversion of pregnenolone to hormonal steroids.

In addition to its adrenal actions, ACTH also has some extra-adrenal actions including the promotion of lipolysis in fat cells, stimulation of amino acid and glucose uptake in muscle, stimulation of the pancreatic β-cells to secrete insulin, and the somatotroph cells of the pituitary to secrete GH (27).

Actions of Adrenal Steroids

Glucocorticoid is a term applied to steriods that have effects on carbohydrate metabolism

TABLE 5.1
Relative Potencies of Steroids

Steroid	Glucocorticoid Activity	Mineralocorticoid Activity
Cortisol	1	1
Cortisone	0.7	0.7
Corticosterone	0.2	2
11-Deoxycorticosterone	nil	20
Aldosterone	0.1	400
Fludrocortisone	10	400
Prednisone	4	0.7
Prednisolone	4	0.7
Dexamethasone	30	2
Triamcinolone	3	nil
6α-Methylprednisolone	5	0.5

including promotion of gluconeogenesis, increased liver glycogen deposition, and elevation of blood glucose concentrations. Cortisol is the most potent naturally occurring glucocorticoid. Mineralocorticoid is a term applied to steroids that effect ion transport by epithelial cells, resulting in sodium conservation and loss of potassium. Aldosterone is the most potent naturally occurring mineralocorticoid. The relative glucocorticoid and mineralocorticoid activities of various naturally occurring and synthetic steroids are given in Table 5.1.

All of the glucocorticoids have the following biologic properties, some of which have significant clinical importance:

Protein-wasting Activity. Glucocorticoids accelerate the breakdown of certain proteins and inhibit the uptake of amino acids by certain extrahepatic tissues. Glucocorticoids also accelerate gluconeogenesis in which amino acids are deaminated by the liver to form urea and substrates for energy metabolism.

ACTH-Suppressing Activity. All glucocorticoids inhibit the secretion of ACTH by the pituitary gland.

Anti-inflammatory Activity. Glucocorticoids, when present in supraphysiologic amounts, inhibit the inflammatory response at several points. They have been shown to stabilize lysosomal membranes, thus preventing the release of proteolytic enzymes from lysosomes. Glucocorticoids inhibit the diapedesis of white blood cells across capillary walls and migration through tissues. They inhibit granuloma formation. Consequent upon these actions, glucocorticoids may interfere with host responses to bacterial infections. Closely related to these anti-inflammatory actions are immunosuppressive properties of glucocorticoids. Such steroids are lympholytic, cause a reduction in the number of circulating lymphocytes, diminish the size of the lymph nodes, spleen and thymus, and decrease antibody production.

Therapeutic Activity. These anti-inflammatory and immunosuppressive properties of supraphysiologic doses of glucocorticoids have made them useful therapeutic agents in a wide variety of diseases. The undesired side effects of corticosteroids are generally related to prolonged usage and include promotion of protein wasting, insulin antagonism, stimulation of fat deposition in facial, cervical and truncal regions, involution of lymphoid tissues and inhibition of antibody production. Certain groups of patients are particularly vulnerable to the untoward effects of corticosteroids. Elderly, debilitated, and poorly nourished patients are susceptible to the protein-wasting effects of steroids. In children, growth retardation may result from supraphysiologic doses of steroids. Patients with subclinical diabetes mellitus may become frankly diabetic while under corticosteroid therapy. Postmenopausal women are susceptible to the development of osteoporosis during treatment with glucocorticoids and these drugs may contribute to the perforation or hemorrhage of peptic ulcers. The use of corticosteroids in these particular patients should be for clear indications and therapy should be maintained for as short a period of time as necessary, with as low a dosage as possible.

After prolonged administration of corticosteroids, abrupt withdrawal may result in adrenal insufficiency due to the inactivation of the pituitary-adrenal axis by the inhibitory effect of the exogenous steroids. Thus, gradual tapering of the steroid is recommended.

Effects of Stress on Adrenal Function

The normal individual responds to a major stress with a brisk increase in ACTH secretion and a consequent increase in cortisol secretion. Stresses which have been shown to initiate increased pituitary-adrenal activity include, among others, severe trauma, acute hypoglycemia, sepsis, acute anxiety, and electroconvulsive therapy. In general, the level of ACTH achieved is directly related to the degree of stress. Also, the lower the plasma cortisol at the time of the stress, the greater the amount of ACTH secretion. The significant fact is that the brain is capable of responding to actual or perceived danger by altering various glandular activities.

Acute Adrenal Insufficiency

Acute adrenal insufficiency, or "Addisonian crisis" is a life-threatening condition in which a patient's physiologic requirement for glucocorticoid and mineralocorticoid steroid hormones exceeds the available supply. With the increased use of glucocorticoid therapy, acute adrenal insufficiency has become more commonly recognized among patients with bilateral adrenalectomy, hypophysectomy, and in those on long-term glucocorticoid therapy for various disorders (52).

Primary adrenal insufficiency (Addison's disease) results from the destruction or impairment of the adrenal cortex, regardless of the underlying process. The major clinical manifestations are due to the deficiencies of aldosterone and cortisol. Lack of aldosterone impairs the patient's ability to conserve sodium and excrete potassium. This situation can be exacerbated by anorexia, vomiting, diarrhea, or excessive sweating. Excretion of sodium in excess of intake results in weight loss, decreased plasma volume, hypotension, decreased cardiac output, decreased heart size, increased renin production, decreased renal blood flow, azotemia, and generalized weakness. Lack of cortisol results in anorexia, abdominal pain, wasting of fat depots, apathy, weakness, fasting hypoglycemia, and hyponatremia.

Secondary adrenal insufficiency, or ACTH deficiency, is a more common occurrence in neurosurgical practice. Any cause of hypopituitarism (Table 5.2) may result in secondary adrenal insufficiency. There are some important distinctions to be made between primary and secondary adrenal insufficiency (71). First, in secondary adrenal insufficiency, the aldosterone-secretory mechanism is usually intact and mineralocorticoid replacement is not required unlike primary adrenal insufficiency where cortisol deficiency is accompanied by aldosterone deficiency. Second, ACTH deficiency should alert the physician to the possibility that the patient may have multiple pituitary hormone deficiencies and should stimulate a search for the cause of pituitary destruction. Early treatment of the primary pituitary disorder may not only save a portion of the gland, but may spare adjacent neural structures from damage.

Secondary hypocortisolism may occur in patients with chronic suppression of ACTH by exogenous steroids, a cortisol-producing adrenal neoplasm or in patients with ectopic or pituitary ACTH hypersecretion (Cushing's syndrome). Once the underlying disorder is treated, the pituitary-adrenal axis will usually recover, but this may take as long as 1 year. During that time, replacement glucocorticoid therapy is essential and protective doses during major stresses are required.

Precipitating events of acute adrenal insufficiency are various stressful situations—surgery, severe infection, trauma, drugs, fasting—where the requirement for corticosteroids is increased but not met by the fixed dose the patient is taking.

Acute adrenal insufficiency, either primary or secondary, is relatively easy to manage. The difficult aspect is thinking of the possibility of its existence. It is generally characterized by one or more of the following nonspecific signs and symptoms: (*a*) hypotension, (*b*) nausea and vomiting, (*c*) severe weakness and fatigue, (*d*) anorexia, (*e*) hypothermia. Common laboratory findings include hyponatremia, hyperkalemia, and azotemia. Less frequent are anemia, eosinophilia, lymphocytosis, hypoglycemia, and hypercalcemia. The plasma cortisol is low.

In the acute situation, the diagnosis of adrenal insufficiency must be empirical as there is no time to confirm the clinical impression. Before treatment is initiated, blood should be drawn for a complete blood cell count with differential white count and measurement of elec-

TABLE 5.2
Causes of Hypopituitarism*

Pituitary tumors
Functional
Nonfunctional
Vascular disorders
Intracranial aneurysm
Sheehan's syndrome
Arteritides
Wernicke's encephalopathy
Atheroma
Physical agents
Trauma, head injury
Radiation
Surgery
Alcohol injection
Infectious and granulomatous processes
Tuberculosis, mycoses, syphilis, virus infections
Sarcoidosis
Histiocytosis X
Demyelinating conditions
Hypothalamic and parasellar tumors
Craniopharyngioma
Glioma, including optic nerve glioma
Meningioma
Pinealoma
Metastasis, especially breast and lung
Leukemia, lymphoma
Hamartoma
Congenital-familial
Diabetes Insipidus (DI)
Hypogonadotrophic hypogonadism
Isolated growth hormone (GH) deficiency
Prader-Willi syndrome
Laurence-Moon-Biedl syndrome
Miscellaneous
Idiopathic DI
Iron overload, hemochromatosis, multiple transfusions
"Empty sella" syndrome

*Modified from P. E. Belchetz, Hypopituitarism. In: *Management of Pituitary Disease*, edited by P. E. Belchetz, John Wiley & Sons, New York, 1984.

trolytes, glucose level, blood urea nitrogen level, and plasma cortisol and ACTH levels (52). The plasma cortisol level will later confirm the clinical impression. A normal plasma cortisol level in the face of severe clinical stress is inappropriately low and strongly suggests adrenal insufficiency.

Therapy is begun immediately after the above blood work is drawn without waiting for any laboratory results. Treatment requires the rapid intravenous infusion of physiologic saline, parenteral administration of glucocorticoids, and specific treatment for any recognizable precipitating cause.

A large intravenous line is used to give 1 to 2 liters of normal saline-dextrose 5% over the first 2 hours. An adult may require as much as 3 liters of saline over a period of a few hours; a child will require proportionately less in terms of volume, but vigorous therapy is just as urgent (71). The blood pressure will usually respond to hydration but occasionally vasopressors are necessary. Phenylephrine hydrochloride 0.25 to 0.5 mg may be given as an intravenous bolus or phenylephrine can be continuously infused in a concentration of 4 mg/1,000 ml of saline at a rate of 4 μg/minute.

Hydrocortisone sodium succinate should be given in an intravenous bolus of 100 mg as soon as possible and 100 mg administered by intravenous infusion every 8 hours for at least 36 to 48 hours. After the patient's condition has stabilized, oral glucocorticoid therapy can be initiated with hydrocortisone or cortisone acetate, 5.0 mg every 6 hours and tapered 20% to 30% daily until the maintenance dose has been obtained (52).

Hyperkalemia that accompanies acute adrenal insufficiency usually does not require specific therapy and will return to normal following rehydration and institution of steroid therapy. However, if the serum potassium level is >6.54 mEq/liter in the presence of cardiac arrhythmias, one or two ampules of 44.5 mEq of sodium bicarbonate can be given intravenously every 1 to 2 hours as needed.

Steroids and Brain Edema

Corticosteroids have been used extensively in the treatment of various neurologic conditions. The use of steroids in the treatment of brain edema, however, has received considerable experimental and clinical attention.

Types of Brain Edema

Edema is an abnormal accumulation of fluid in a tissue. The two possible locations of such fluid are intra- or extracellular. The crucial pathologic event required for the development of intracellular edema is a disturbance in cell membrane permeability of individual cells resulting in cellular inhibition, whereby in the development of extracellular edema an increased vascular permeability allows passage of fluid from the intravascular space (61).

On the basis of extensive animal experimentation, Klatzo (60) in his classical paper on the neuropathologic aspects of brain edema distinguished two types of edema: a vasogenic and a cytotoxic type. Vasogenic edema results from a breakdown of the blood-brain barrier to macromolecules with leakage of protein-rich edema fluid into the extracellular space, particularly in the white matter. Cytotoxic edema develops in the absence of blood-brain barrier damage, the water increase being due to a disturbance in cell metabolism. Vasogenic edema is responsible for brain swelling associated with brain tumors, brain abscesses, and trauma. Brain swelling associated with ischemic or anoxic conditions provides clinical examples of cytotoxic brain edema (58). The vasogenic type of brain edema is clinically the most important and more common.

Spread and Resolution of Vasogenic Brain Edema

After penetration of the blood-brain barrier, edema fluid migrates through the extracellular space, the extent and speed of which is dependent upon two factors: (*a*) the level of the systolic blood pressure, and (*b*) the duration of vascular injury and opening of the blood-brain barrier (62). The spread of vasogenic edema has a striking predilection for the white matter, regardless of the etiology of primary vascular damage. This may be due to the fact that an advancing front of edema fluid encounters less resistance by migrating through extracellular channels of the orderly arranged nerve fibers of the white matter than through the more tangled cytoarchitecture of the gray matter (61). Once the blood-brain barrier permeability resolves, the edema fluid moves by bulk flow toward the ventricular system as it resolves.

Effects of Steroids on Brain Edema

There is much experimental evidence to suggest that the brain is a target organ for corticosteroid hormones. For example, the presence of specific steroid receptors in the brain (6), the induction of enzymes by steroids, development of brain edema secondary to adrenalectomy and its prevention by steroid replacement (6), inhibition of CSF production by steroids (104), and attenuation of gross blood-brain barrier damage by steroids (15, 34, 89, 103) all indicate that steroids may somehow interfere with brain edema mechanisms. The method(s) by which exogenously administered steroids affect brain edema are unclear. They may have an affect on the initial cause of the edema, restrict its development, hasten its resolution or a combination of all of these mechanisms. Cerebral edema, regardless of the initiating cause, ultimately represents a pertubation of membrane biomolecules that maintain water and solute compartments (29). The edema and accompanying dysfunctions are benefited by exogenously administered steroids, possibly by effects on separate membrane systems (29). Influx of vasogenic edema may be curtailed by limiting the period of barrier dysfunction (6). Stabilization of membranes by steroids may limit damage due to radical peroxidation (29). Induction of enzymes and stimulation of blood flow and metabolism by steroids may enhance clearance of vasogenic edema fluid from the extracellular space or may reverse the primary or secondary cell swelling that occurs with cytotoxic cerebral edema (6). Edema resolution may be hastened through steroid-induced inhibition of CSF production, thus enhancing the flow of edema fluid through the extracellular space to the CSF spaces (97). One or more of these mechanisms or others could play a role in the beneficial effects on brain swelling seen with the use of exogenous corticosteroids.

The clinical response to steroids varies with different causes of brain edema. The dramatic success of steroids in reducing edema associated with brain tumors, initially reported by Galicich and French (43), stimulated much of the interest in using these agents. Since the early 1960s, steroids have been used extensively to help manage the edema associated with intracranial tumors and abscesses (9, 38, 43, 94, 98, 118). Some experimental studies on traumatic brain edema have shown that steroids have a favorable effect (63, 73, 74, 87, 88, 91, 110), while others have failed to show a benefit (11, 22, 30, 85, 113). The relationship of these experiments to clinical situations is unclear. Equally ambiguous results have resulted from certain clinical studies on the effect of steroids on traumatic brain edema (2, 35, 37, 39, 45, 48, 54, 93, 108). The studies of Fraupel *et al.* (37) and Gobiet *et al.* (45), both indicated that high doses of dexamethasone favorably influenced the outcome of severe head injuries and stimulated further interest in the use of steroids in this situation.

Drawing conclusions regarding the efficacy of steroids in head injury from these early studies is difficult (80). The overall management varied, the treatment schedules were different, the time of onset of therapy was difficult to assess, the severity of the initial injury and final outcomes were not measured uniformly, and few attempts were made to analyze carefully the etiology of death in the fatal cases (80).

Beginning with the report by Cooper *et al.* (24) in 1979, there have been a series of well-controlled studies that have attempted to deal with these problems (16, 44, 46, 105). An analysis of these well-controlled, prospective, double-blind studies indicates that there is no improvement in the outcome of severely head-injured patients as a result of treatment with corticosteroids. Certain of these studies indicate that steroid-treated patients have a significantly higher incidence of steroid-related complications (gastric hemorrhage, hyperglycemia, infections) while other fail to show an increased complication rate (16, 24, 44, 46).

Another unsettled issue raised by these important studies is whether subsets of head-injured patients exist that could benefit from high-dose corticosteroid therapy. These might include patients under the age of 40 years and those with Glasgow coma scores of 6 to 8 (44, 105).

Neurohypophysis—Physiology and Disorders of Secretion

As discussed earlier, vasopressin (antidiuretic hormone, ADH), and oxytocin along with their related neurophysins, are synthesized as prohormones in the cell bodies of the supraoptic and paraventricular neurons. The prohormones are transported in membrane-bound vesicles through the axons to the neural lobe where they are stored until released. Processing of the prohormone to the secreted products—vasopressin, oxytocin, and the two neurophysins—takes place in the granules during the course of transport. Nerve action potentials arising in the cell body are propagated along the axon and trigger hormone discharge. The neurohypophysial hormones leave the cell together with their neurophysin in a fixed ratio.

Regulation of ADH Secretion

Verney (116) in the early 1930s demonstrated the influence of hyperosmolar stimuli on antidiuresis by perfusing the carotid artery of experimental animals with hypertonic saline. He concluded that the brain was sensitive to alterations in osmolarity and localized the region of the brain critical for this antidiuretic effect to the anterior hypothalamus, in the region of the supraoptic and paraventricular nuclei. As a consequence of Verney's work, the term *osmoreceptor* was applied to cells within the brain which monitor extracellular osmolality.

The most important factors regulating vasopressin secretion are plasma osmolarity and circulating blood volume. Blood pressure, nausea, and various forms of stress also influence vasopressin release (51, 79, 81, 96, 100).

Osmolarity. Maintenance of normal blood water concentration is the major homeostatic function of the neurohypophysis. Blood osmolality is closely maintained within a relatively narrow range (±1.8%). Detailed studies of osmotic control of vasopressin release show that the set point of plasma osmolality for normal individuals is 280 mOsm/kg and that vasopressin release is initiated after infusion of hypertonic saline has led to an increase to 287.3 mOsm/kg, a value termed the osmotic threshold (79, 81, 82, 100). Plasma ADH levels are 2 pg/ml at this plasma osmolality. Above this value, vasopressin secretion increases rapidly with increasing plasma osmolarity. On the other hand, water loading inhibits vasopressin release. The exquisite sensitivity of the osmoreceptor-ADH-renal reflex can be demonstrated by comparing radioimmunoassay measurements of ADH in blood with plasma osmolality determinations. An increase in total body water by 1% causes a fall of 2.8 mOsm/kg, a decrease in ADH levels to 1 pg/ml, and a fall in urine osmolality from 500 to 250 mOsm/kg. An increase in total body water by 2% suppresses ADH maximally (0.25 pg/ml). A 2% decrease in total body water will increase plasma osmolality by 2% (5.6 mOsm/kg), plasma ADH will rise from 2 to 4 pg/ml and urine will be maximally concentrated (>1000 mOsm/kg) (4). This precise osmotic regulatory system operates through a hypothalamic osmoreceptor neuron system. Minor irregularities may have profound effects on body fluid homeostasis.

Volume Regulation. Decreased blood volume from any cause is followed by vasopressin release. The change in volume must be relatively large (e.g., an acute blood volume change >10%) (82). Although under normal conditions plasma osmolality is the main determinant of vasopressin secretion, severe volume depletion can over-ride the osmoreceptor control. What this means is that in the volume-depleted subject there is a shift of the "osmotic set point" so that a lower osmotic threshold is required to trigger vasopressin secretion in the volume-depleted subject. Receptors for volume control are located in the left atrium and in the baroreceptors of the carotid sinus and perhaps elsewhere. Modest degrees of volume depletion, insufficient to lower blood pressure, activate the atrial receptors, while depletion sufficient to cause hypotension mobilizes baroreceptor reflexes.

Glucocorticoids also modulate the "set-point" of neurohypophysial control. Adrenal insufficiency raises it and thereby induces a relative increase in vasopressin secretion which may contribute to the lower serum sodium seen in patients with this disorder (5).

Neuropharmacology of ADH

In addition to the direct osmotic control of ADH by osmoreceptors, there is evidence that cholinergic and adrenergic inputs to the neurons of the supraoptic and paraventricular nuclei influence cellular activity and mediate reflex control of secretion (8, 32, 83). Cholinergic agents (acetylcholine) cause an excitatory effect while adrenergic drugs such as norepinephrine inhibit the release of ADH (8, 83). Systemic administration of epinephrine or norepinephrine causes inhibition of ADH release, predominantly by effects mediated through peripheral baroreceptor mechanisms, but central adrenergic mechanisms are also important. Acetylcholine also stimulates oxytocin secretion.

Secretion of vasopressin is also affected by certain neuropeptides. For instance, direct intrahypothalamic application of angiotensin II releases vasopressin and influences drinking behavior (42). Neurohypophysial neurons are also stimulated by endogenous opioids (endorphins). That the endorphins may be involved in vasopressin secretion regulation is further supported by the observation that naloxone, an opiate antagonist, reverses neurogenically inappropriate ADH secretion in some cases (76).

TABLE 5.3
Drugs Effecting ADH Release

ADH Stimulators	ADH Inhibitors
Nicotine	Chlorpromazine
Morphine	Reserpine
Barbiturates	Diphenylhydantoin (dilantin)
Vincristine	Ethanol
Cyclophosphamide	
Tricyclic antidepressants	
Certain anticonvulsants	

A large number of drugs exert important effects on ADH secretion. Many of these are listed in Table 5.3. Alcohol inhibits ADH release, both decreasing basal levels and preventing normal ADH responses to stimuli such as reduced blood volume. Phenytoin also inhibits ADH release transiently. ADH release is *stimulated* by morphine, barbiturates, and other hypnotics. Drug-induced ADH release leads to impaired water excretion and may be responsible in part for water intoxication sometimes seen in hospitalized patients given intravenous fluids. Pain and stress, which also stimulate ADH secretion, can intensify the impaired water clearance.

In summary, the normal human subject synthesizes ADH in certain hypothalamic nuclei from which it gains access to the neurohypophysis by way of axons extending down the supraopticoneurohypophysial tract. After proper stimulation, ADH is released from these axons into the blood stream and carried to the kidneys where it acts to conserve water and concentrate urine by enhancing the reabsorption of water from the collecting tubules into the medullary interstitium. In the kidney, the ADH molecule attaches to a specific vasopressin receptor on the contraluminal side of the renal medullary tubular cell. A resultant activation of renal medullary adenyl cyclase stimulates the production of cyclic AMP which activates a protein kinase on the luminal side of the cell. Phosphorylation of membrane proteins results in increased permeability of the cell to water. Water is thus transported from the collecting tubules into the intercellular spaces, renomedullary circulation, and back into the systemic circulation.

Diabetes Insipidus

Diabetes insipidus (DI) is a disorder characterized by excessive renal water loss and is due to a deficiency in production or release of ADH. DI can also result from an inability of the kidney to respond appropriately to ADH (nephrogenic DI).

Etiology. DI may result from a variety of lesions at any of several sites along the pathway including ADH production, transport, release into the circulation, and action on the kidney. For instance, there may be a deficiency or absence of ADH production or synthesis may be intact but the ability to release ADH following appropriate stimulation may be impaired. ADH release may occur but only after plasma osmolality has reached extremely high levels. Randall *et al.* (92), proposed a useful etiologic classification of DI and a modification of their classification is shown in Table 5.4.

TABLE 5.4
Principal Causes of Diabetes Insipidus*

Primary diabetes insipidus
Idiopathic
Familial or congenital
Secondary diabetes insipidus
Post-traumatic—head injury (e.g., basal skull fractures), neurosurgical operations
Neoplastic
Infections and granulomatous lesions—sarcoidosis, tuberculosis, cryptococcosis, meningovascular syphilis, pyrogenic meningitis
Histiocytosis X
Vascular lesions

*Modified from Randall *et al.* (92).

Idiopathic DI is a disease of unknown etiology and may occur at any age and can affect either gender. The disorder which accounts for approximately half of the acquired cases is characterized by the typical clinical features of DI in the absence of other signs of hypothalamic or pituitary dysfunction.

Familial (congenital) DI is a rare disease and constitutes probably $<1\%$ of all cases. The condition occurs in infancy and childhood and affects both genders. Failure of development of the supraoptic and/or paraventricular neurons appears to be the underlying cause.

Traumatic (or surgery) has become a relatively common cause of DI due to the increasing number of head injuries caused by automobile accidents as well as surgical procedures in the parasellar region. Traumatic cases often exhibit a classic three-stage response which begins with severe DI that transiently abates as the neurohypophysis degenerates and releases excessive ADH into the circulation. In the third stage, permanent DI usually follows, although varying degrees of water imbalance may result.

Neoplastic and granulomatous DI is usually caused by destruction of the upper pituitary stalk and median eminence, where the neurohypophysial neurons converge in a relatively superficial position as they course to the neural lobe. Almost any tumor metastatic to the brain may occur in the infundibulum or upper stalk and cause DI. Both breast and lung cancer appear to have a special predilection for metastatic involvement of the hypothalamic-pituitary region. Sarcoidosis is the most common of the granulomatous lesions causing DI, but tuberculosis, syphilis, and cryptococcosis may also produce the disorder. As with the granulomatous and neoplastic disorders, *histiocytosis X* may result in DI when the disease involves the hypothalamus, infundibulum, and/or upper pituitary stalk.

Vascular lesions can cause DI in several ways. Intracranial aneurysms, particularly of the anterior communicating artery, can cause the condition either from mass effect due to progressive enlargement of the lesion or from rupture with resultant subarachnoid hemorrhage. Subarachnoid hemorrhage may damage the hypothalamic nuclei and/or the infundibulum either during the actual bleed or later as a result of ischemia due to the vasospasm that often follows aneurysmal subarachnoid hemorrhage. Postpartum pituitary necrosis (Sheehan's syndrome) occasionally causes DI in addition to adenohypophysial deficiency, presumably through vascular damage to the upper portion of the stalk.

Clinical and Laboratory Findings. The patient with DI will have polyuria and polydipsia usually with a urine specific gravity <1.005. In patients with large volumes of dilute urine, hypercalcemia, hypokalemia or drug toxicity (e.g., lithium) should be considered. Those with unexplained hypotonic polyuria should have osmolality and sodium determinations. If low, the patient is water overloaded and if high, the patient has DI. Barlow and de Wardener (7) found that the plasma osmolalities of patients suffering from DI average 295 ± 15 mOsm/kg whereas that for normal subjects averaged 280 ± 16 mOsm/kg. As this difference is associated with considerable overlap, the determination of plasma osmolality is of little help diagnostically in certain individual cases. As long as the patient maintains normal thirst mechanisms, the total solute concentration of the body fluids will be preserved close to the normal limits albeit accompanied by the polydipsia and polyuria associated with this condition. However, if there is a defect in the normal thirst mechanism (e.g., coma) in a patient with DI, the clinical situation may become serious. Under these circumstances, the resulting dehydration with accompanying hypovolemia and hyperosmolality may even prove fatal unless the clinical condition is recognized and corrected. If the patient with hypotonic polyuria has a normal random plasma osmolality or sodium level, dehydration tests should be done.

The water deprivation test will determine whether the patient can respond to an osmotic stimulus by elaboration of a concentrated urine. In the test, water intake is restricted and changes in urine volume and plasma concentration measured for a period of 6 to 8 hours. In normal individuals, water deprivation causes a dehydration that produces a fall in urine volume and a rise in urine osmolality. After 6 to 8 hours of fluid deprivation, the urine flow will reduce to <0.5 ml/min, urine osmolality plateaus anywhere between 500 and 1,400 mOsm/kg, and plasma osmolality rises to the range of 288 to 291 mOsm/kg. The subcutaneous administration of 5 u of aqueous vasopressin will not cause a further increase in urine osmolality, indicating that the maximum ability of the kidney to concentrate the urine has been reached.

The patient with severe DI is able to concentrate the urine to only 200 mOsm/kg after dehydration and plasma osmolality may rise as high as 320 to 330 mOsm/kg. The administration of 5 u of aqueous Pitressin will cause the urine osmolality to approximately double, indicating that the inability to concentrate the urine is due to a deficiency of circulating ADH.

Patients with milder DI will exhibit levels of plasma and urine osmolalities of intermediate values following dehydration. Vasopressin will, however, cause a further increase in urine osmolality, signifying a limited capacity for ADH release. In severe dehydration, even DI patients may show a modest increase in urine concentration and a decline in urinary volume due to contraction of blood volume with decreased renal plasma flow. One of the more difficult diagnostic problems can be differentiating the compulsive water drinker from the patient with DI. In this situation, it may be necessary to extend the dehydration period for as long as 18 hours, by which time the compulsive water drinkers are always able to exhibit normal urinary concentration.

Another situation where errors can be made in interpreting the results of a dehydration test is in a patient with mild DI who is able to secrete enough ADH to prevent diuresis, but only at the expense of a higher than normal plasma osmolality. After dehydration and the urine osmolality plateaus, plasma osmolality will be evaluated and vasopressin administration will not cause a further concentration of urine. This patient's response to the water deprivation test will appear to be normal unless the plasma osmolality is measured and found to be high. Therefore, the determination of plasma osmolality should be made after the urine osmolality plateaus and before giving vasopressin.

In patients with marked polyuria and polydipsia, a water deprivation test should not be carried out overnight because of the risk of severe dehydration and hypovolemic shock. Instead, these patients should begin water deprivation in the morning with urine collected hourly until the osmolality plateaus as determined by three consecutive samples. Plasma osmolality is then measured and 5 u aqueous vasopressin is administered subcutaneously. Urine is collected at two consecutive 30-minute intervals and urine osmolality measured in each. Patients with DI will show an increase in urine osmolality of 9% or more after the administration of vasopressin.

Other tests for DI are available and include the hypertonic saline infusion test and the nicotine test (69). In the former, the patient is hydrated initially with an infusion of dextrose and water at a rate (approximately 10 ml/min) to induce diuresis (>5 ml/min). The intravenous solution is then switched to a 2.5% solution of NaCl at a rate of 0.25 ml/min/kg body weight and continued for 45 minutes. Urine flow is measured by voiding every 15 minutes. If both neurohypophysial and renal function are normal, urine flow may be expected to fall sharply with the infusion of hypertonic saline whereas in DI, urine flow is unaffected. Nicotine, which causes ADH release in normal subjects by its stimulating action on the supraoptic neurons, can be used to assess neurohypophysial function. The test is performed by inducing a water diuresis and then administering nicotine intravenously. In normal subjects, a sharp fall in urine flow will occur, whereas in patients with DI little or no antidiuresis will be observed.

Management. Patients with mild to moderate DI, who have an intact thirst mechanism and a readily available supply of water, are usually in no danger. The marked polydipsia and polyuria are annoying, and usually prevent sleep at night. Thus, for reasons of convenience, therapy usually is justified (111).

In clinical practice, there are varying degrees of ADH impairment and treatment must be tailored for the individual patient. In institutions where a large volume of pituitary surgery is performed, varying degrees of DI will frequently be encountered. Postoperatively, in patients with pituitary tumors, the condition is usually transient, whereas in patients undergoing ablative hypophysectomy, as many as 70% or more will experience postoperative DI, many of which will be permanent (111).

A number of effective therapeutic preparations are available for treating DI (81) (Table 5.5). As with other peptide hormones, the oral administration of vasopressin is ineffective. Oral treatment with nonhormonal drugs may be efficacious in patients who have some residual capacity to release ADH.

Chlorpropamide induces an antidiuresis in patients with DI in proportion to their ability to release ADH. A dose of 200 to 500 mg once daily is usually sufficient for 24 hours. The drug also facilitates the action of ADH on the kidney by increasing the ADH-induced activation of adenylate cyclase. It is not effective in patients with nephrogenic DI. A potential side-effect of chlorpropamide administration is hypoglycemia which can be avoided by eating regular meals.

Clofibrate is another oral agent effective in the treatment of DI which acts centrally by releasing ADH from the neurohypophysis. It does not have any intrinsic ADH activity of its own and does not potentiate the peripheral action of ADH, so it is only useful in patients with some ADH reserve. The usual dosage is 500 mg four times a day. Some patients who do not respond to chlorpropamide or clofibrate alone will respond to a combination of the two drugs. In this situation, a regimen of chlorpropamide 100

TABLE 5.5
Agents Used to Treat Diabetes Insipidus (DI)*

Agent	Usual Dose	Duration of Action	Clinical Indication
Hormone Replacement			
8-Lysine vasopressin (Lypressin) (5 ml bottle, 50 U/ml)	10–20 U IN†	4–6 hr.	Severe transient or permanent DI
1-Deamino-8-D-arginine vasopressin (DDAVP) (3.5 ml bottle, 200 μg/ml)	10–20 μg IN	12–24 hr.	Severe, transient or permanent DI
Aqueous vasopressin (5 U/ml ampule)	5–10 U SC	3–6 hr.	DI in unconscious patient
Vasopressin tannate in oil (5 U/ml ampule)	5 U IM	24–72 hr.	Severe idiopathic DI
Nonhormonal Agents			
Chlorpropamide (100 & 250 mg tablets)	200–500 mg/day	24 hr.	Some residual ADH function
Clofibrate (500 mg capsules)	500 mg QID	24 hr.	Some residual ADH function
Carbamazepine (200 mg tablets)	400–600 mg/day	24 hr.	Some residual ADH function
Thiazide Diuretics			
Hydrochlorothiazide	50–100 mg/day	24 hr.	Nephrogenic DI

*Adapted from A. M. Moses (81).

†IN, intranasal; IM, intramuscular; SC, subcutaneous; QID, 4 times daily; ADH, antidiuretic hormone.

to 150 mg twice daily and clofibrate 1.5 to 2 g in daily divided doses is used.

Carbamazepine, a tricyclic anticonvulsant, also stimulates endogenous ADH. It will induce an antidiuresis in patients with partial DI at doses of 400 to 600 mg daily. Because of its potential toxicity, it is not used as frequently as the other oral agents.

Synthetic 8-lysine vasopressin is available as a nasal spray but has several disadvantages. A single application produces antidiuresis for only 4 to 6 hours and its absorption is impaired under various circumstances including allergic rhinitis, respiratory infections, trans-sphenoidal surgery and other conditions that produce edema of the nasal mucosa.

1-Desamino-8-D-arginine vasopressin (DDAVP), which is the synthetic analogue of vasopressin, is a more satisfactory replacement. It is also available as a nasal spray and has an antidiuretic effect for 12 to 24 hours, with no pressor activity.

Injectable vasopressin is available in an aqueous solution or as Pitressin tannate in oil. The short duration of aqueous Pitressin is advantageous in treating patients receiving intravenous fluids, especially unconscious patients, because it minimizes the risk of water intoxication. In patients with an altered level of consciousness with DI from head trauma or neurosurgery, we treat with aqueous Pitressin administered intramuscularly or subcutaneously in doses of 5 to 10 u. Pitressin tannate in oil is used in similar doses for more chronic treatment of DI.

The only useful treatment of nephrogenic DI is the use of a thiazide diuretic with sodium restriction. Although this appears paradoxical, the drugs cause a depletion of sodium which decreases the delivery of sodium to the ascending limb of the loop of Henle and a consequent reduction in the ability to dilute the urine. The glomerular filtration rate is reduced and reabsorption of fluid in the proximal nephron is enhanced.

Inappropriate Secretion of ADH (Schwartz-Bartter Syndrome)

The syndrome of inappropriate secretion of antidiuretic hormone (SIADH) results from the continuous, and thus, inappropriate secretion of ADH despite an abnormally low serum osmolarity and an expanded extracellular fluid volume. The term "inappropriate" is used because under these conditions, the hypothalamic neurons should be inhibited and the secretion of ADH suppressed. In SIADH, however, ADH excess induces water retention by the kidney to the point of hyponatremic expansion of the extracellular fluid volume and a secondary natriuresis.

Etiology. Dilutional hyponatremia due to excessive water retention is a common disorder seen in many unrelated clinical states. The main causes of SIADH (Table 5.6) include: (*a*) suprahypothalamic brain disease causing excessive release of ADH from the neurohypophysial system; (*b*) hypothalamic damage which leads to ADH "leakage" from the supraoptic neurons; (*c*) ADH release due to persistent drive from baro- or volume-receptors as a result of cardiac or pulmonary disease; (*d*) ectopic production of ADH by neoplastic tissue (e.g., oat-cell tumor of the lung); and (*e*) administration of drugs that stimulate ADH release (Table 5.3).

TABLE 5.6
Causes of Inappropriate Antidiuretic Hormone (ADH) Secretion*

Central hypersecretion of ADH
Hypothalamic disorders
Trauma
Surgery
Metabolic encephalopathy
Acute intermittent porphyria
Myxedema
Subarachnoid hemorrhage
Vascular lesions
Suprahypothalamic disorders
Cerebral infarcts
Subdural hematoma
Infections, meningitis (tuberculosis)
Peripheral hypersecretion
Excessive stimulation in recumbant posture (coma)
Excessive production from nonhypothalamic sites (ectopic ADH)
Pulmonary infections—TB
Tumors—lung, etc.
Drugs
Vincristine
Chlorpromazine
Chlorothiazide
Cyclophosphamide
Carbamazepine
Clofibrate
Chlorpromazine

*From Martin *et al.* (75) with permission.

A variety of intracranial disorders are associated with SIADH. Subarachnoid hemorrhage, head injury, craniotomy, brain tumors, cerebral infarction, and meningitis are among the long list of CNS entities associated with the syndrome. Fox *et al.* (36) showed that 30% of neurosurgical patients developed SIADH at some time during hospitalization. The large variety and lack of anatomic specificity of lesions associated with SIADH have not been adequately explained. The assumption that an insult to the suprahypothalamic brain reduces the normal, predominantly inhibitory effect of these centers on ADH secretion has not been supported by experimental studies.

Clinical Manifestations. The signs and symptoms of SIADH are related to the water retention and correlate to some extent with the degree of resultant hyponatremia and the rapidity with which it develops. A slow drop of serum sodium to a value near 124 mEq/liter results in nonspecific symptoms such as anorexia, nausea, vomiting, diffuse weakness, and mental alteration (3). A more rapid fall in sodium to levels below 120 mEq/liter may be associated with seizures, stupor, or coma (3). Patients with underlying neurologic disease may have symptoms at higher sodium levels than patients with normal brains. Focal signs such as pseudobulbar palsy, reflex changes, Babinski sign, or extrapyramidal signs may be associated with hyponatremia.

Pathophysiology. Some investigators believe that water retention and hyponatremia produce a cytotoxic cerebral edema that is responsible for the neurologic manifestations. Severe hyponatremia and water intoxication, however, are not associated with a significant increase in intracranial pressure and corticosteroids have no effect on the condition. Dila and Pappius (31) have investigated changes in cerebral electrolyte values in a rat model of SIADH and found diminished levels of potassium as well as sodium with the potassium depletion related to the level of consciousness. This work was expanded by Holliday *et al.* (53) who found that brain potassium depletion was associated with hyponatremia but not with acute changes in brain intracellular volume.

Diagnosis and Management. Hyponatremia may be due to sodium depletion as seen in prolonged vomiting, adrenal insufficiency, or the cerebral salt-wasting syndrome (see below). These disorders require distinctly different treatments. The laboratory criteria for SIADH are: (*a*) a serum sodium <135 mEq/liter; (*b*) urinary sodium >25 mEq/liter; (*c*) serum osmolality <280 mOsm/kg; and (*d*) urine osmolality inappropriately concentrated compared to serum osmolality. To make the diagnosis of SIADH, the patient must be in a normal state of hydration, not be on diuretics, and have normal renal, thyroid and adrenal function. In this syndrome, blood volume and peripheral circulation (pulse and blood pressure) are normal. Hyponatremia due to sodium depletion is accompanied by contraction of blood volume and decreased renal blood flow with elevation of BUN and creatinine (prerenal azotemia).

As water retention is the source of symptoms and signs of SIADH, fluid restriction is the mainstay of therapy. For mild symptoms, daily water restriction of 400 to 800 ml is usually adequate. For more severe symptoms (i.e., seizures or coma) the use of 3% saline (500 ml over 6 to 8 hours) plus a forced diuresis with furosemide (20 to 40 mg) eliminates free water and rapidly corrects the hyponatremia. Because furosemide induces a natriuresis, urinary electrolytes become important and sodium losses may need to be replaced. Once the hyponatremia has been corrected, institution of fluid restriction is important in preventing recurrence of water intoxication.

Certain drugs that inhibit the secretion or action of ADH have been used to treat SIADH. Dilantin and alcohol both inhibit ADH release but large doses are usually required. Lithium carbonate inhibits the action of ADH at the kidney but is not used frequently because of renal toxicity. Dimethylchlortetracycline, a tetracycline antibiotic, has been used more widely in doses from 600 to 1,200 mg/day for the same pharmacologic property of ADH inhibition at the kidney.

Nelson *et al.* (84) have described 10 of 12 unselected neurosurgical patients with intracranial disease who fulfilled the laboratory criteria for SIADH but had significant decreases in their red blood cell mass, plasma volume, and total blood volume. These authors believe this finding indicates that there is a spectrum of abnormalities in the hyponatremic, natriuretic patient from true SIADH to a "cerebral salt-wasting syndrome". The latter disorder may result from an inability of the kidney to conserve sodium, perhaps due to an undefined natriuretic factor in the brain (59). Blood volume determinations are necessary to differentiate the two causes of hyponatremia as fluid restriction would exacerbate a cerebral salt-wasting syndrome associated with volume depletion. This group of patients require volume replacement with packed red blood cells and colloids to replace both the volume and sodium deficits.

Trauma to the Hypothalamus and Pituitary

Traumatic lesions may occur in the pituitary gland, stalk, and/or hypothalamus in association with closed head injury (1, 25). If studied carefully, over two-thirds of patients dying with closed head injuries will have lesions in the hypothalamus or pituitary (77, 78). The most common autopsy findings in the pituitary are hemorrhages in the posterior lobe or infarction in the anterior lobe although anterior lobe hemorrhages, stalk hemorrhages, or lacerations also occur. Hypothalamic injuries include both infarction and hemorrhages (25, 26).

Injuries to the pituitary and hypothalamus may be the result of direct trauma or secondary to elevated intracranial pressure. Pituitary ischemia and infarction may be due to stalk damage with interruption of the hypothalamic-hypophysial portal system. Damage to the pituitary and hypothalamus rarely occurs in isolation, but rather as a part of multifocal brain damage. Associated skull fractures are common (1, 26).

Clinically, traumatic hypothalamic and/or pituitary lesions manifest themselves most commonly as disorders of systemic water balance (DI or SIADH). Hypopituitarism, ranging from panhypopituitarism to selective deficiency of a single hormone, occurs less commonly. Deficiencies of nearly all the adenohypophysial hormones have been reported (90). DI may be associated with anterior pituitary dysfunction, but interestingly, may be masked by TSH and ACTH deficiency and not be clinically apparent until glucocorticoid therapy is instituted (90). Traumatic adenohypophysial hormone deficiencies are usually not recognized until long after the injury.

Higher than normal levels of circulating cortisol exist following head injuries, in part due to the liberation of CRF from the median eminence, causing release of ACTH which, in turn, stimulates cortisol secretion. Normally, the increased cortisol would inhibit further ACTH secretion by negative feedback. There is, however, interruption of the normal circadian rhythm of ACTH and loss of responsiveness in the negative feedback system (90). Even if the negative feedback system remains intact, dexamethasone suppression tests indicate that it appears to be set at a higher level, also accounting for the lack of inhibition of ACTH by cortisol (109). A negative nitrogen balance occurs in head-injured patients which may be steroid-related (23).

REFERENCES

1. Adams, J. H., Gennarelli, T. A., and Graham, D.I. Brain damage in nonmissle head injury: Observations in man and subhuman primates. In: *Recent Advances in Neuropathology*, No. 2, edited by W. T. Smith and J. B. Cavanaugh, pp. 165–190. Churchill-Livingstone, Edinburgh, 1982.
2. Alexander, E., Jr. Medical management of closed head injuries. Clin. Neurosurg., *19:* 240–243, 1972.
3. Arieff, A., Llach, F., and Massey, S. G. Neurological manifestations and morbidity of hyponatremia: Correlation with brain water and electrolytes. Medicine, *55:* 121, 1976.
4. Arnaud, E., Cirino, M., Layton, B. S., and Renaud, L. P. Contrasting actions of amino acids, acetylcholine, noradrenaline and leucine enkephalin on the excitability of supraoptic vasopressin-secreting neurons: A microiontophoretic study in the rat. Neuroendocrinology, *36:* 187, 1983.
5. Aubry, R. H., Nankin, H. R., Moses, A. M., and Streeten, D. H. P. Measurement of the osmotic threshold for vasopressin release in human subjects, and its modification by cortisol. J. Clin. Endocrinol. Metab., *25:* 1481, 1965.
6. Baethmann, A., Oettinger, W., Moritake, K., Chaussy, L., and Jesch, F. Metabolic effects of corticosteroids in central nervous tissue. In: *Treatment of Cerebral Edema,* edited by A. Hartmann and M. Broch, pp. 24–30. Springer-Verlag, Berlin, Heidelberg, New York, 1982.
7. Barlow, E. D., and de Wardener, H. E. Compulsive water drinking. Quart. J. Med., *28:* 235, 1959.
8. Barker, J. L., Crayton, J. W., and Nicoll, R. A. Noradrenaline and acetylcholine responses of supraoptic neurosecretory cells. J. Physiol. (Lond.), *218:* 19, 1971.
9. Beks, J. W. F., Doorenbos, H., and Walstra, G. J. M. Clinical experiences with steroids in neurosurgical patients. In: *Steroids and Brain Edema,* H. J. Reulen and K. Schürmann, pp. 233–238. Springer-Verlag, Berlin, Heidelberg, New York, 1972.

10. Ben-Jonathan, M., Mical, R. S., and Porter, J. C. Transport of LRF from CSF to hypophysial portal systemic blood and the release of LH. Endocrinology, *95:* 18–25, 1974.
11. Benson, V. M., McLaurin, R. L., and Foulkes, E. C. Traumatic cerebral edema. An experimental model with evaluation of dexamethasone. Arch. Neurol., *23:* 179–186, 1970.
12. Bergland, R. M., and Page, R. B. Can the pituitary secrete directly to the brain? (Affirmative anatomical evidence.) Endocrinology, *102:* 1325–1338, 1978.
13. Bergland, R. M., and Page, R. B. Pituitary-brain vascular relations: A new paradigm. Science, *204:* 18–24, 1979.
14. Biron, R., Burger, A., *et al.* Thyroid hormones and the energetics of active sodium-potassium transport in mammalian skeletal muscles. J. Physiol. (Lond.), *297:* 47, 1979.
15. Blomstrand, C., Johansson, B., and Rosengren, B. Dexamethasone effect on blood-brain barrier damage caused by acute hypertension in X-irradiated rabbits. Acta Neurol Scand., *52:* 331–334, 1975.
16. Braakman, R., Schouten, H. J. A., Dishoeck, M. B., and Minderhoud, J. M. Megadose steroids in severe head injury. Results of a double-blind clinical trial. J. Neurosurg., *58:* 326–330, 1983.
17. Brandt, M. R., Skorsted, L., Kehlet, H., and Hansen, J. M. Rapid decrease in plasma-triiodothyronine during surgery and epidural analgesia independent of afferent neurogenic stimuli and of cortisol. Lancet, *2:* 1333, 1976.
18. Brazeau, P., Vale, W., Burgus, R., *et al.* Hypothalamic polypeptide that inhibits the secretion of immunoreactive pituitary growth hormone. Science, *179:* 77–79, 1973.
19. Brownstein, M. J., Russell, J. T., and Gainer, H. Synthesis, transport, and release of posterior pituitary hormones. Science, *207:* 373, 1980.
20. Burman, K. D., Dimond, R. C., Harvey, G. S., O'Brien, J. T., George, L. P., Bruton, J., Wright, F. D., and Wartofsky, L. Glucose modulation of alterations in serum iodothyronine concentrations induced by fasting. Metabolism, *28:* 291, 1979.
21. Chan, V., Wang, C., and Yeung, R. T. T. Pituitary-thyroid responses to surgical stress. Acta Endocrinol. (Copenh.), *88:* 490, 1978.
22. Clasen, R. A., Cooke, P. M., Pandolfi, S., Carnecki, G., and Hass, G. M. Steroid-antihistamine therapy in experimental cerebral edema. Arch. Neurol., *13:* 504–592, 1965.
23. Clifton, G. L., Robertson, C. S., Grossman, R. G., Hodge, S., Foltz, R., and Garza, C. The metabolic response to severe head injury. J. Neurosurg., *60:* 687–696, 1984.
24. Cooper, P. R., Moody, S., Clark, W. K., Kirkpatrick, J., Maravilla, K., Gould, A. L., Drane, W. Dexamethasone and severe head injury. A prospective double-blind study. J. Neurosurg., *51:* 307–316, 1979.
25. Crompton, M. R. Hypothalamic lesions following closed head injury. Brain, *94:* 165–172, 1971.
26. Crompton, M. R. Hypothalamic and pituitary lesions. In: *Handbook of Clinical Neurology*, vol. 23, edited by P. J. Vinken and G. W. Bruyn, pp. 465–469. North-Holland, Amsterdam, 1975.
27. Daughaday, W. H. The adenohypophysis. In: *Textbook of Endocrinology*, edited by H. Williams, 6th ed., pp. 73–116. W. B. Saunders, Philadelphia, 1981.
28. De Groot, L. J., Larsen, P. R., Refetoff, S., and Stanbury, J. B. Physiology of the hypothalamus, pituitary and thyroid. In: *The Thyroid and Its Diseases*, 5th ed., pp. 118–163. John Wiley, New York, 1984.
29. Demopoulos, H. B., Milvy, P., Kakari, S., and Ransohoff, J. Molecular aspects of membrane structure in cerebral edema. In: *Steroids and Brain Edema*, edited by H. J. Reuben and K. Schürmann, pp. 29–39. Springer-Verlag, New York, Heidelburg, Berlin, 1972.
30. Dick, A. R., McCallum, M. E., Maxwell, J. A., and Nelson, S. R. Effect of dexamethasone on experimental brain edema in cats. J. Neurosurg., *45:* 141–147, 1976.
31. Dila, C. J., and Pappius, H. M. Cerebral water and electrolytes, an experimental model of inappropriate secretion of antidiuretic hormone. Arch. Neurol., *256:* 85, 1972.
32. Dreifuss, J. J., and Kelly, J. S. The activity of identified supraoptic neurones and their response to acetylcholine applied by iontophoresis. J. Physiol. (Lond.), *220:* 105, 1972.
33. Dupont, A., *et al.* Effect of hippocampal stimulation on the plasma thyrotropin (TSH) and corticosterone responses to acute cold exposure in the rat. Can. J. Physiol. Pharmacol., *50:* 364, 1972.
34. Eisenberg, H. M., Barlow, C. F., and Lorenzo, A. V. Effect of dexamethasone on altered brain vascular permeability. Arch. Neurol. *23:* 18–22, 1970.
35. Fox, J. L. Use of methylprednisolone in intracranial surgery. Med. Ann. DC, *34:* 261–266, 1965.
36. Fox, J. L., Falik, J. L., and Shalhoub, R. J. Neurosurgical hyponatremia: The role of inappropriate antidiuresis. J. Neurosurg., *34:* 506, 1971.
37. Fraupel, G., Reulen, J. H., Müller, D., and Schürmann, K. Double-blind study on the effects of steroids in severe closed head injury. In: *Dynamics of Brain Edema*, edited by H. Pappius and W. Feindel, pp. 337–343. Springer-Verlag, Berlin, Heidelberg, New York, 1976.
38. French, L. A., and Galicich, J. H. The use of steroids for control of cerebral edema. Clin. Neurosurg., *10:* 169–174, 1964.
39. French, L. A. The use of steroids in the treatment of cerebral edema. Bull. N.Y. Acad. Med., *42:* 301–311, 1966.
40. Furutani, Y., Morimoto, Y., Shibahara, S., *et al.* Cloning and sequence analysis of cDNA for ovine corticotropin-releasing factor precursor. Nature (Lond.), *301:* 537–540, 1983.
41. Gainer, H. Biosynthesis of vasopressin and neurophysin. In: *The Neurohypophysis: Physiological and Clinical Aspects*, edited by S. Reichlin, pp. 35–50. Plenum, New York, 1984.
42. Ganten, D., Fuxe, K., Phillips, M. I., *et al.* The brain isorenin-angiotensin system: Biochemistry,

localization, and possible role in drinking and blood pressure regulation. Front. Neuroendocrinol., *5:* 61, 1978.

43. Galicich, J. H., and French, L. A. Use of dexamethasone in the treatment of cerebral edema resulting from brain tumors and brain surgery. Ann. Pract., *12:* 169–174, 1961.
44. Giannotta, S. L., Weiss, M. H., Apuzzo, M. L. J., and Martin, E. High dose glucocorticoids in the management of severe head injury. Neurosurgery, *15:* 497–501, 1984.
45. Gobiet, W., Bock, W. J., Liesegang, J., *et al.* Treatment of acute cerebral edema with high dose of dexamethasone. In: *Intracranial Pressure III*, edited by J. W. F. Beks, D. A. Bosch, and M. Brock, pp. 231–235. Springer-Verlag, Berlin, Heidelberg, New York, 1976.
46. Gudeman, S. K., Miller, J. D., and Becker, D. P. Failure of high-dose steroid therapy to influence intracranial pressure in patients with severe head injury. J. Neurosurg., *51:* 301–306, 1979.
47. Guillemin, R., Braxeau, P., Böhlen, P., *et al.* Growth hormone-releasing factor from a human pancreatic tumor that caused acromegaly. Science, *218:* 585–587, 1982.
48. Gutterman, P., and Shenkin, H. A. Prognostic features in recovery from traumatic decerebration. J. Neurosurg., *32:* 201–210, 1977.
49. Hagenfeldt, I., Melander, A., Thorell, J., Tibblin, S., and Westgren, U. Active and inactive thyroid hormone levels in elective and acute surgery. Acta Chir. Scand., *145:* 77, 1979.
50. Haiback, H., and McKenzie, J. M. Increased free thyroxine postoperatively in the rat. Endocrinology, *81:* 435, 1967.
51. Hayward, J. N. Functional and morphological aspects of hypothalamic neurons. Physiol. Rev., *57:* 574, 1977.
52. Himathongkam, T., Newmark, S. R., Greenfield, M., and Dluhy, R. G. Acute adrenal insufficiency. J.A.M.A., *230:* 1317–1318, 1974.
53. Holliday, M. A., Kalacyi, M. N., and Harrah, H. Factors that limit brain volume changes in response to acute and sustained hyper- and hyponatremia. J. Clin. Invest., *47:* 1916, 1968.
54. Hoyt, H. J., Goldstein, F. P., Reigel, D. H., and Holst, R. Clinical evaluation of highly-soluble steroids in the treatment of cerebral edema of traumatic origin (a double-blind study). Clin. Pharmacol. Ther. *13:* 141, 1972.
55. Horvath, E., and Kovacs, K. Pathology of the pituitary gland. In: *Pituitary Diseases*, edited by C. Ezrin, E. Horvath, B. Kaufman, *et al.* pp. 1–84. CRC Press, Boca Raton, FL, 1980.
56. Ingbar, S. H., and Woeber, K. A. The thyroid gland. In: *Textbook of Endocrinology*, 6th ed., edited by R. H. Williams, pp. 117–247. W. B. Saunders, Philadelphia, 1981.
57. Itoh, N., Obata, K., Yanaihara, N., and Okamoto, H. Human preprovasoactive intestinal polypeptide contains a novel PHI-27-like peptide, PHM-27. Nature (Lond.), *304:* 547–549, 1983.
58. Katzman, R., Clasen, R., Klatzo, I., Meyer, J. S., Pappius, J. M., and Waltz, A. G. Report of joint committee for stroke resources. 4. Brain edema in stroke. Stroke *8:* 512–540, 1977.
59. Klahr, S., and Rodriguez, H. J. Natriuretic hormone. Nephron, *15:* 387, 1975.
60. Klatzo, I. Presidential Address: Neuropathological aspects of brain edema. J. Neuropath. Exp. Neurol. *26:* 1–14, 1967.
61. Klatzo, I. Pathophysiological aspects of brain edema. In: *Steroids and Brain Edema*, edited by H. J. Reulen and K. Schürmann, pp. 1–8. Springer-Verlag, New York, Heidelberg, Berlin, 1972.
62. Klatzo, I., Wisniewski, H., Steinwall, O., and Streicker, E. Dynamics of cold injury edema. In: *Brain Edema*, edited by I. Klatzo and F. Seitelberger, pp. 554–563. Springer-Verlag, Berlin, Heidelberg, New York, 1967.
63. Kobrine, A. I., and Kempe, L. G. Studies in head injury. Part II: Effect of dexamethasone on traumatic brain swelling. Surg. Neurol. *1:* 38–42, 1973.
64. Kovacs, K., and Horvath, E. Pituitary tumors: Pathologic aspects, In: *Clinical Neuroendocrinology: A Pathophysiological Approach*, edited by G. Tolis, F. Labrie, J. B. Martin, and F. Naftolin, pp. 367–384. Raven Press, New York, 1979.
65. Kovacs, K., and Horvath, E. Pathology of pituitary adenomas. In: *Hormone-Secreting Pituitary Tumors*, edited by J. R. Givens, pp. 97–119. Year Book Medical Publishers, Chicago, 1982.
66. Krieger, D. T., and Martin J. B. Brain peptides (first of two parts). N. Engl. J. Med., *304:* 876, 1981.
67. Krieger, D. T., and Martin, J. B. Brain peptides (second of two parts). N. Engl. J. Med., *304:* 944, 1981.
68. Land, H., Schultz, G., Schmale, H., and Richter, D. Nucleotide sequence of cloned cDNA encoding bovine arginine vasopressin-neurophysin 11 precursor. Nature (Lond.), *295:* 299, 1983.
69. Leaf, A., and Coggins, C. H. The neurohypophysis. In: *Textbook of Endocrinology*, 5th ed., edited by R. H. Williams, pp. 80–94. W. B. Saunders, Philadelphia, 1974.
70. Lechan, R. M., Nestler, J. L., Jacobson, S., and Reichlin, S. The hypothalamic 'tuberoinfundibular' system of the rat as demonstrated by horseradish peroxidase (HRP) microiontophoresis. Brain Res. *195:* 13–27, 1980.
71. Liddle, G. W. The adrenals. In: *Textbook of Endocrinology*, 6th ed., edited by R. H. Williams, pp. 249–292. W. B. Saunders, Philadelphia, 1981.
72. Ling, N., Esch, F., Bohlen, P., *et al.* Isolation, primary structure, and synthesis of human hypothalamic somatocrinin: Growth hormone-releasing factor. Proc. Natl. Acad. Sci. U. S. A., *81:* 4302–4306, 1984.
73. Long, D. M., Maxwell, R. E., and French, L. A. The effects of glucosteroids upon experimental brain edema. In: *Steroids and Brain Edema*, edited by J. H. Reulen and K. Schürmann, pp. 65–76. Springer-Verlag, New York, 1972.
74. Long, D. M., Maxwell, R. E., Choi, K. S., Cole, H. O., and French, L. A. Multiple therapeutic approaches in the treatment of brain edema induced by a standard cold lesion. In: *Steroids and Brain*

Edema, edited by J. H. Reulen and K. Schürmann, pp. 87-94. Springer-Verlag, Berlin, Heidelberg, New York, 1972.

75. Martin, J. B., Reichlin, S., and Brown, G. M. *Clinical Neuroendocrinology*. F. A. Davis, Philadelphia, 1977.
76. Martin, J. B. Neuroendocrinology. In: *Disorders of the Pituitary*, by G. T. Tindall and D. L. Barrow, pp. 23-63. C. V. Mosby, St. Louis, 1986.
77. McCormick, W. F. Trauma. In: *Clinical Neurosciences*, Vol. 3, edited by S. S. Schochet, Jr. pp. 241-283. Churchill-Livingstone, New York, 1983.
78. McCormick, W. F. Pathology of closed head injury. In: *Neurosurgery*, Vol. 3, edited by R. H. Wilkins and S. S. Rengachary, pp. 1544-1570. McGraw-Hill, New York, 1985.
79. Miller, M., and Moses, A. M. Clinical states due to alteration of ADH release and action. In: *Neurohypophysis*, edited by A. M. Moses and L. Share, pp. 153-161. S. Karger, Basel, 1977.
80. Molofsky, W. J. Steroids and head trauma. Neurosurgery, *15:* 424-426, 1984.
81. Moses, A. M. Diabetes insipidus and ADH regulation. In: *Neuroendocrinology*, edited by D. T. Krieger and J. C. Hughes, Chap. 15, p. 141. Sinauer Assoc., Sunderland, MA, 1980.
82. Moses, A. M. Clinical and laboratory features of central and nephrogenic diabetes insipidus and primary polydipsia. In: *The Neurohypophysis: Physiological and Clinical Aspects*, edited by S. Reichlin, pp. 115-138. Plenum, New York, 1984.
83. Moss, R. L., Dyball, R. E. J., and Cross, B. A. Responses of antidromically identified supraoptic and paraventricular units to acetylcholine, noradrenaline and glutamate applied iontophoretically. Brain Res., *35:* 573, 1971.
84. Nelson, P. B., Seif, S. M., Maroon, J. C., and Robinson, A. G. Hyponatremia in intracranial disease: Perhaps not the syndrome of inappropriate secretion of antidiuretic hormone (SIADH). J. Neurosurg., *55:* 938, 1981.
85. Nelson, S. R. Effects of drugs on experimental brain edema in mice. J. Neurosurg., *41:* 193-199, 1974.
86. Page, R. B., and Bergland, R. M. The neurohypophyseal capillary bed. I. Anatomy and arterial supply. Am. J. Anat., *148:* 345-358, 1977.
87. Pappius, H. M. Effects of steroids on cold injury edema. In: *Steroids and Brain Edema*, edited by J. H. Reulen and K. Schürmann, pp. 57-63. Springer-Verlag, Berlin, Heidelberg, New York, 1972.
88. Pappius, H. M., and McCann, W. P. Effect of steroids on cerebral edema in cats. Arch. Neurol., *20:* 207-216, 1969.
89. Pappius, H. M., and McCann, W. P. Effects of steroids on cerebral edema in cats. Arch. Neurol., *20:* 207-216, 1969.
90. Popp, A. J., and Bourke, R. S. Pathophysiology of head injury. In: *Neurosurgery*, edited by R. H. Wilkins and S. S. Rengachary, pp. 1536-1543. McGraw-Hill, New York, 1985.
91. Raimondi, A. J., Clasen, R. A., Beattie, E. J., and Taylor, C. B. The effect of hypothermia and steroid therapy on experimental cerebral injury. Surg. Gynecol. Obstet., *108:* 333-338, 1959.
92. Randall, R. V., Clark, E. C., and Bahn, R. C. Classification of the causes of diabetes insipidus. Proc. Mayo Clin. *34:* 299, 1959.
93. Ransohoff, J. The effects of steroids in brain edema in man. In: *Steroids and Brain Edema*, edited by J. H. Reulen and K. Schürmann, pp. 211-217. Springer-Verlag, Berlin, Heidelberg, New York, 1972.
94. Rasmussen, T., and Gulati, D. R. Cortisone in the treatment of postoperative cerebral edema. J. Neurosurg., *19:* 535-544, 1962.
95. Reichlin, S. Neuroendocrinology. In: *Textbook of Endocrinology*, 6th ed., edited by R. H. Williams, pp. 589-645. W. B. Saunders, Philadelphia, 1981.
96. Reichlin, S. The neurohypophysis: Historical overview. In: *The Neurohypophysis: Physiological and Clinical Aspects*, edited by S. Reichlin, pp. 1-4. Plenum, New York, 1984.
97. Reulen, H. J., Tsuyumu, M., Tack, A., Fenske, A. R., and Prioleau, G. R. Clearance of edema fluid into cerebrospinal fluid. J. Neurosurg. *48:* 754-764, 1978.
98. Reulen, H. J., Hadjidemos, A., and Schürmann, K. The effect of dexamethasone on water and electrolyte content and on rCBF in perifocal brain edema in man. In: *Steroids and Brain Edema*, edited by J. H. Reulen and K. Schurmann, pp. 239-252. Springer-Verlag, Berlin, Heidelberg, New York, 1972.
99. Rivier, J., Spiess, J., Thorner, M., and Vale, W. Characterization of a growth hormone-releasing factor from a human pancreatic islet tumor. Nature (Lond.), *300:* 276-278, 1982.
100. Robertson, G. L. The regulation of vasopressin function in health and disease. Recent Prog. Hormone Res., *33:* 333, 1977.
101. Robinson, A. G. Neurophysins. In: *Clinical Neuroendocrinology*, edited by L. Martini and G. M. Besser, pp. 585, 602. Academic Press, New York, 1977.
102. Robinson, A. G. The contribution of measured secretion of neurophysins to our understanding of neurohypophyseal function. In: *The Neurohypophysis: Physiological and Clinical Aspects*, edited by S. Reichlin, pp. 65-94. Plenum, New York, 1984.
103. Rovit, R. L., and Hagan, R. Steroids and cerebral edema: The effect of glucocorticosteroids on abnormal capillary permeability following cerebral injury in cats. J. Neuropath. Exp. Neurol., *27:* 277-299, 1968.
104. Sato, O., Hara, M., Asai, T., Tsugane, R., and Kageyama, M. The effect of dexamethasone phosphate on the production rate of cerebrospinal fluid in the spinal subarachnoid space of dogs. J. Neurosurg., *39:* 480-484, 1973.
105. Saul, T. G., Ducker, T. B., Salcman, M., and Carro, E. Steroids in severe head injury. J. Neurosurg., *54:* 596-600, 1981.
106. Smith, T. J., and Edelman, I. S. The role of sodium transport in thyroid thermogenesis. Fed. Proc., *38:* 2150, 1979.
107. Snyder, S. H. Drug and neurotransmitter receptors in the brain. Science, *224:* 22, 1984.

108. Sparacio, R. R., Lin, T. H., and Cook, A. W. Methylprednisolone sodium succinate in acute craniocerebral trauma. Surg. Gynecol. Obstet., *121:* 513–516, 1965.

109. Steinbok, P., and Thompson, G. Serum cortisol abnormalities after craniocerebral trauma. Neurosurgery, *5:* 559–565, 1979.

110. Taylor, J. M., Levy, W. A., Herzog, I., and Scheinberg, L. C. Prevention of experimental cerebral edema by corticosteroids. Biochemical and ultrastructural studies. Neurology (Minneap.), *15:* 667–674, 1965.

111. Tindall, G. T., and Barrow, D. L. *Disorders of the Pituitary*, C. V. Mosby, St. Louis, 1986.

112. Tobin, R., Berdanier, C. D. *et al.* Effects of thyroxine treatment on the hepatic membrane ATPase activity in rats. J. Environ. Pathol. Toxicol. *2:* 1235, 1979.

113. Tornheim,, P. A., and McLaurin, R. H. Effect of dexamethasone on cerebral edema from cranial impact in the cat. J. Neurosurg., *48:* 220–227, 1978.

114. Vale, W., Spiess, J., and Rivier, J. Characterization of a 41-residue ovine hypothalamic peptide that stimulates secretion of corticotropin and β-endorphin. Science, *213:* 1394–1397, 1981.

115. Valverder, C., Chieffo, V., and Reichlin, S. Prolactin-releasing factor in porcine and rat hypothalamic tissue. Endocrinology, *91:* 982–993, 1972.

116. Verney, E. B. Croonian Lecture. The antidiuretic hormone and the factors which determine its release. Proc. R. Soc. Lond. (Biol.), *135:* 25, 1947.

117. Weche, J. Circadian variation of the serum thyrotropin level in normal subjects. Scand. J. Clin. Lab. Invest., *32:* 337, 1973.

118. Weinstein, J. D., Toy, F. J., Jaffe, M. E., and Goldberg, H. I. The effect of dexamethasone on brain edema in patients with metastatic brain tumors. *Neurology* (Minneap.), *23:* 121–129, 1973.

119. Werner, S., Hulting, A. L., Hokfelt, T., *et al.* Effect of the peptide PHI-27 on prolactin release in vitro. Neuroendocrinology, *37:* 476–478, 1983.

120. Weigand, S. J., and Price J. L. Cells of origin of the afferent fibers to the median eminence in the rat. J. Comp. Neurol., *192:* 1–19, 1980.

121. Wilber, J. F., and Baum, D. Elevation of plasma TSH during surgical hypothermia. J. Clin. Endocrinol., *31:* 372, 1970.

CHAPTER 6

Hematology and Coagulation: Physiology, Pathophysiology, and Management

WARREN R. SELMAN, M.D., and
CAROLE A. MILLER, M.D.

INTRODUCTION

The neurosurgeon must understand normal hematologic physiology and the diagnostic evaluation and manifestations of hematologic disorders. This knowledge is necessary to estimate the risk of surgical intervention, determine the proper timing of surgery, and to manage critically ill patients in a Neurosurgical Intensive Care Unit (NICU). The neurosurgeon must also be aware of the potential effects of hematologic therapeutics upon the Central Nervous System (CNS). Although the advice of experts in hematology is necessary, the effect of volume management and component replacement therapy must be assessed by the neurosurgeon with reference to disease processes of the CNS such as edema, vasospasm, and increased intracranial pressure.

This chapter is divided into three parts: Hematologic Physiology, Hemostasis, and Transfusion. Pathologic conditions of particular interest to neurosurgeons are reviewed. A scheme for evaluating and managing patients with these disorders, particularly as they relate to NICU patients is presented.

HEMATOLOGIC PHYSIOLOGY

Circulating blood consists of formed elements, erythrocytes, leukocytes, and platelets suspended in native plasma. Disease states can produce diverse changes in blood composition. Some changes affect the cellular component of blood, others the chemical composition of the plasma, and still others the physical properties of blood as a fluid. Alterations of blood composition may critically affect neurologic function, particularly when brain function is already compromised (36). Although whole blood is a functional unit, it is most helpful to analyze changes in its various components separately.

Red Blood Cell Function: Oxygen Delivery

One basic function of blood with respect to the CNS is to provide the steady supply of oxygen needed to support metabolism. The oxygen-carrying capacity of blood is determined largely by the red cell mass. Tissue hypoxia occurs when the oxygen tension in the capillaries is insufficient for metabolic needs. The normal cerebral oxygen demand of 3.5 ml/100 g/min can be met by physiologic oxygen delivery (57). The oxygen-carrying capacity of normal blood is 1.34 ml/g of hemoglobin or, at 97% saturation approximately 19.4 ml of O_2/dl. At the venous end of the capillary, blood contains 14.4 ml of O_2/dl. Thus, 5 ml of O_2/dl is delivered to the tissue, or 25% of the oxygen content is extracted. Oxygen demand may increase greatly with stress or disease. A 20-fold increase in oxygen delivery can be provided by an increase of the oxygen extraction to 75% and a 6- to 7-fold increase in cardiac output (25).

Anemia, regardless of etiology, results in a decreased red cell mass. In anemia, the normal extraction of oxygen leads to greater hemoglobin desaturation and a lower oxygen tension at the venous end. This results in destructive cellular hypoxia in the immediate vicinity. Compensatory adjustment in the supply of blood and oxygen must occur to prevent tissue damage in vital organs.

Since the blood volume in anemia is not changed significantly, increased tissue perfusion has to be performed selectively with blood shunted from presumably nonvital donor areas to oxygen-sensitive recipient organs. In chronic anemia the donor areas are the cutaneous tissue and the kidneys. Vasoconstriction and oxygen deprivation in the subcutaneous tissue is well tolerated. Although the kidney is hardly nonvital, its oxygen supply under normal conditions exceeds oxygen demands. The kidney has a small arterial-venous oxygen content difference. This implies that oxygen extraction is low relative to flow, and that metabolism is fairly independent of flow. In contrast, the brain's arterial-venous difference is six to seven times greater than that of the kidney, and thus metabolism is more sensitive to changes in blood flow (36). The benefit of redistribution is that organs with the most pressing need for oxygen, such as the brain, will be largely unhampered by a moderate reduction in oxygen-carrying capacity. Pre-existing CNS disorders such as edema or spasm, however, can render the brain more susceptible to even minor changes in oxygen-carrying capacity and as such should be aggressively treated.

Severely injured patients may be less tolerant of the systemic consequences of compensatory mechanisms. An increase in cardiac output by decreasing the required oxygen extraction is an excellent but metabolically expensive compensatory device. A measurable increase in resting cardiac output does not occur until the hemoglobin concentration is below 7 g/dl and clinical signs of cardiac hyperactivity are present only at lower hemoglobin levels (28, 50). While the normal myocardium can tolerate a prolonged period of sustained hyperactivity, patients with heart disease may not be able to increase cardiac output sufficiently to maintain compensatory mechanisms. If compensation fails, CNS symptoms including a decreased level of consciousness or a new or worsened focal deficit may appear (43). Treatment of the CNS manifestations requires correction of cardiomegaly and pulmonary edema with oxygen, intravenous furosemide, and transfusion of red blood cells.

The medical etiologies of anemia are diverse, but the neurosurgeon should be alert to common causes which may affect patient management. Anemia is one of the characteristic features of chronic renal failure (37). The degree of anemia is roughly proportional to the degree of uremia. A blood urea nitrogen concentration in excess of 100 mg/dl is always associated with a hematocrit below 30%. The anemia is caused by a failure of renal excretory function, which leads to hemolysis, blood loss, and impaired erythropoietin production secondary to failure of renal endocrine function (22, 54, 68).

Chronic alcohol ingestion is often associated with anemia. The anemia may be due to folic acid and iron deficiency, or a result of the direct toxic affect of alcohol on erythropoiesis. There are myriad hematologic complications of alcoholism (12). While both uremia and alcohol abuse result in anemia, these disorders also produce coagulation abnormalities that may require more immediate attention (18, 38). The therapy and diagnosis of coagulation disorders is discussed in a separate section.

Sickle cell anemia has several unique characteristics that can affect neurosurgical management. The gene for hemoglobin S is common in black populations. Ten percent of American blacks have a single hemoglobin S gene (27). Clinical manifestations of sickling disorders vary in severity from the virtually symptomless trait to the potentially lethal state characteristic of sickle cell anemia. The majority of CNS symptoms are caused by vascular occlusion that results from the altered red blood cells. Deoxygenation is the most important factor determining the sickling in a red cell containing hemoglobin S (46). The degree of deoxygenation required to produce sickling varies with the percentage of hemoglobin S in the cells. Sickle trait cells will sickle at an oxygen tension of 15 mm Hg, while those from a patient with sickle cell anemia may begin to sickle at an oxygen tension of 40 mm Hg (46). Changes that impair adequate oxygenation of blood may be extremely deleterious to people with sickle hemoglobin, particularly if they have an associated CNS problem. This factor should be a consideration in the acute management of any black patient and may account for otherwise unexplained neurologic complications.

Patients with sickle cell disease are at increased risks during anesthesia. Factors known to precipitate crisis including hypoxia, dehydration, acidosis, hypothermia, and infection must be scrupulously avoided. Pre- and postoperative transfusion with packed cells may help prevent such complications. Partial exchange transfusion for patients undergoing angiography can prevent crises precipitated by deleterious changes in pH (26).

Blood as a Fluid: Rheologic Considerations

Reduced cerebral blood flow—ischemia as opposed to hypoxia—may be caused by decreased cardiac output, acute hypovolemia, vessel occlusion, stenosis or spasm, or raised intracranial pressure. In the presence of a normal oxygen-carrying capacity, neurologic function and viability are related to certain thresholds of cerebral blood flow (3). Normal function occurs with flows between 20 and 50 ml/100 g/min. At flows between 12 and 20 ml/100 g/min, the EEG becomes isoelectric and clinical deficits may be manifested but the cells remain viable. With further flow reductions, cell membrane integrity is disrupted and cell death ensues. Whatever the etiology of the decreased blood flow, changes in the fluid component of blood may be needed to prevent neurologic sequelae.

The most dramatic cause of ischemia, an acute decrease in blood volume, can be seen after multiple trauma or major surgery. Immediately following an acute hemorrhage, hematocrit and erythrocyte counts may be normal despite a markedly reduced blood volume. Thus even with a normal hematocrit, there may be a need to replace both red cell mass and volume. During the recovery phase, re-institution of blood volume is produced by an increase in plasma volume and the hematocrit and erythrocyte counts are reduced. The treatment of red blood cell and volume loss is discussed further in the section on replacement therapy.

More subtle changes in the fluid component of blood may be helpful in the therapy of stenosis or spasm. The rheologic properties of blood as a fluid become important when considering therapeutic maneuvers. The relationship between relative viscosity of blood and the hematocrit is nearly linear for hematocrits below 40%; above 40%, the relative viscosity becomes greater. While other factors, such as fibrinogen concentration, affect blood viscosity, the hematocrit is the dominant factor and most amenable to therapeutic alteration. Increased blood viscosity caused by high hematocrit may aggravate neurologic deficits on the basis of a decrease in regional cerebral blood flow (36). Conversely, neurologic deficits may be improved by acute hematocrit reduction (65). Hemodilution may be accomplished by the infusion of volume expanders such as dextran 40 or hydroxyethyl starch in normal saline, either alone or in combination with venesection. The beneficial effects of flow improvement in hemodilution should be tempered by the theoretical risk of altered metabolism secondary to a decreased oxygen-carrying capacity. Particular attention should be paid to central venous pressure or pulmonary capillary wedge pressure to avoid systemic hemodynamic consequences. Recent reviews suggest that an hematocrit of 33% may be ideal to improve flow without producing untoward sequelae (34).

Hemodilution therapy may be used alone or in combination with induced hypertension to produce an increase in regional cerebral blood flow. The safest method to achieve this goal is by an infusion of isotonic fluid or volume expanders. Hypotonic solutions should be avoided to prevent exacerbation of cerebral edema. The addition of pressor agents should be used only if the desired pressure increase cannot be achieved by volume expansion alone. The advantages of improved flow by induced hypertension must be tempered by the theoretical risk of aggravating cerebral edema in the presence of disordered autoregulation. Again systemic complications can be avoided by monitoring central venous pressure or pulmonary capillary wedge pressure, cardiac output, and peripheral resistance.

HEMOSTASIS

Alterations of the Hemostatic Mechanism

Normal hemostatic mechanisms are dependent on the integrity of the vessel wall, platelet function, coagulation factors (Table 6.1), and the fibrinolytic system (21, 44, 51). Abnormalities in any component of this complex may be responsible for hemorrhage or thrombosis. Either of these conditions may require intervention in patients with neurologic disorders. While all these elements interact to maintain normal hemostasis, it is best to analyze each independently.

Most of the life-threatening disorders of hemostasis result from excessive hemorrhage. The neurosurgeon should be aware of the presentation of bleeding disorders to direct an expedient work-up to prevent or treat hemostatic abnormalities. The history of a bleeding disorder, easy bruising, current medications, and familial bleeding tendencies are essential parts of patient evaluation.

Bleeding from platelet deficiencies presents a clinical picture distinct from that due to deficiencies or abnormalities of coagulation factors. Platelets are responsible for cessation of bleeding in small vessels. Prolonged bleeding time and petechial hemorrhages are the hallmarks of platelet disorders. Coagulation factor abnormalities, in contrast, cause hemorrhages in deeper structures such as subcutaneous tissue, muscle, or joint spaces. In these disorders, both platelet function and bleeding times are normal. Bleeding, in the absence of major trauma, is characteristic of severe plasma coagulation factor disorders. External bleeding associated with abnormalities of plasma coagulation factors responds only slowly to local pressure and recurs after the pressure is removed (44).

The distinction between superficial bleeding with platelet disorders and deeper bleeding with coagulation disorders is a clinically useful point, but platelets and plasma coagulation factors are interdependent in hemostasis (52). A severe coagulation defect may interfere with thrombin formation and give rise to abnormalities of platelet function and petechial bleeding. Defects in the platelet system and in plasma coagulation factors may co-exist as, for example, in patients with von Willebrand's disease (33) or defibrination syndromes (17), and in people who suffer severe hemorrhage with replacement by banked blood that is deficient in factors V and VIII and in platelets (70).

Hemostasis results from the interaction of several mechanisms at the site of injury. The primary mechanism in hemostasis is the reaction of the platelets, endothelium, and subendothelial tissues (29). The first reaction is vasoconstriction initiated by serotonin released from platelets. Next is activation of blood coagulation mechanisms in the micro-environment of the platelet aggregate, resulting in the deposition of fibrin and formation of a "white thrombus." A later effect, activation of the fibrinolytic system, dissolves the formed fibrin and restores partial or complete patency of the blood vessel (44, 57).

TABLE 6.1
Coagulation Factors

Factor	Synonyms
Factor I	Fibrinogen
Factor II	Prothrombin
Factor III	Thromboplastin, tissue factor
Factor IV	Calcium
Factor V	Proaccelerin
Factor VI (obsolete)	
Factor VII	Serum prothrombin conversion accelerator (SPCA)
Factor VIII*	Antihemophilic globulin (AHG) Antihemophilic factor (AHG)
Factor IX	Plasma thromboplastin component (PTC) Christmas factor
Factor X	Stuart factor Autoprothrombin III
Factor XI	Plasma thromboplastin antecedent (PTA)
Factor XII	Hageman factor
Factor XIII	Fibrin-stabilizing factor
—+	Prekallikrein (Fletcher factor)
—‡	High molecular weight kininogen (Fitzgerald factor)

*Also designated as factor VIII von Willebrand factor.
+No numerical designation.
‡No numerical designation.

The sequence of events that terminate with the polymerization of fibrinogen can be represented in several ways. One method is to divide the sequence into four clinical phases (Fig. 6.1). These four phases or sets of reactions represent the major clinical categories of hemostatic abnormalities (45). Within this system, the concept of an intrinsic and extrinsic mechanism for the initiation of clotting is useful (Fig. 6.2), although the traditional distinction between intrinsic and extrinsic pathways may not be as sharp as once believed (32, 40, 51). The cata-

Reactants	Activators / Catalysts	Products / Inhibitors
Phase I: The Initiater (Contact) Reaction		
Platelets	Contact	Platelet factor 3 (phospholipid)
	→	
"Inactive" contact Factors (XI and XII)	(thrombin)	"Activated" contact Factors (XI and XII) Inhibitor: normal Endothelial surface
Phase II: Thromboplastinogenesis		
Platelet phospholipid Factor VIII	Activated XI and XII Ca^{2+}	Plasma thromboplastin
	→	
Factor IX Factor X	(Thrombin)	Inhibitor: antithromboplastin (S)
Phase III: Thrombinogenesis		
Prothrombin	Thromboplastin Ca^{2+} → Factor V Factor VII Factor X (Thrombin)	Thrombin Inhibitor: antithrombin
Phase IV: Fibrin Formation		
Fibrinogen	Thrombin →	Fibrin (Stabilizer: Factor XIII) Inhibitor: Fibrinogenolysins, fibrinolysins, and fibrin split products

Figure 6.1 Schematic representation of the process of blood coagulation. The division into four phases is arbitrary and is used only as a convenient scheme for classifying the hemorrhagic disorders and the tests used to study them. Thrombin in parentheses in phases I, II, and III indicates that it acts as a catalyst rather than a reactant. (From J. B. Miale, *Laboratory Medicine Hematology.* C. V. Mosby, St. Louis, 1982.)

lytic action of thrombin in phases I and II and its action as an autocatalyst in phase III, provides a biochemical amplifier. Following a series of complex and poorly understood events (44), the conversion of fibrinogen to fibrin occurs very rapidly when a critical concentration of thrombin is reached. Inhibitory mechanisms are present at each phase to counteract uncontrolled reactions (29). In phase I, normal endothelium (containing heparinoids) prevents the platelets and contact factors from triggering the coagulation sequence. In phase II, naturally occurring antithromboplastins can inhibit the reaction. In phase III, antithrombins are inhibitory. In phase IV, there are no known physiologic inhibitors of fibrin formation, but the reaction is stopped by fibrinopeptides and by absorption of excess thrombin into the fibrin clot. The fibrinolytic system, while not inhibitory, does provide a way to dissolve fibrin and re-establish the patency of a vessel occluded by thrombus. These inhibitory mechanisms may be viewed from two perspectives. First, when these systems are pathologically hyperactive, they can cause excessive hemorrhage (27). Second, modification of the inhibitory systems may be an important avenue for therapy designed to prevent or treat thromboembolic disease.

The interaction of platelets with the endothelial cell lining of the blood vessel represents the first phase of hemostasis. Phase I arbitrarily separates the role of platelets in hemostasis from subsequent reactions, although platelet phospholipids are required in some reactions involving blood coagulation factors, and the "contact factors" XI and XII are stimuli for initiating the reactions of platelet adhesiveness

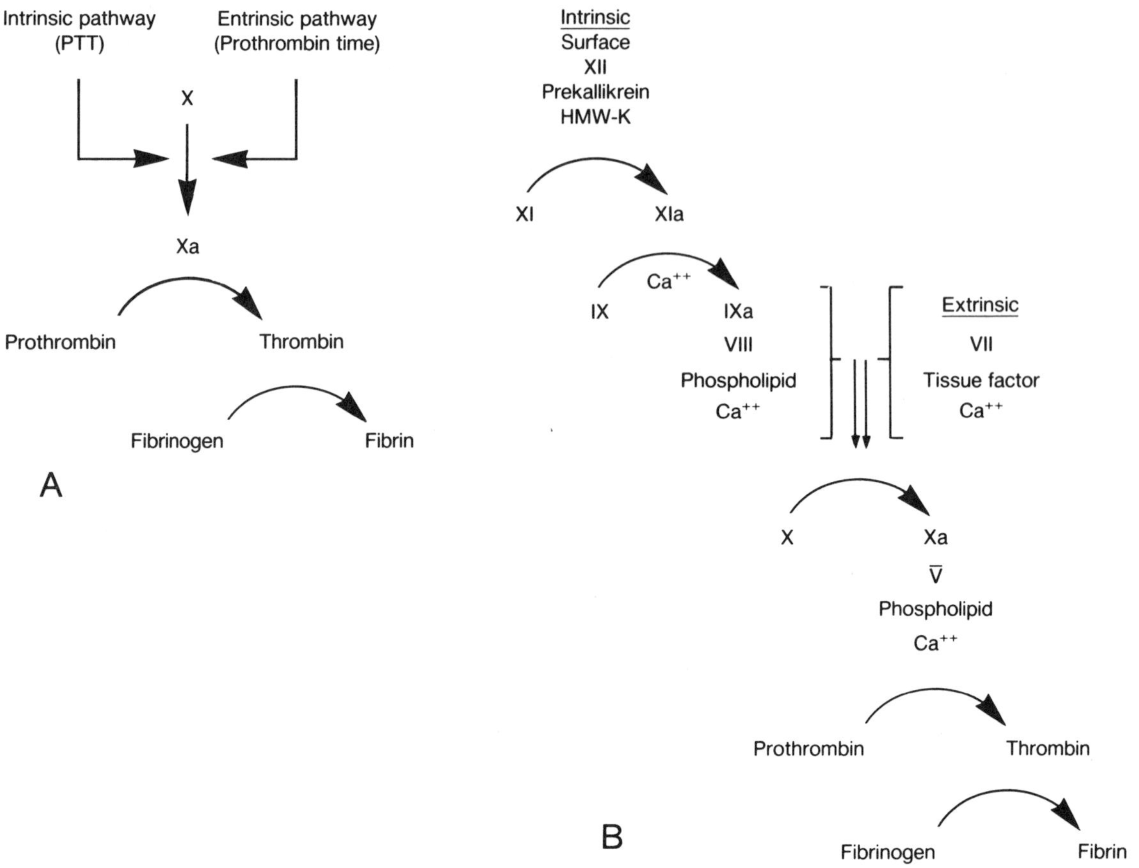

Figure 6.2 *A*. A simplified scheme of blood coagulation. PTT, partial thromboplastin time. *B*. Details of intrinsic and extrinsic pathology as a scheme of blood coagulation.

and aggregation (52, 61, 73). Disorders of phase I result from quantitative and qualitative platelet abnormalities. Patients with phase I problems have a history of purpura, ecchymosis, and a prolonged bleeding time. Platelets normally range from 150,000 to 400,000/mm^3. The mean range is 250,000/mm^3. The lower the platelet count, the greater the probability of serious hemorrhage. Major hemorrhages are unusual even with platelet counts less than 20,000/mm^3. Platelet counts of about 50,000 to 60,000/mm^3 prevent hemorrhage during surgical procedures *if* the platelets are functioning *normally* (70). Elevated platelet counts may also be accompanied by bleeding, particularly in patients with myeloproliferative disorders. The patient with a markedly elevated platelet count may either bleed or develop thrombosis (62, 70).

The platelet performs its hemostatic function by responding to a variety of stimuli and undergoing a predictable sequence of reactions: (*a*) shape change; (*b*) adhesion; (*c*) primary aggregation; (*d*) secondary aggregation; and (*e*) release reaction (44). The entire sequence is completed if the stimulus produced is sufficiently strong and no inhibitors are operative. All inducers of platelet adhesion and aggregation cause the platelet shape to change from a disc to a spiny sphere (7). The spiny processes promote adherence to foreign surfaces, i.e., adhesion, as well as cell-to-cell bonding, i.e., aggregation (16, 51, 11, 31). The release reaction refers to the release of platelet substances into the surrounding medium. The primary sequence of adhesion-aggregation-release reaction is accompanied by the release of adenosine 5-diphosphate (ADP) and other substances which initiates a second sequence of adhesion-aggregation-release reactions.

Both adequate numbers and normally functioning platelets are essential in phase I. Bleeding time is an in vivo measure of hemostatic efficiency. It should be performed according to the Ivy technique, as modified by Mielke (average 2.3 to 9.5 min $\pm$ 2 SD) or with the bleeding time device template (General Diagnostics). In platelet functional disorders, the bleeding time is prolonged and in thrombocytopenic states, it is inversely proportional to the platelet count when the latter is below 60,000/mm^3. The bleeding time is also prolonged in von Willebrand's disease (55). Bleeding time is determined by the interaction of the platelets with the subendothelial tissues and not by the integrity of the coagulation mechanisms; however, patients on long-term anticoagulant therapy may have a moderately prolonged bleeding time (19). Aspirin prolongs bleeding time 2 to 3 minutes in most persons and to a greater degree in patients with von Willebrand's disease (69). Aspirin inhibits platelet aggregation and secretion by preventing the synthesis of prostaglandins. This inhibition is only partial, but may be detected in the blood from 3 to 7 days after the ingestion of 0.3 to 1.2 gm of the drug (71).

Phase I abnormalities secondary to quantitative or qualitative platelet disorders may make management of a postoperative patient or NICU patient quite difficult. Specific treatment should be directed toward the correction of the particular problem. The effect of any medication the patient is receiving must be investigated and platelet transfusion may be required (48, 63).

The coagulation process may be viewed as a waterfall or cascade sequence, in which there is sequential proenzyme to enzyme transformation. (Fig. 6.1) (58). A numerical system for identifying accepted coagulation factors has been recommended (Table 6.2). The activated coagulation factor (denoted by the lower case letter *a*) at each step in turn activates the next proenzyme. Such a scheme is helpful, but should not be interpreted to mean that these reactions apply to all coagulation factors (44, 52).

Phase II involves reactions that lead to the formation of plasma intrinsic thromboplastic activity. Development of this intrinsic thromboplastic activity involves the interaction of several coagulation factors: platelet phospholipid (platelet factor 3) made available during platelet reactions in phase one, factors V, VIII, IX, X, XI, and XII. When any factor is reduced below a certain critical limit, there is less plasma thromboplastin formed and the conversion of prothrombin to thrombin is incomplete (10, 44). The sequence is initiated in vivo by the interaction of platelets with subendothelial tissues with the liberation of tissue thromboplastin, which bypasses the "contact" reactions and utilizes factor VII (19). Factor XIIa activates factor XI. Thromboplastin generation involves the activation of factor X to Xa. Factors XI, VIII, and platelet factor 3 form a lipid protein complex in the presence of calcium ions that activate factor X to Xa (67). The formation of a prothrombin activator, plasma thromboplastin, involves the formation of a complex between factor Xa, factor V, and platelet factor 3 in the presence of calcium ions (70). Assuming that sufficient platelet factor 3 is made available from phase I, the disorders in phase II are caused by a deficiency of the factors involved in the generation of plasma thromboplastin or the development of pathologic antithromboplastic activity. The deficiency of factor VIII causes hemophilia. The deficiency of factors IX, X, XI, and XII cause hemorrhagic states, sometimes called the hemophilioid diseases. A severe deficiency in factor V also leads to defective generation of plasma thromboplastin.

The partial thromboplastin time (PTT) of plasma is the coagulation time when a "partial thromboplastin" is used, and is a measure of the integrity of the intrinsic system (13). It is most sensitive to the levels of factors VIII, IX, X, XI, or XII, although the PTT is prolonged in severe deficiency of factor V. The PTT is prolonged in prothrombin deficiency only when the factor is almost completely absent. The PTT is most useful, therefore, as a screening test to detect the deficiency of factor VIII, IX, X, XI, or XII. The addition of an activating agent to the partial thromboplastin agent provides maximum activation of factors XI and XII (APTT). As in other tests that depend on the formation of fibrin as the end point, the PTT and APTT will be prolonged in afibrinogenemia. The tests are also abnormal in the presence of the anticoagulant, heparin, and as such are used to monitor heparin therapy (35). The PTT and APTT may be slightly prolonged in intensive oral anticoagulant therapy because of reduction in factors IX and X. Because partial thromboplastin is a substitute for platelet factor 3, the PTT and APTT are normal in quantitative and qualitative platelet defects (4). The test will be abnormal in von Willebrand's disease if the level of factor VIII is very low (44). The one-stage prothrombin time (PT) of plasma using tissue thromboplastin is normal in uncomplicated deficiencies of factors VIII, IX, or XII.

In phase III "thrombinogenesis", prothrombin is converted to thrombin (44). Abnormalities in phase III are characterized by a prolonged prothrombin time. The conversion of prothrombin to thrombin is preceded by a prothrombin activator complex of factor Xa, factor V, and platelet factor 3. Prothrombin activator complex converts prothrombin to thrombin in the presence of calcium ions (44). Prothrombin activator complex is common to both the intrinsic and extrinsic pathways. The extrinsic pathways involve the interaction of tissue factor with factor VII. Congenital deficiencies or deficiencies caused by oral anticoagulants or factors needed for phase III are detected by the one-stage prothrombin time. A prolonged PT can result from other factors such as a fibrinogen concentration below 60 ml/dl, or pathologic circulating anticoagulants against thrombin, factor X or factor V (19, 20). A prolonged PT and a prolonged partial thromboplastin time are characteristic of factor X deficiency. A similar pattern is seen in factor V deficiency, different only in that the PT is much more abnormal than the partial thromboplastin time. The PT and PTT are prolonged in afibrinogenemia and in the presence of pathologic or administered anticoagulants and inhibitors (44, 51). The administration of heparin causes only a slight elevation of the PT.

One unique feature of phase III is that the synthesis of several factors involved in the PT test is vitamin-K-dependent. These vitamin-K-dependent factors include prothrombin and factors VII, IX, and X. Their production may be abnormal secondary to oral anticoagulation therapy. Bishydroxycoumadin (dicumarol) and related compounds are used extensively in the treatment of acute and chronic thrombotic disease (19). Coumadin drugs result in the formation of variant, nonactive coagulation factors. Synthesis of the vitamin-K-dependent factor is inhibited by oral anticoagulants, and the PT test is used principally for the control of oral anticoagulant therapy (19). Some patients are resistant to coumadin drugs, presumably on the basis of a deficient enzyme system (30). The influence of various drugs, such as barbiturates, which decrease, and phenylbutazone, which potentiates the effect of anticoagulants is related to effects on the enzyme system (52).

Vitamin K deficiency secondary to deficient nutritional intake, defective synthesis or absorption in the bowel, or lack of utilization by a diseased liver also affects synthesis of the same coagulation factors (6). Treatment of acquired prothrombin and factor VII deficiency with vitamin K must take into account the pathogenesis of the deficiency (31). Oral administration of vitamin K is not effective in obstructive jaundice. The defective absorption mechanism can be bypassed by giving vitamin K parenterally. If the hemorrhagic diathesis is secondary to hepatocellular disease, vitamin K will not be effective regardless of the route of admistration (8). In this event, it is necessary to depend on blood transfusions to supply sufficient coagulation factors.

In phase IV, thrombin brings about the polymerization of fibrinogen to fibrin. The abnormalities in this phase include quantitative and qualitative alterations in fibrinogen, a deficiency of fibrin-stabilizing factor (XIII), increased fibrinolytic activity, or interference with fibrinogen polymerization (44). Thrombin acts as a hydrolytic enzyme causing a degradation of the fibrinogen molecule into fibrin monomer and polypeptides A and B (52). Molecules of fibrin monomer join to form larger molecules of fibrin polymer to initiate clotting (44).

Minute amounts of thrombin will clot a very large amount of fibrinogen. Thrombin initiates the reactions, after which polymerization of the fibrin takes place independently. The properties of the fibrin clot depend on the pH and ionic concentrations of the medium. If these conditions are not favorable, ultimate polymerization may not occur and the intermediate polymer molecules will remain in solution without forming a gel. The presence of macroglobulins in the blood or an abnormal amount of globulin, as in multiple myeloma, causes a gelatinous clot to form that shows no retraction (9, 23, 52).

The hemorrhagic diseases caused by deficient function in phase IV fall into four categories: (*a*) Those caused by afibrinogenemia, hypofibrinogenemia, or dysfibrinogenemia; (*b*) those caused by excessive fibrinolytic activity; (*c*) those caused by dysproteinemia in which there is an interference with the formation of fibrin; and (*d*) those caused by deficiency of factor XIII, fibrin stabilizing factor.

Diffuse Intravascular Coagulation (DIC)

The diffuse intravascular coagulation (DIC) syndrome is the constellation of signs associated with the intravascular deposition of fibrin, and resulting depletion of coagulation factors and platelets (14, 26, 41, 47, 56, 64, 74). The etiology of DIC syndrome is varied.

The Intrinsic Form of DIC

Endotoxemia or other septicemias can activate factor XII which through the intrinsic system leads to formation of thrombin. Both specific and nonspecific immune reactions can be involved in DIC. Specific antiplatelet antibodies produce a breakdown of platelets, liberation of platelet factor 3, and activation of the intrinsic coagulation system. Immunologic lysis of erythrocytes by antibodies, specific for red cell antigens, also activates the intrinsic coagulation mechanism through the release of active phospholipids. The classic example of the latter is the massive intravascular hemolysis with subsequent shock that results from the transfusion of incompatible blood (27).

The Extrinsic or Fibrinolytic Form of DIC

The extrinsic system can be primarily responsible for DIC when tissue thromboplastin enters the blood stream producing widely disseminated thrombosis. Large carcinomas with central necrosis can incite DIC if the products of tumor necrosis enter the blood and act as activators of the extrinsic system (60).

Severe head injury may be associated with coagulation abnormalities which correlate best with the extent of brain injury. There is a correlation between the increase of fibrin/fibrinogen degradation products (FDP) and the clinical neurologic condition and clinical course, the latter reflecting to some extent the structural brain damage (24, 59).

Laboratory Diagnosis of DIC

The laboratory findings in acute DIC syndrome are characteristic of a profound hemostatic defect that involves abnormalities in all four phases of blood coagulation. Single tests ordered without understanding the pathophysiology are certain to be misleading (60). Given an understanding of the pathogenesis of the syndrome, the laboratory data can be cogently interpreted.

Plasma fibrinogen may be reduced to extremely low levels. Examination of blood clotting may demonstrate inability to form a clot or the lack of clot retraction. Fibrinogen screening tests may show a reduced concentration of fibrinogen which can be confirmed by the chemical determination (59). Factors II, V, and VIII are reduced in conjunction with the low concentration of fibrinogen. Factor XIII is always diminished in proportion to the reduction of fibrinogen (27). The PT and PTT demonstrate a prolonged clotting time or may show no end point at all.

The platelet count is universally reduced, sometimes to extremely low levels and at times out of proportion to the reduction of coagulation factors (59). This results from platelet aggregation and increased sequestration of aggregated platelets aggregates in the fibrin network.

Clotting of fibrinogen is accompanied by the release of fibrinopeptide split products. Their physiologic role is considerable but their diagnostic importance has been exaggerated. They contribute to the pathogenesis of DIC by their action as inhibitors of fibrinogen polymerization. Split products also interfere with platelet aggregation but this would not seem to be an adverse effect in this situation.

Differential Diagnosis

The acute syndrome of DIC usually presents little problem in diagnosis. Laboratory tests, however, must be interpreted in light of the severity and stage of the disease process. Early in the syndrome, thrombocytopenia and afibrinogenemia may be the most abnormal findings. During recovery, assuming that the initial cause of DIC has been removed, the abnormalities may return to normal at different rates. The platelet count may be higher than normal and there may be accelerated clotting during the recovery phase (39).

Hyperfibrinolytic states may resemble DIC. Increased fibrinolytic activity is seen in shock, acute hemorrhage, cirrhosis of the liver, barbiturate poisoning, methyl alcohol intoxication, and severe anxiety states, or it may be physiologic in some individuals. Hyperfibrinolysis reduced the level of factors I, II, and V. As a result, a pattern similar to that in DIC is demonstrated by hyperfibrinogenemia, a prolongation of the PT and PTT, and the presence of fibrin split products. The clotting tests are seldom as prolonged in hyperfibrinolysis as they are in DIC as the consumption of factors II and V is not as great as in intravascular coagulation. Factor VIII levels are normal in hyperfibrinolysis but decreased in DIC. The presence of fibrin split products does not distinguish one condition from the other. DIC is usually accompanied by moderate to severe thrombocytopenia. In hyperfibrinolysis syndromes the platelet count is usually normal but there is an important exception. Fibrinogen split products can cause platelet aggregation and it is possible to have thrombocytopenia when the fibrinolytic process is so severe that there is a high concentration of fibrinogen split products (42).

Therapy for DIC

Since there are many disorders and presentations associated with DIC, there is no single approach to managing these patients. The management of DIC has been re-evaluated in recent years. It remains axiomatic that treatment of the underlying disorder is essential. More emphasis has been placed on blood component replacement therapy in selected cases, while heparin therapy remains controversial. There is no controlled prospective study that demonstrates the efficacy of heparin in acute severe DIC.

Acute severe DIC associated with profound coagulation factor depletion may require selective factor repletion in order to gain time to direct therapy against the underlying disorder. The usual argument against blood component therapy in DIC is that coagulation factor repletion will fuel the fire of DIC. A distinction should be made between acute, severe coagulopathy with clotting factor depletion where factor replacement may be appropriate versus chronic compensated continuing intravascular coagulation where factor repletion is not indicated. Clotting factor assays can be done to differentiate these two conditions and to determine the need for fresh frozen plasma replacement.

It has been reported that ϵ-aminocaproic acid (EACA) blocks plasminogen activation and also neutralizes plasma. This substance has been tested in vivo in fibrinolytic states and the results are encouraging. This therapy is indicated only when the extrinsic or primary fibrinolytic syndrome is present and absolutely contraindicated when fibrinolysis is secondary to the intrinsic form of DIC.

The Prethrombotic (Hypercoagulable) State

While it would be ideal to detect patients who are at risk for thrombosis, a sensitive and specific test for a hypercoagulable state is not yet available (5, 27, 49). Some of the abnormalities in blood parameters found in established thrombosis are the result, not the cause, of thrombus formation.

The two most common situations predisposing to venous thrombosis with the risk of pulmonary embolism are malignancies and surgical procedures. The association of malignancy with thrombosis has been reported many times, especially in carcinoma of the pancreas where the incidence of venous thromosis may be as high at 50%. Cancer of the lung, ovary, or stomach also have a high incidence of venous thromosis. The high incidence of thrombosis in mucin-producing carcinomas is attributed to the activation of factor X by mucin. Tumor extracts other than mucin also activate factor X directly (66).

Thrombosis is one of the complications of the postoperative state. The incidence following neurosurgical procedures may be as high as 25%. Predisposing factors are previous venous thrombosis, varicose veins, obesity, malignancy, and age (47).

Thrombocytosis is an indication of a prethrombotic state and may in fact be the only platelet abnormality unequivocally related to thrombosis. Platelet adhesiveness and platelet aggregation are difficult to evaluate. With respect to coagulation factors no consistent relationship has been found between increased levels and either established or impending thrombosis.

The APTT may have some predictive value. An APTT of less than 28 seconds, with a reagent giving a mean normal of 30 seconds, is a good indication that there is a risk of thrombosis in postoperative patients (27).

Activation of the fibrinolytic system is one of the natural mechanisms for minimizing thrombus or for dissolving thrombi. There is normally a balance between fibrinogen, fibrin, and fibrin monomers which is shifted toward fibrin monomers at sites of incipient fibrin deposition. Reduced fibrinolytic activity then favors thrombus deposition. Reduced fibrinolytic activity may be caused by an increase in inhibitors of plasmin. There is good evidence that reduced fibrinolytic activity may precede thrombosis and thus may be useful in detecting the prethrombotic state. Decreased fibrinolytic activity has been found in women taking oral contraceptives, in pregnancy, in postoperative patients, and in obesity.

Venous thrombosis is not the only risk to neurosurgical patients. Arterial thrombosis and subsequent embolization may severely compromise neurologic function. Antithrombotic therapy and therapy designed to selectively "dissolve" arterial thrombi are areas of intensive investigation.

TRANSFUSIONS

A blood group system is a series of antigens controlled by allelic genes inherited independently of other genes. Blood group antigens are clinically significant if they elicit antibodies following transfusion, or if they react with antibodies in such a way that in vivo hemolysis occurs. The ABO and Rh systems dominate, and although others exist, they rarely cause clinical problems (53).

Transfusions of whole blood or various blood components should be administered to correct the exact deficiencies needed by the patient. Tables 6.2 and 6.3 summarize the use of blood and components in transfusion therapy (44).

Circulating blood consists of plasma, red cells, white cells, and platelets. Modern blood bank technology permits the separation of individual components from whole blood, so the indiscriminant use of whole blood is no longer required nor justified. The blood component most likely to correct a specific deficiency can be administered. The distinction between red blood cell loss and volume loss must be recognized in order to minimize the dangers of transfusion. In severe hemorrhage, there may be a severe reduction in red blood cell mass that impairs oxygen-carrying capacity. In the majority of cases, however, correction of hypovolemia alone is effective therapy for hemorrhagic shock. Volume replacement alone is usually sufficient unless the hematocrit is less than 30%. Solutions of albumin or of less purified plasma proteins are used for volume expansion. When properly prepared, they carry virtually no risk of hepatitis. Volume expansion can also be accomplished with colloid "plasma expanders" such as dextran 40 and hydroxyethyl starch suspended in normal saline. These agents have no risk of transmitting hepatitis, but can be associated with platelet dysfunction and the total volume administered should not exceed the recommended maximum allowance over a 24-hour period.

Since neither white cells nor platelets survive refrigeration, stored whole blood consists functionally of red cells in plasma. Patients with adequate blood volume, but deficient hemoglobin, derive little benefit from plasma or transfused whole blood. Patients whose cardiac function is precarious may suffer congestive heart failure if given whole blood (44). A red cell preparation has the oxygen-carrying capacity of the original unit without plasma. Transfused red cells must lack antigens to which the recipient has antibodies. If anti-A is present, A or AB cells cannot be given. The same applies to B or AB cells in a patient with anti-B. The concept of group O as the universal donor applies to red cells but not whole blood. It is good practice to give group specific blood at all times. When this is impractical, group A or group B recipients can receive O red cells and AB recipients can receive cells of any type. O recipients can receive only group O blood. Since Rh antibodies are not naturally occurring, no immediate harm will result in giving Rh positive blood to an Rh negative patient.

Glycerol is commonly used to prevent damage to red cell membranes. Glycerol removes all traces of plasma and nearly all the platelets and white cells. Patients severely immunized to plasma proteins or white blood cells usually tolerate transfusion of deglycerolized red cells (44).

Two kinds of platelet preparations are available. One is a single unit of concentrate that contains approximately 70% of the original platelets suspended in a small amount of plasma, and the other is a thrombocytophoresis concentrate that contains platelets from the equivalent of six units of blood, all obtained from a single donor by means of hemophoresis procedures (43, 63).

When platelets are given to a bleeding patient, the therapeutic effect is measured by im-

TABLE 6.2
Treatment of Acute Coagulation Disorders

Disorder	Specific Therapy	Dose
Thrombocytopenia (patient not receiving heparin)	Platelet concentrate	1 donor unit/kg of body weight
Thrombocytopenia (heparin-induced)		
Without new thrombosis	Discontinue heparin	As above
	Platelet concentrate (if bleeding not controlled by discontinuing heparin)	
With new thrombosis or abnormal platelet aggregation response to heparin	Discontinue heparin [including intravenous (IV) capping solutions and flushes]	
	Start one of the following anti-aggregates:	
	Dextran	25 ml/hr continuous IV
	Acetylsalicylic acid	5 gr every 12 hr
	Dipyridamole (Persantine)	50 mg three times daily
	Sulfinpyrazone (Anturane)	200 mg three times daily
Multiple plasma coagulation factor deficiencies	Fresh frozen plasma	As needed
Disseminated intravascular coagulation (DIC)	Whole blood, crystalloid, or packed red blood cells	As needed to restore blood volume, red cell mass
	Definitive therapy of underlying cause, e.g. antibiotics for sepsis, uterine evacuation for abruptio placenta	
	Heparin (if DIC not controlled by definitive therapy)	2,000 units every 4 hr IV
	Fresh frozen plasma	As needed
	Platelet concentrate	As needed
Primary fibrinolysis	ϵ-Aminocaproic acid (Amicar)	5 g IV, followed by 1 g/hr IV for 2–3 hr, then 1 g/2 hr per os or IV
	Note: Amicar is absolutely contraindicated in DIC	
Heparin	Protamine sulfate	25–50 mg/vol control if thrombin time remains prolonged, repeat initial dose.
Warfarin (Coumadin)	Phytonadione (Aquamephyton)	25–50 mg
Platelet anti-aggregates	Discontinue drug(s)	
	Platelet concentrate (if bleeding is not controlled by discontinuing drug	1 donor unit/kg of body weight
Vitamin K deficiency	Menadiol sodium disphosphate (Synkayvite)	10–15 mg 4 times daily for 7 days
	Phytonadione	10–15 mg 4 times daily for 7 days
Antithrombin III deficiency	Fresh frozen plasma	2 units, followed by 1 unit every 12 hr
	Heparin	Usual systemic treatment

TABLE 6.3
Blood Components for Transfusion (Widmann)

Component	Composition	Indication	Special Considerations
Whole blood	450 ml of blood 63 ml of coagulant	Volume deficit associated with hypoxia or low red cells mass	Must be ABO compatible Must be cross-matched Risk of volume overload
Red blood cells (RBC)	250–350 ml Hematocrit 70–80%	Symptomatic anemia Low red cell mass	Must be ABO compatible Must be cross-matched
Deglycerolized frozen red cells	−200 ml of red cells Few white cells or platelets	Red cell transfusion in patients with RBC antibodies, or reactions to white blood cells	Must be ABO compatible Must be cross-matched Very high cost
Fresh frozen plasma	200–300 ml of plasma All coagulation factors No platelets	Coagulation disorders	Should be ABO compatible Risk of allergic reaction
Cryoprecipitate	80–100 units factor VIII in 10–15 ml of plasma −250 mg of fibrinogen 10	Factor VIII deficiency von Willebrand's disease Fibrinogen deficiency	Many units needed to provide massive factor replacement
Platelet concentrate	5.5 × 10 platelets in −50 ml of plasma (random donor) 11 3 × 10 platelets in −300 ml of plasma (single donor thrombocytopheresis) 10	Platelet deficiency	Preferably ABO compatible May elicit HLA antibodies
Granulocyte concentrate	10 granulocytes in 300–500 ml of plasma −25 ml RBCs	Bacterial sepsis severely granulocytopenic patient	Should be ABO compatible Frequent occurrence in febrile reactions

proved hemostasis, not solely by improved laboratory values. If DIC has caused bleeding and a low platelet count, transfused platelets will suffer the same entrapment and destruction. Platelet transfusions produce only slight clinical improvement, if any, in DIC. Similarly, patients with large spleens or with autoimmune platelet destruction derive little benefit from transfused platelets. Infection or high fever from any cause also reduces the survival of transfused platelets. It is desirable, but not essential, that platelets and platelet plasma be ABO compatible. HLA antibodies elicited from past transfusions damage platelets far more than do ABO antibodies (63).

Coagulation factor deficiencies require specific replacement. Fresh frozen plasma is a good source of labile coagulation factors (44). It has the same hepatitis risk as whole blood and may contain antibodies against the recipients' white blood cells or plasma proteins. Coagulation factor concentrates carry a substantial risk of hepatitis and autoimmune deficiency syndrome (AIDS) because pooling plasma from a large number of donors multiplies the risk. Factor VIII concentrates have a moderately high risk while concentration of the "liver factors" (factor IX concentrate, prothrombin concentrate) carries a very high risk. Transfusion products from plasma of individual donors have a low risk of disease transmission. Cryoprecipitate is a residue obtained by freezing and slowly thawing freshly drawn plasma that contains 80 to 100 IU of factor VIII and about 250 mg of fibrinogen in a volume of 10 to 15 ml. Cryoprecipitate is used for treating minor or moderate bleeds in patients with factor VIII deficiency. If very high factor VIII concentrates are needed, as for life-threatening hemorrhage or surgical procedures, the commercial concentrates are more convenient and more effective. Cryoprecipitate is the only transfusion product that contains concentrated fibrinogen. It is also the best available source of von Willebrand factor, which is not present in commercial concentrates of factor VIII (44).

Adverse Reactions of Transfusions

Despite major advances in transfusion technology, most blood components and products remain capable of inflicting serious and occasionally lethal harm upon the recipient. Even careful adherence to current standards and use of the most sophisticated tests will not completely prevent such complications as hepatitis, delayed hemolytic reactions, AIDS, or anaphylaxis (72).

Most complications can be categorized by etiology as immunologic, infectious, metabolic, physical, or thromboembolic. Acute hemolytic transfusion reactions (AHTR) are among the worst transfusion complications. Human error is primarily responsible for these avoidable immunologic mishaps. The frequency of AHTRs has been reported to be from 1 per 541 units to 1 per 6,200 units transfused and mortality varies from 17% to 53% (72).

AHTRs are heralded by subjective complaints of palpitations, substernal pressure or flank pain, and objective changes of an increase in temperature and decrease in blood pressure. These symptoms result from widespread interaction between antibodies and antigens. DIC and a generalized bleeding tendency may develop. As red cells are destroyed, hemoglobin is released into the plasma and excreted in the urine. Hemoglobinuria, by itself, does not damage the kidney, but renal failure can result from the combined effects of sudden hypotension, massive antigen-antibody reaction, and the presence of hemoglobin in the glomerular filtrate. Damage is especially likely if flow rates are low and the urine is highly concentrated. Urine output should be maintained at a level of 1,000 ml/hr for 6 to 24 hours. Furosemide, 80 to 120 mg intravenously (IV) may be superior to mannitol because it increases renal cortical blood flow and thus lessens the risk of vascular stasis and thrombosis. For the treatment of severe shock, dopamine hydrochloride is useful in doses of 0.1 μg/kg/min IV. Dopamine acts as an α-adrenergic vasopressor that restores blood pressure and its β-adrenergic function increases cardiac output. It has the capacity to enhance renal cortical blood flow, resulting in increased sodium ion excretion, increased glomerular filtration rate (GFR), and elevated renal plasma flow (72).

The term, delayed hemolytic transfusion reaction (DHTR), should be restricted to hemolysis resulting from a secondary anamnestic antibody response, although both acute hemolytic reactions and primary immunization are occasionally labeled as DHTRs. The antibody screen or indirect antiglobulin (Coombs') test becomes positive near the time that clinical hemolysis is noted (15). The most important finding is a positive direct antiglobulin [Coombs' test (direct antiglobulin test)] on the patient's post-transfusion red cell sample. Usually within 4 to 8 days after the transfusion, the red cell antibody attains sufficient levels in the peripheral circulation to produce clinical and laboratory evidence of hemolysis.

The classic febrile nonhemolytic (FNA) episode results from infusion of donor leukocytes into a patient whose plasma contains leukoagglutinins. Patients receiving granulocyte transfusions are particularly at risk. A second form of reaction to antileukocyte antibodies results from the passive administration of donor plasma containing high titered leukoagglutinins incompatable with recipient's leukocytes. White blood cells, FFP, and pheresis products contain antibodies that induce severe and occasionally fatal reactions, characterized by fever, chills, dyspnea, and a nonproductive cough. The accumulation of pulmonary interstitial fluid is demonstrated by chest x-ray.

Urticaria is a very common but benign transfusion reaction consisting of a purpuric rash with irregular raised red blotches that vary in size and extent. Simple reactions do not require laboratory investigation. The transfusion should be slowed or stopped and an intramuscular injection of antihistamine administered prior to resumption in 15 to 30 minutes. In most cases the etiology is unknown (72).

Although anaphylactic transfusion reactions are fortunately rare, the outcome may be fatal. In a typical reaction, a transfusion of only a few milliliters leads to the sudden onset of generalized flushing, bronchospasm, laryngeal edema, difficulty breathing, dyspnea, cyanosis, substernal pain, severe gastrointestinal distress with abdominal cramps, vomiting or diarrhea, transient mild hypertension followed by extreme hypotension, shock, and chills without fever. The rapid onset of gastrointestinal symptoms, with or without shock in the absence of a fever, helps distinguish anaphylactic reactions from those due to leukoagglutinins, hemolysis, or bacterial sepsis. In contrast to many other types of transfusion reactions, such events often occur in patients with no previous history of transfusion. The most frequently recognized cause is an interaction between infused IgA and a class specific anti-IgA in the patient's plasma. Laboratory evaluation is difficult because demonstration of anti-IgA requires agglutination of red cells coated with chromic chloride coupled IgA monoclonal antibody (72).

Prompt treatment is imperative when clinical findings indicate anaphylaxis. The transfusion must be stopped immediately, but the IV line must be kept open and maintained with continuous infusion of isotonic fluids. Epinephrine may be administered subcutaneously as 0.4 mg of a 1:1,000 solution or intravenously over 10 minutes as 0.1 ml of 1:1,000 solution diluted into 10 mg of normal saline or Ringer's lactate.

Other complications of blood transfusion include hypothermia, circulatory overload, congestive heart failure, and potentially lethal pulmonary edema. These complications occur particularly in patients with long-standing severe anemia or borderline myocardial function, who are transfused too rapidly. Onset may be immediate or delayed up to 24 hours.

Hepatitis has been a major complication of transfusion reactions. Three types are identified. Hepatitis A or infectious hepatitis, hepatitis B, and non-A, non-B hepatitis (NANB). NANB hepatitis emerged as the major agent in post-transfusion hepatitis during the late 1970's and early 1980's. Efforts to identify specific serologic markers or to isolate the virus have proven unsuccessful to date. The incidence is reported as high as 10% after transfusion. It is usually mild and requires no treatment (1, 2). An important and striking feature of NANB hepatitis is the marked tendency for variable and often chronic elevations of trans-amylase levels, frequently accompanied by morphologic evidence suggesting chronic liver disease. Until specific tests are available, the recognition of NANB hepatitis remains a diagnosis of exclusion with more than one causative organism probably responsible for the spectrum of the disease (72).

AIDS has recently emerged as a major concern with regard to transmission by transfusion. The HTLV-III screening test may lessen the incidence of transmission by contaminated blood.

The administration of blood and its various components are a critical part of the management of the neurosurgical intensive care patient. Blood flow and oxygen-carrying capacity as it relates to various intracranial processes have been central to this discussion. An understanding of what is being given, why it is being given, plus a thorough understanding of the patient's overall condition is critical to appropriate management. Only the neurosurgeon is in a position to weigh the risks and benefits in these various conditions as it relates to the functional outcome of CNS activity.

REFERENCES

1. Aach, R. D., and Kahn, R. A. Post transfusion hepatitis: Current perspectives. Ann. Intern. Med., *92:* 539, 1980.
2. Alter, H. J., *et al.* Non-A non-B hepatitis: A review and interim report of an ongoing prospective study. In: *Viral Hepatitis*, edited by G. N. Vyas, S. N. Cohen, and R. Schmid, pp. 359–369. Franklin Institute Press, Philadelphia, 1978.
3. Astrup, J., Siesjo, B. K., and Symon, L. Thresholds in cerebral ischemia—the ischemic penumbra. Stroke *12:* 723–725, 1981.
4. Bailey, E. L., Harper, R. A., and Pinkerton, P. H. The therapeutic range of the one-stage prothrombin time in the control of anticoagulant therapy: The effect of different thromboplastic preparations. Can. Med. Assoc. J., *105:* 1044, 1971.
5. Barritt, D. W., and Jordon, S. C. Anticoagulant drugs in the treatment of thromboembolism. Lancet, *1:* 1309–1312, 1960.
6. Beck, W. S. Folic acid deficiency. In: *Hematology*, edited by W. J. Williams, *et al.*, Ed. 3, pp. 334–355. McGraw-Hill, New York, 1983.
7. Bentley, A. S. A. An overview of granulopoiesis laboratory hemology. In: *Hematology*, edited by W. J. Williams, *et al.*, Ed. 3, Chapt. 9, Book 2. McGraw-Hill, New York, 1983.
8. Blanchard, R. A., Furie, B. C., Jorgensen, M., *et al.* Acquired vitamin-K-dependent carboxylation deficiency in liver disease. N. Engl. J. Med., *305:* 242–248, 1981.
9. Cash, J. D. Control mechanisms of activator release. In: *Progress in Chemical Fibrinolysis and Thrombolysis*, edited by J. F. Davison, R. M. Rowan, M. M. Samama, and P. C. Desnoyer, Vol. 3, p. 65. Raven Press, New York, 1978.
10. Chesney, C. M., Pifer, D., and Colman, R. W. Subcellular localization and secretion of factor V from human platelets. Proc. Natl. Acad. Sci. U.S.A., *78:* 5180, 1981.
11. Coller, B. S., and Grainick, H. R. Studies on the mechanism of restocetin-induced platelet aggregation. J. Clin. Invest., *60:* 302, 1977.
12. Colman, N., and Herbert, V. Hematologic complications of alcoholism: Overview. Semin. Hematol., *17:* 164, 1980.
13. Colman, R. W. Activation of plasminogen by human plasma kallikrein. Biochem. Biophys. Res. Comm., *31:* 273, 1969.
14. Colman, R. W., Robboy, S. J., and Ninna, J. D. Disseminated intravascular coagulation: A reappraisal. Am. Rev. Med., *30:* 359, 1979.
15. Coombs, R. R. A., Mourant, A. E., and Race, R. R. A new test for the detection of weak and "incomplete" Rh agglutinins. Br. J. Exp. Pathol., *16:* 255, 1945.
16. Cooper, H. A., Clementson, J. J., and Luscherm, E. F. Human platelet membrane receptor for bovine von Willebrand factor (platelet aggregating factor): An integral membrane glycoprotein. Proc. Natl. Acad. Sci. U.S.A., *76:* 1069, 1979.
17. Damus, P. S., Hicks, M., and Rosenberg, R. D. Anticoagulant action of heparin. Nature (Lond.), *246:* 355, 1973.
18. Deck, P., and O'Grady, L. F., Anemia associated with liver disease and endocrine disorders. In: *Laboratory Hematology*, edited by J. A. Koepke, Chap. 5, Book 2. Churchill, Livingstone, New York, 1984.
19. Douglas, A. S., and McNicol, G. P. Anticoagulant therapy. In: *Human Blood Coagulation. Haemostasis and Thrombosis,* edited by R. Biggs, Ed. 2, p. 557. Blackwell, Oxford, 1976.
20. Egan, E. L., Bowie, E. J. W., Kasimer, F. J., *et al.* Effect of surgical operations on certain tests used to diagnose intravascular coagulation fibrinolysis. Mayo Clin. Proc., *49:* 658, 1974.
21. Fauci, A. S., Haynes, B. F., and Katz, P. The spectrum of vasculitis: Clinical, pathologic, immunologic, and therapeutic considerations. Ann. Intern. Med., *89:* 660, 1978.
22. Fisher, J. W., Lertora, J. J. L., Lindholm, D. D. *et al.* Erythropoietin production and inhibitors in serum in the anemia of uremia. Proc. Clin. Dial. Transplant Forum, *3:* 22, 1973.
23. Frick, P. G. Acute hemorrhagic syndrome with hypofibrinogenemia in metastatic cancer. Acta Haematol., *16:* 11, 1956.
24. Goodnight, W. S., Kenoyer, G., Rapaport, S. I., *et al.* Definition after brain-tissue destruction. N. Engl. J. Med., *290:* 1043, 1974.
25. Guyton, A. C. *Textbook of Medical Physiology*, Ed. 7, pp. 493–502. W. B. Saunders, Philadelphia, 1986.
26. Harkness, D. R. Hematological and clinical factors of sickle cell diseases: A review. Hemoglobin, *4:* 313, 1980.
27. Harlan, J. M., and Harker, L. A. Hemostasis, thrombosis and thromboembolic disorders. Med. Clin. North Am., *65:* 855, 1981.
28. Hillman, R. S. Acute blood loss. In: *Hematology*, edited by W. J. Williams, *et al.*, Ed. 3, pp. 618–623. McGraw-Hill, New York, 1983.
29. Holsen, H. Mechanisms of platelet secretion. In: *Platelets Cellular Response Mechanisms and Their Biological Significance*, edited by A. Rotman, F. A. Meyer, C. Gitler, and A. Silberberg, p. 249. Wiley, New York, 1980.
30. Jackson, C. M., and Suttie, J. W. Recent developments in understanding the mechanisms of vitamin K and vitamin K antagonist drug action and the consequences of vitamin K action in blood coagulation. In: *Progress in Haematology*, edited by E. B. Brown, pp. 333–359. Grune & Stratton, New York, 1977.
31. Jaffe, R., and Deykin, D. Platelet aggregation by different types of collagen. Circulation, *49–50* (suppl. 3)*:* 289, 1974.
32. Jesty J., Maynard, J. B., Radcliff, R. D., *et al.* Intiation and control of the extrinsic pathway of blood coagulation. In: *Proteases and Biological Control*, edited by E. Riech, D. B. Rifkin, and E. Shaw, p.

171. Cold Spring Harbor Laboratory, Cold Spring Harbor, New York, 1975.

33. Kao, K. J., Pizzo, S. V., and McKee, P. A. Demonstration and characterization of specific binding sites for Factor VIII/von Willebrand factor on human platelets. J. Clin. Invest., *63:* 656, 1979.

34. Kee, D. B. Jr., and Wood, J. H. Rheology of the cerebral circulation. Neurosurgy, *15:* 125–131, 1984.

35. Kepke, J. A., Triplett, D. A., and Banez, G. The partial thromboplastin time for monitoring heparin therapy. In: *Chemistry and Biology of Heparin*, edited by R. Lindblad, *et al.*, p. 625. Elsevier North-Holland, New York, 1981.

36. Lewis, J. P. An overview of erythropoiesis. In: *Laboratory Hematology*, edited by J. K. Koepke, Chap. 1. Churchill Livingstone, New York, Edinburgh, London, and Melbourne, 1984.

37. Lewis, J. P., and Meyers, F. J. The anemia of renal insufficiency. In: *Laboratory Hematology*, edited by J. K. Koepke, Chap. 4. Churchill Livingstone, New York, Edinburgh, London, and Melbourne, 1984.

38. Lindebaum, J. Folate and vitamin B_{12} deficiencies in alcoholism. Semin. Hematol., *17:* 119, 1980.

39. Mant, M. J., and King, E. G. Severe acute disseminated intravascular coagulation. A reappraisal of its pathophysiology, clinical significance and therapy based on 47 patients. Am. J. Med., *67:* 557, 1979.

40. McConnell, D. J. Inhibitors of kallikrein in human plasma. J. Clin. Invest., *51:* 1611, 1972.

41. Merskey, C., Johnson, A. J., Kleiner, G. J., *et al.* The defibrination syndrome, clinical features and laboratory diagnosis. Br. J. Haematol., *13:* 529, 1967.

42. Merskey, C., Kleiner, G. J., and Johnson, A. J. Quantitative estimation of split products of fibrinogen in human serum, relation to diagnosis and treatment. Blood *28:* 1, 1966.

43. Miale, J. B. *Laboratory Medicine Hematology*, Chap. 12. C. V. Mosby Company, St. Louis, Toronto, London, 1982.

44. Miale, J. B. *Laboratory Medicine Hematology* Chap. 17. C. V. Mosby Company, St. Louis, Toronto, London, 1982.

45. Mills, D. C. B. Adenylate cyclase system in human platelets. In: *Platelets and Thrombosis*, edited by S. Sherry and A. Scriabine, p. 45. University Park Press, Baltimore, 1974.

46. Milner, P. F. The clinical effects of HbS, an overview. In: *The Function of Red Blood Cells: Erythrocyte Pathobiology*, edited by D. F. H. Wallach, pp. 297-300. Alan R. Liss, New York, 1981.

47. Minna, J. D., Robboy, S. J., and Coman, R. W. *Disseminated Intravascular Coagulation in Man.* Charles C Thomas, Springfield, IL, 1974.

48. Myhre, B. A., and Nakasako, R. Graphs to facilitate the computation of patient response to platelet concentrates or antihemophiliac concentrate. Transfusion *17:* 179, 1977.

49. Penner, J. A. Hypercoagulation and thrombosis. Med. Clin. North Am., *64:* 743, 1980.

50. Petz, L. D. Drug induced immune haemolytic anemia. Clin. Haematol., *9:* 455, 1980.

51. Phillips, D. R. An overview of coagulation. In: *Laboratory Hematology*, edited by J. K. Koepke, Chap. 20. Churchill, Livingstone, New York, Edinburgh, London and Melbournc, 1984.

52. Pizzo, S. V. *An Overview of Coagulation in Laboratory Hematology*, edited by J. K. Koepke, Chap. 20. Churchill, Livingstone, New York, Edinburgh, London, Melbourne, 1984.

53. Race, R. R., and Sanger, R. *Blood Groups in Man*, Ed. 6. Blackwell Scientific Publications, Oxford, 1975.

54. Radtke, H. W., Claussner, A., Erbes, P. M. *et al.* Serum erythropoietin concentration in chronic renal failure: Relationship to degree of anemia and excretory renal function. Blood, *54:* 877, 1979.

55. Reisner, H. Diagnosis and therapy of von Willebrand's disease. In: *Laboratory Hematology*, edited by J. K. Koepke, Chap. 22. Churchill Livingstone, New York, Edinburgh, London, and Melbourne, 1984.

56. Robboy, S. J., Colman, R. W., and Minna, J. D. Pathology of disseminated intravascular coagulation (DIC): Analysis of twenty-six cases. Hum. Pathol., *3:* 327, 1972.

57. Rosse, W. F. The hemolytic anemias. In: *Laboratory Hematology*, edited by J. K. Koepke, Chap. 7. Churchill Livingstone, New York, Edinburgh, London and Melbourne, 1984.

58. Saito, H. Normal hemostatic mechanisms. In: *Disorders of Hemostasis*. edited by O. D. Ratnoff, C. D. Forbes, pp. 22–42. Grune & Stratton, New York, 1984.

59. Sande, J. J., van der, Veltkamp, J. J., Boekhout, Mussert, F. J., *et al.* Head injury and coagulation disorders. J. Neurosurg., *94:* 357, 1978.

60. Schmaier, A. H., and Colman, R. W. Disseminated intravascular coagulation: An approach to management including the use of blood component therapy. Standardization of coagulation assays. In: *College of American Pathologists*, edited by D. A. Triplett, p. 353. In: American Society of Clinical Pathologists: "Laboratory Evaluation of Coagulation," Skokie, IL, 1982.

61. Schmaier, A. H., Shapira, M., and Colman, R. W. Methodology to study the proteins of the contact phase of coagulation. In: *Disorders of Thrombin Formation*, edited by R. W. Colman. Churchill Livingstone, New York, 1982.

62. Shattil, S. J., and Bennett, J. S. Platelets and their membranes in hemostasis: Physiology and pathophysiology. Ann. Intern. Med., *94:* 108–118, 1981.

63. Slichter, S. J. Controversies in platelet transfusion therapy. Annu. Rev. Med., *31:* 509–540, 1980.

64. Spero, J. A., Lewis, J. H., and Hasiba, U. Disseminated intravascular coagulation. Findings in 346 patients. Thromb. Haemost., *43:* 28, 1980.

65. Strand, T., Splund, K., Eriksson, S., Haag, E., Lithner, F., and Wester, P. O. A randomized controlled trial of hemodilution therapy in acute ischemic stroke. Stroke, *15:* 980–989, 1984.

66. Sun, N. C. J., Bowie, E. J. W., Kazmer, F. J., *et al.* Blood coagulation studies in patients with cancer. Mayo Clin. Proc., *49:* 626, 1974.

67. Taylor, F. G. (Eds.). *The Regulation of Coagulation.* Elsevier/North-Holland, New York, 1980.

68. Wallner, S. F., and Vautrin, R. M., Evidence that inhibition of erythropoiesis is important in the anemia of chronic renal failure. J. Lab. Clin. Med., *87:* 170, 1981.
69. Weinstein, M., and Deykin, D. Comparison of factor VIII-related von Willebrand factor proteins prepared from human cryoprecipitate and factor VIII concentrate. Blood, *53:* 1095, 1979.
70. Weiss, H. J. Platelet physiology and abnormalities of platelet function. N. Engl. J. Med., *293:* 531, 1975.
71. Weiss, H. J. Antiplatelet therapy. N. Engl. J. Med., *298:* 1344–1347, 1981.
72. Widman, F. K. Immunohematology and blood banking In: Clinical Interpretation of Laboratory Tests, edited by F. K. Widman, Ed. 9, Chap. 7. F. A. Davis, Philadelphia, 1983.
73. Wiggens, R. C., Bouma, B. N., Cochrane, C. G., and Griffin, J. H. Role of high molecular-weight kininogen in surface-binding and activation of coagulation factor XI and prekallikrein. Proc. Natl. Acad. Sci. U.S.A., *74:* 4636, 1977.
74. Yoshikawa, T., Kouichi, R., Tanaka, M. D., *et al.* Infection and disseminated intravascular coagulation. Medicine, *50:* 237, 1971.

CHAPTER 7

Infection: Prevention and Management

JULIAN T. HOFF, M.D., DENNIS SCHABERG, M.D. and JOHN McGILLICUDDY, M.D.

HOST-ORGANISM RELATIONSHIPS

Whether an infection develops after exposure to an organism depends upon the resistance of the host and the virulence of the organism (30). If the host has a competent immune system and the quantity and quality of the inoculum is insufficient to overcome that system, then infection fails to develop. Conversely, if the host is unusually susceptible, because of an underlying illness or a depressed immune system, then infection may occur (9). Sometimes infection will develop if the normal host is exposed to large quantities of virulent organisms that simply overwhelm host defences, or sometimes ubiquitous and nonvirulent organisms under normal circumstances become pathogenic when they multiply in hosts with compromised immunity. Microbial resistance to antibiotics is an evolving and persistent problem, indicating that infections will continue to develop from increasingly resistant organisms (42).

Debilitating illnesses, massive trauma, the injudicious use of steroids and antibiotics, and the increasing use of immunosuppressant drugs all contribute to the imbalance that is necessary for many infections to develop. Acquired immune deficiency syndrome (AIDS) and chemotherapeutic regimens for malignancies also contribute significantly to the increasing spectrum of CNS infections encountered by neurosurgical practitioners. Thus, mixed bacterial infections are diagnosed more often today than ever before, and infections by ubiquitous organisms such as fungi and some viruses are no longer rare (62).

PREDISPOSING FACTORS FOR SYSTEMIC INFECTION IN CRITICALLY ILL PATIENTS

Due to the severity of underlying illness, a variety of indwelling devices are necessary for management of critically ill patients to ensure optimum care. Unfortunately, important components of modern therapy such as endotracheal tubes, intravenous pressure monitoring lines, Foley catheters, and intracranial pressure monitors carry risks of microbial invasion. The specialized care these patients require also contributes to increased risks for infection. The demands of caring for the critically ill patient have led to the development of intensive care units (ICUs), functionally concentrating high risk patients in small geographic areas. This concentration of ill patients contributes to the spread of organisms from patient to patient, especially multiple-drug-resistant pathogens such as *Serratia marcescens* and *Pseudomonas aeruginosa* (18). The approach to control infection thus involves efforts to minimize risk, prevent cross-infection, ensure optimum aseptic technique, and institute prompt therapy when infection develops.

Respiratory Infections

Pneumonia can be the most serious infection in the ICU setting. Depressed levels of consciousness coupled with the need for endotracheal intubation frequently encountered in the neurosurgical setting predispose to the development of pulmonary infection. Gram-negative bacilli, often resistant to many antimicrobial drugs, emerge as important pathogens further complicating management. Aspiration of oropharyngeal organisms is generally the route of infection. Critically ill patients acquire Gram-negative organisms in the oropharynx soon after admission to the hospital. This consistent acquisition of potential pathogens reduces the reliability of sputum culture alone for the diagnosis of specific varieties of pneumonia (35).

Fever, rales, and peripheral leukocytosis are usually noted. Cough is rare due to the depressed level of consciousness. Increasing hypoxemia is common. Chest roentgenograms may show a new infiltrate, but other underlying pulmonary processes make x-ray interpretation difficult. A good sputum Gram stain with few contaminating squamous epithelial cells is essential and often provides valuable information for management. The presence of a large number of neutrophils supports the diagnosis of pneumonia and a predominant organism can usually be seen. *Staphylococcus aureus* can be encountered as a cause of pulmonary infection in this setting and the presence of organisms morphologically compatible with *S. aureus* influences the choice of antibiotics. Regimens selected for the more commonly encountered Gram-negative pathogens are not usually optimum for staphylococcal disease.

Although not helpful in diagnosis, treatment of pneumonia can be guided by sputum culture results. Pending culture results, knowledge of local epidemiology is often useful in selecting initial therapy. As Gram-negative organisms usually predominate on sputum stains, a variety of pathogens are possible. Often a particular organism will "circulate" in an ICU; awareness of its expected antimicrobial susceptibility should guide early therapy. If no predominant organism is encountered in a particular ICU, a common approach is to treat empirically for the most difficult possible organism, *P. aeruginosa*, pending culture results. Thus, an antipseudomonal penicillin in combination with an aminoglycoside is recommended. Vigorous pulmonary toilet and adequate hydration are important adjunctive measures. Despite aggressive therapy, mortality remains high for ICU-acquired pneumonia. Attempts to prevent pulmonary infection may often be unsuccessful.

Sinusitus can be a difficult process to diagnose in critically ill patients unable to complain of pain or tenderness. Thus, nosocomial sinusitus should be considered in patients at risk with unexplained fever and leukocytosis (11). Major risk factors include nasotracheal and nasogastric tubes, especially if intubation is prolonged. A transnasal tube can cause disease by blockage of sinus ostia. Skull fractures and nasal packing also contribute through the same mechanism. Traditional upper respiratory pathogens *Haemophilus influenzae* and *Streptococcus pneumoniae* can be involved, but nosocomial Gram-negative pathogens are also common.

Genitourinary Infections

Infections of the urinary tract are common in the ICU setting and may be the focus for secondary bacteremia. Bladder catheterization and urinary instrumentation are the prime factors responsible for the development of bacteriuria. The risk of infection is correlated with the duration of bladder catheterization and lack of maintenance of a closed urinary drainage system (39). Every effort should be made to minimize the duration of catheterization. Urine specimens should be aspirated from the proximal portion of the catheter and the collecting bag should be dependent to minimize infection risk. The use of prophylactic antimicrobials and antibiotics are not effective for maintaining sterility of indwelling catheters. Urinalysis and culture remain the cornerstones of diagnosis. The most common infecting pathogens are the enteric Gram-negative rods, *P. aeruginosa* and the enterococci. Therapy for *P. aeruginosa* is generally adequate for the other commonly encountered pathogens until culture results indicate more selective antibiotic treatment.

Bacteremia

Bacteremia in the severely ill patient is most often secondary to a focus in the urinary tract, skin, soft tissue, or lungs. When no obvious focus can be identified, it is sometimes termed "primary" bacteremia. An infected intravascular device should be suspected. Organisms such as *S. aureus*, *Staphylococcus epidermidis*, and Candida species should especially suggest "line" sepsis.

Intravascular catheters are easily overlooked as a cause of sepsis in the complicated patient. Many infections are preventable. The time a peripheral line is in place at one site is directly related to the chance of sepsis. The care in placement is also a factor (56). Central lines are commonly placed under emergency conditions. If so, note should be made and the line replaced under more controlled, aseptic conditions as soon as feasible.

The diagnosis of catheter-associated bacteremia is likely when the organism clears from the bloodstream on removal of the device, but newer culture methods provide even better supporting evidence. The semiquantitative culture methods proposed by Maki et al. (47), consisting of rolling the catheter tip on solid agar media, is very helpful. If more than 15 colonies are identified on the plate, the withdrawn catheter is highly likely to be the source of the bacteremia. Common causes of bacteremia in this setting include Gram-negative bacilli and Staphylococcus species. One approach to presumptive therapy for suspected bacteremia due to an intravascular device combines an aminoglycoside with vancomycin, the latter agent to provide activity for *S. epidermidis* as well as the increasingly important methicillin-resistant *S. aureus* isolates encountered in many hospitals. Therapy is then adjusted when culture and sensitivity results are available.

BACTERIAL INFECTIONS OF THE CENTRAL NERVOUS SYSTEM

Subgaleal Abscess

Localized infection between the galea of the scalp and the pericranium constitutes a subgaleal abscess. Usually the process is initated by contamination of an open scalp wound by staphylococci, streptococci, or anaerobic organisms. Localized scalp tenderness and heat and swelling adjacent to the wound are signs of abscess formation. Signs of regional and systemic spread include fever, lymphadenopathy, and diffuse scalp and facial swelling. Subgaleal infections rarely extend intracranially unless the skull beneath has been penetrated. Osteomyelitis of the skull occasionally occurs secondarily. Treatment includes open drainage and debridement, coupled with systemic antibiotics.

Osteomyelitis

Osteomyelitis of the skull may develop from extension of a localized infection, such as sinusitis or mastoiditis, from direct contamination of the skull at operation or after trauma, or rarely, by hematogenous spread from a distant source such as the respiratory or urinary tract (3, 69). Chronic exposure of the skull because of scalp loss predisposes the patient to osteomyelitis. An established skull infection may extend inward to produce an epidural abscess or outward into the subgaleal space, causing a "puffy tumor" originally described by Potts (69). The usual osteomyelitis pathogens are staphylococci and anaerobic streptococci. Occasionally, Gram-negative organisms and fungi are responsible. Treatment consists of drainage, debridement of infected bone, and appropriate antibiotics for a prolonged period.

Epidural Abscess

This localized infection results from a preexisting osteomyelitis adjacent to it or secondarily from contamination of epidural tissue at operation or after trauma. If the dura is intact, infection rarely extends transdurally. Treatment consists of drainage, debridement, and systemic antibiotics. True intracranial epidural abscess is rare (64).

Spinal epidural abscess is more common and is usually a medical and surgical emergency. It is characterized by fever, local spinal tenderness, and rapid progression of neurologic deficits. Radicular pain and impairment of cord function, with early motor and sensory deficits including sphincter disturbances, occur within a few days. Most epidural abscesses are caused by local extension of vertebral osteomyelitis or by hematogenous spread from a distant suppurative focus. The cerebrospinal fluid (CSF) often has markedly elevated protein levels and mild pleocytosis. A myelogram defines the extent of the epidural mass. The most common causative organisms are staphylococci and the streptococci. The tubercle bacillus is still a principal cause of epidural abscess in many parts of the world. Treatment should be urgent, including laminectomy and drainage of the abscess. Specific antibiotic therapy should be initiated and continued for a prolonged period of time. Recovery of neurologic function is directly related to the duration and severity of impairment prior to surgery (71).

Subdural Empyema

Subdural empyema is a purulent infection of the subdural space. It accounts for approximately 25% of all intracranial infections and is usually a complication of sinusitis, meningitis, or open contamination of the subdural space at operation or after trauma (32).

When paranasal sinusitis is the source, infection spreads intracranially from the sinus by transcranial emissary vein thrombophlebitis. Staphylococci, streptococci, and anaerobic cocci are commonly responsible (78). Once the subdural space is violated, infection spreads over the convexity of the brain and into the interhemispheric and Sylvian fissures. The accumulation of pus may be sufficient to produce an intracranial mass. The intense inflammatory response provokes brain swelling and edema. The clinical result is rapid neurologic deterioration, often with lateralizing signs (50%), coma, and death. Mortality from acute fulminant subdural empyema from a paranasal source remains about 25% (37). Treatment is emergent, including evacuation of the empyema by craniotomy, drainage, debridement, and antibiotic administration for an extended period.

Subdural empyema may develop in association with meningitis, particularly from *H. influenzae* in infants (43). This variety of extracerebral infection may evolve into subdural effusions during treatment for meningitis. The effusions are commonly bilateral. Organisms may or may not be cultured from these chronic, postmeningitic subdural fluid collections. Treatment consists of drainage and prolonged antibiotic administration. Communicating hydrocephalus may appear if CSF resorption over the cerebral convexities is disrupted by the infection. Drainage of subdural effusions in infancy may be accomplished by subdural aspiration, craniotomy, or both. The course of Haemophilus subdural effusion is usually less fulminant than that typical of subdural empyema from sinusitis.

Subdural empyema is a serious postoperative complication after burr hole exploration or craniotomy. The infection is usually confined to the operative site, and is caused by contamination during operation or afterwards. *S. aureus* and *S. epidermidis* are common pathogenic organisms. The infection is rarely fulminant, and is often detected by its subgaleal extension. Sometimes the empyema is sufficiently large to distort the underlying brain, causing progressive neurologic deterioration. Treatment includes debridement, drainage, and antibiotics. The source of the infection, wherever it is, must be treated aggressively (37). A sinus or mastoid drainage procedure is often required if paranasal sinuses are involved. If a bone plate exists, it should be removed.

The diagnosis of intracranial subdural empyema is made readily by computed tomography (CT) scan. The mass itself may be isodense, necessitating contrast enhancement. Sometimes angiography is required to demonstrate it despite the use of contrast material during CT scanning (20). Skull and paranasal sinus plain radiographs often show that sinus or mastoid infection is responsible for the empyema. Spinal fluid analysis is rarely diagnostic, but may show nonspecific inflammatory changes (45). The risk of lumbar puncture in a patient suspected of harboring an intracranial mass is sufficiently great to countermand the test until CT scanning has confirmed the absence of intracranial mass effect.

Spinal subdural empyema is rare. It usually develops from local extension transdurally or through the arachnoid in the presence of meningitis. Spinal cord compression and transverse myelitis may develop. Treatment is emergent, consisting of drainage by laminectomy and prolonged antibiotic administration.

Bacterial Meningitis

Bacterial meningitis is a purulent infection of the subarachnoid space. It is usually an acute, fulminating illness characterized by fever, headache, nausea, vomiting, and nuchal rigidity. Coma occurs in about 5% to 10% of cases and its development carries a poor prognosis. Seizures occur in approximately 20% of patients, and cranial nerve palsies in 5%. Untreated bacterial meningitis is almost always fatal. CSF cultures provide a diagnosis in 90% of cases. Blood cultures may be positive and thereby are helpful in the diagnosis, particularly with infections caused by *S. pneumoniae* and *Neisseria meningitidis*. In 75% of cases a Gram stain of the CSF will demonstrate bacteria that subsequently will be shown to be the causative organism. CSF pleocytosis, with a preponderance of polymorphonuclear cells, is typical of untreated bacterial meningitis.

The organisms responsible for bacterial meningitis are characteristic for certain age groups and may reflect the antecedent condition necessary for bacterial meningitis to occur (43). Table 7.1 demonstrates some of the organisms

TABLE 7.1.
Meningitis—Causative Organisms in Age Groups

Age	Common organisms
2 months	Enterobacteriaceae (50%) (Mostly *Escherichia coli*)
	Streptococcus group B (10%) *Haemophilus influenzae* (1%)
2 months to 5 years	*H. influenzae* (50%)
	Neisseria meningitidis *Streptococcus pneumoniae*
5 years to adult	*N. meningitidis* *S. pneumoniae* Other streptococci Gram-negative organisms
	Staphylococcus aureus

commonly associated with meningitis in different age categories.

Meningitis that develops following a penetrating wound or a neurosurgical procedure is usually caused by staphylococcal, streptococcal, or Gram-negative organisms, whereas meningitis occurring after closed-head trauma with either a skull fracture or CSF rhinorrhea is most often caused by *S. pneumoniae* (31). CSF shunt and reservoir infections that cause meningitis are likely to occur from *S. epidermidis* or *S. aureus*.

The treatment for acute bacterial meningitis depends on the causative organism, its antibiotic sensitivity, and the primary source of the infection from which the meninges were seeded. Treatment should be directed to both the CSF infection and the primary source. Bacterial endocarditis, pneumonia, sinusitis, concurrent subdural empyema, and brain abscess are common associates of meningitis.

Brain Abscess

Brain abscess is a purulent infection of brain tissue. It begins as a focal infection usually in the white matter surrounded by a typical inflammatory response within brain parenchyma. Sequential changes occur during abscess formation. Acute inflammation develops, then necrosis and liquefaction. The blood-brain barrier is disrupted. Eventually the process is encapsulated by fibrous granulation tissue or the infection spreads through the parenchyma to the subarachnoid spaces and the ventricular system (76). Whether cerebritis evolves into abscess depends upon the host-organism interaction and the effect of treatment rendered.

Brain abscess often occurs secondary to a focal infection elsewhere, particularly in the ear or paranasal sinuses (Table 7.2) (54, 77). Abscesses that develop secondarily by direct intracranial extension are usually solitary and are typically found in the frontal and temporal lobes. Multiple brain abscesses may develop in the presence of sepsis (63). Common systemic infections that provide a source for brain abscesses are bacterial endocarditis, pneumonia, and diverticulitis. Cyanotic congenital heart disease with concurrent infection is an increasingly frequent source of mulitiple brain abscess. Direct contamination of the brain through a penetrating brain wound is another cause of abscess, particularly in times of war (59). Indriven bone fragments and other debris are commonly found in the abscesses of patients with traumatic brain infection. Abscess formation is infrequent during the course of bacterial meningitis. Conversely, brain abscess is frequent among patients with compromised immunity from an underlying illness or with treatment during organ transplantation (17).

Signs and symptoms of brain abscess are commonly related to its mass effect. Headache,

TABLE 7.2.
Brain Abscess

Predisposing cause	Usual location	Common organism
Otitis Mastoiditis	Temporal lobe Subdural abscess	Streptococcus Bacteriodes *Haemophilus influenzae* Gram-negative organisms
Sinusitis	Frontal lobe Subdural abscess	Streptococcus Staphyloccus
Pneumonia Endocarditis Diverticulitis	Multiple brain abscesses	Various organisms (depends on source)
Penetrating wound Neurosurgical postoperative infection	Site of trauma	Staphylococcus

focal or lateralizing neurologic deficits, and impaired mentation are often seen. There may be little or no evidence of systemic infection, the patient may be afebrile, and seizures may occur. Because of the mass effect, brain shifts can develop, and may be exaggerated by changes in CSF pressure. Hence, a lumbar puncture should not be performed until a definitive study of the intracranial contents has excluded a mass (12).

CT scanning is highly accurate for detecting a brain abscess and, if possible, should be done before the CSF is sampled (53). The CSF of patients with a brain abscess may be entirely normal. The causative organism can be identified and cultured from the abscess itself in 60% to 80% of cases, provided that cultures are processed carefully for both aerobic and anaerobic organisms. Blood cultures are also helpful, particularly if the abscess is secondary to systemic infection.

The most effective therapy for brain abscess continues to be drainage of the pus and administration of appropriate antibiotics (33). Surgical drainage reduces the mass effect and thereby reduces the most critical and dangerous aspect of this infection (57).

When abscess formation is in an early stage, medical therapy with the appropriate parenteral antibiotic may be sufficient (8, 61). Otherwise, the preferred course of treatment is aspiration or excision of the abscess, in addition to appropriate antibiotic therapy administered for a minimum of 4 weeks (67). In certain cases of high surgical risk, medical treatment of formed abscesses may be effective, provided the causative organism is known (10, 60).

The results of treatment for a brain abscess depend on the patient's neurologic status when treatment is begun, the appropriateness of the antibiotic used and its CNS penetration, the extent to which the intracranial mass is controlled by surgery, and effective treatment of the primary source of the abscess. Despite aggressive surgical and medical treatment, mortality rates associated with brain abscess are still in the range of 20% to 40% (2).

Postoperative Infection

Any or all of the pyogenic infections described earlier may develop after operation. Once identified, characterized, and treated with appropriate antibiotics, the infection almost always subsides. While drainage of an infected wound is a time-honored surgical principle, that method must be modified when applied to infections of the CNS. Generally, the dura must be closed tight to maintain an effective barrier between the CSF and the external environment in order to heal the wound and prevent or control meningitis. Drainage of an infected wound involving the CNS cannot be instituted unless the dura is sealed.

If a foreign body is involved, eradicating the infection becomes more difficult (27). In general the foreign body, including prosthetic materials and shunt apparatus, should be removed when infection is discovered. Sometimes, however, infections can be cleared in the presence of retained foreign materials, such as a shunt, provided the infection is indolent and the shunt essential (29). Common organisms involved in postoperative infections are *S. aureus* and *S. epidermidis*. Combined systemic and intrathecal antibiotics are usually necessary to cure the infection and salvage the shunt or prosthetic material.

Current therapy for shunt infections caused by Gram-negative enteric bacilli includes intravenous nafcillin (12 g/day or 300 mg/kg/day) and a third generation cephalosporin such as cefotaxime (12 g/day or 200 mg/kg/day). For infections caused by methicillin-resistant *S. epidermidis*, a combination of intravenous vancomycin (2 g/day or 40 mg/kg/day), gentamicin (5 mg/kg/day), and rifampin (200 mg/day or 20 mg/kg/day) is recommended.

In patients whose infected shunt is not removed, intraventricular antibiotics via the shunt reservoir are often used. Cefazolin (1 to 2 mg/kg up to a maximum dose of 50 mg/day) or gentamicin (0.5 to 5 mg total dose) administered daily for 2 to 3 weeks, in combination with systemic antibiotics, is often adequate to sterilize the shunt and the CSF.

When the patient fails to respond to antibiotic therapy promptly, removal of the shunt, external drainage, and appropriate antibiotics administered in the absence of a shunt may be required to eradicate the infection.

VIRAL INFECTIONS OF THE CENTRAL NERVOUS SYSTEM

Most viral infections of the CNS are caused by viruses common in the general population—mumps, enteroviruses, and herpes simplex.

They are relatively rare and are frequently associated with a benign and self-limited course. Viral meningitis, the most common viral infection of the CNS, is often not brought to medical attention because of the relatively mild and brief nature of the disease. Nonetheless, serious consequences and even death can occur in primary diseases such as herpes simplex encephalitis, the equine encephalytides, and polio. Viruses may also damage the CNS in chronic infections such as subacute sclerosing panencephalitis (SSPE) due to the measles virus, and progressive multifocal leukoencephalopathy (PML), caused by JC papova virus. Jakob-Creutzfeldt disease, a slow virus infection of the CNS, also has severe and eventually fatal consequences.

Antibodies for the common viral causes of CNS infections are widely prevalent. This fact indicates that such infections are not due simply to an encounter with viral agents, but rather to breakdown in the usual host-defense mechanisms. Very few specific drugs for the treatment of viral diseases are available. The major therapeutic advance has been the development of killed and attenuated viral strains for immunization against polio, mumps, and measles.

Some viral diseases are of neurosurgical interest. Acute viral meningitis often presents as aseptic meningitis and must be included in the differential diagnosis of such diseases as subdural empyema, carcinomatous meningitis, fungal meningitis, and brain abscess. Enteroviral meningitis begins abruptly with little or no prodrome; a course occasionally resembling a mild subarachnoid hemorrhage may lead to initial neurosurgical referral. Acute viral encephalitis may present with a wide variety of neurologic findings, including seizures, focal weakness or paralysis and, rarely, cerebellar signs such as ataxia or nystagmus; the level of consciousness is frequently depressed (49).

General Virology

Viruses are obligate intracellular parasites, carrying only one type of nucleic acid. In contrast to all other living organisms, viruses contain either DNA or RNA but not both. They cannot multiply or grow independently; they are completely dependent upon the invaded cell for replication of the nucleic acid and for the synthesis of their protein coat. Unlike all other organisms, viruses do not need to contain DNA for their replication. In fact, most animal viruses contain a single strand of RNA (36).

Viruses are classified according to type of nucleic acid that they contain. These in turn are further subdivided by the size and shape of their protein coat. There are 10 groups of RNA viruses and five groups of DNA viruses. All DNA viruses except poxviruses replicate in the cell nucleus while RNA viruses replicate in the cell cytoplasm. Not every virus-cell contact leads to infection; susceptible cells have appropriate receptor sites on their cytoplasmic membranes to match the polypeptide attachment molecule on the viral surface (14). Selective vulnerability of the species or of a particular cell type to a given virus appears to be dependent upon these receptor sites. A high degree of complexity of CNS cell membranes may explain the discrete vulnerability of certain groups of neurons to a specific virus. For example, rabies virus involves the limbic system neurons but not neocortical neurons.

Viral Entry into the CNS

Viruses usually enter the body through the mucous membranes of the respiratory, gastrointestinal, or urinary tracts. The epidermis is an effective barrier to viral entry; viral infection must depend on a breach in the skin as in animal bites or with hypodermic injections. While some viruses remain confined to the susceptible surfaces, others, such as mumps, rubeola, and rubella, are invasive and capable of wide dissemination through the lymphatic and circulatory systems. Three routes have been postulated for viral entry into the CNS: along peripheral nerve, along the olfactory nerve, and via the bloodstream. A neural route is very important in the movement of rabies virus and of herpes simplex and varicella zoster. Invasion via the olfactory nerve is now largely discredited.

It is clear that most viral infections of the CNS occur as the result of the arrival of bloodborne virus in susceptible areas of the CNS. This in turn depends upon the production of a heavy viremia after invasion through the mucosa. Viruses may multiply in regional lymph nodes and in the reticuloendothelial cells of the liver and spleen. The immune response triggered in the lymph nodes and the ingestion of virus particles by phagocytes in liver and spleen tend to destroy the virus particles. The intensity of the viremia is thus dependent upon the rate of viral replication in the nodes, liver, and spleen and the destruction of virus in these same tissues.

In the presence of a large viremia, viruses can reach brain parenchyma despite the tight junctions between cerebral capillary endothelial cells. They may be transported through the endothelial cells or may attack and infect them. Once the particles have gained entry into the CNS, they must be transported through the parenchyma and must reach susceptible cells which they can successfully attack. Not all cell types of the CNS are vulnerable to attack by a given virus and progression of the disease would thus be halted unless the virus contacts the appropriate cells.

The production of clinical neurologic disease is also dependent on the effects of the virus on the invaded suceptible cells. Herpes simplex causes such profound changes in cellular protein metabolism as to lead to early cell death. Other viruses may produce little change in the essential cellular metabolism but cause alterations in the production of enzymes and neural transmitters leading to major abnormalities of specialized neural physiologic functions. Yet other viruses may persist for long periods in the CNS before producing evidence of disease. This long latency is most commonly seen with DNA viruses and is associated with the so-called slow, chronic, or latent infections.

The wide variation of symptoms in viral diseases is due to the differing vulnerability of CNS cell population to the various viruses. Some viruses, such as herpes simplex, can successfully infect a wide variety of cell types. Others are much more limited in their range, invading and multiplying only in specific cell types. Viral diseases and viral-associated diseases having the most importance to neurosurgeons are herpes simplex encephalitis, Jakob-Creutzfeldt disease, Reye's syndrome, and AIDS. These will be considered in greater detail.

Herpes Simplex Encephalitis

A DNA virus that replicates itself in the nucleus of infected cells, herpes simplex, is best known as the agent of the ubiquitous and benign recurrent cold sore of the oral mucosa. For reasons that are currently unknown, this virus at times can demonstrate a powerful virulence causing a localized necrotizing encephalitis of greater morbidity and mortality than any other viral CNS disease.

There are two antigenically distinct subtypes of herpes simplex virus: type 1, spread by respiratory droplets and saliva and responsible for the common oral mucocutaneous lesions; and type 2, spread by sexual contact and the cause of genital mucosal lesions. The usual adult encephalitis is caused by type 1 herpes. A diffuse encephalitis in newborns may be caused by type 2 herpes; this is but one manifestation of a lethal and widespread involvement of many organs. Neonatal herpes is thought to be transferred during passage through an infected birth canal.

Approximately 90% of adults have antibodies to type 1 herpes virus and about 25% have recurrent cold sores. An important characteristic of the virus is its ability to remain in a dormant, asymptomatic state for long periods of time, reappearing intermittently in the form of mucocutaneous lesions around the mouth. The dormant virus can be reactivated by a variety of stimuli, including fever, injury, exposure to ultraviolet light, and trauma to the sensory root of the trigeminal nerve, to produce a new skin lesion. The virus, in its latent state, appears to reside in the cell bodies of the sensory neurons in the trigeminal ganglia. Interestingly, early findings suggesting this localization came from neurosurgical procedures. The frequent appearance of skin lesions of herpes simplex after retrogasserian rhizotomy for tic douloureux implied that manipulation of the trigeminal nerve could stimulate recurrence. Herpetic lesions were found by Carton and Kilbourne (13) in approximately 90% of patients after section of the proximal trigeminal root for tic. Later studies showed herpes virus could be recovered by tissue culture techniques from a high proportion of trigeminal ganglia removed at autopsy (4). No virus particles or viral antigens, however, can be demonstrated in the trigeminal ganglia between recurrences. The herpes viral genetic material is thus preserved in some way without production of viral particles and without affecting the cellular integrity of metabolism of the sensory neurons. After stimulation, however, viral replication takes place rapidly. Following infection, the virus appears to reach the trigeminal ganglia by moving up the axons supplying the area of the lesion. This presumably occurs by retrograde axoplasmic transport. The later development of skin lesions probably occurs via centrifugal movement of the virus particles down the sensory axon to the mucosa. The relationship of herpes encephalitis to oral herpes infection is unclear. Although some patients have an active oral lesion at the time of onset of encephalitis, this is by no means common. A past history of herpetic lesions is present in 25% of encephalitis cases, but a similar percentage of the general population has the same history.

Herpes simplex encephalitis is as virulent as oral cold sores are benign. The most common form of acute, nonepidemic encephalitis in the Western world, herpes simplex causes 1,000 to 2,000 estimated cases of encephalitis per year in the United States. The mortality rate may be as high as 70% in some series (73).

The encephalitis process is limited to the inferior frontal and temporal lobes and its onset may be rapid or subtle. About 90% of the patients show early neurologic signs, indicating frontotemporal localization—hallucinations, behavioral abnormalities, and personality change. Fever and headache are almost universally present in the early stages, as are seizures, either focal motor, grand mal, or partial complex. Memory impairment, implying bilateral basal temporal involvement, is seen in many patients (19). Focal motor deficits, usually in the face and arm, may occur and aphasia is common if a dominant frontotemporal region is involved. With progression of the disease, the frontotemporal region becomes edematous and acts as an intracranial mass, leading to increased intracranial pressure and often to uncal herniation (1). The course of the disease is frequently one of progressive deterioration to death. Although spontaneous recovery can occur in milder infections, significant residual neurologic deficits usually result.

Laboratory confirmation of the disease is quite difficult. Examination of the CSF is of only modest help; herpes simplex virus has only rarely been recovered from the spinal fluid. White cells in the spinal fluid are most often a mixture of neutrophils and mononuclear cells with the latter predominating; usually less than 1,000 cells/mm^3 are present. Red blood cells, very rare in other encephalytides, are frequently present and constitute a valuable diagnostic clue. Spinal fluid protein is moderately elevated and glucose is normal. There are no reliable early serologic tests of the spinal fluid for herpes simplex. While viral antibodies can eventually be demonstrated in the spinal fluid, this may take many weeks. More recent sensitive radioimmunoassays have a diagnostic accuracy of only 50% the first 10 days of the disease.

The best early diagnostic tests are EEG, the CT scan, and radionuclide scans. No one of these tests is definitely diagnostic, but all may demonstrate a disease process localized to the frontal and temporal lobes and thus add strong support to the clinical diagnosis (21). The EEG may show periodic paroxysmal discharges or slow wave complexes at intervals of less than 4 seconds in one or both temporal lobes (68). The most useful test appears to be the CT scan, which may show decreased attenuation in one or both temporal lobes as early as the third day of the disease. This decreased attenuation represents the edema and necrosis found in areas of encephalitis. The use of contrast agents can also show areas of abnormal enhancement surrounding the low density areas. Radionuclide scans are capable of revealing areas of increased uptake in the temporal lobes and appear to be no more accurate or specific than CT scans. The CT scan has the advantage of being able to demonstrate the mass effect of an edematous area and to follow the evolution of the disease in time. The role of MRI scanning is not yet clear. Full confirmation of the diagnosis of herpes encephalitis ultimately depends on brain biopsy. Demonstration of the intracellular virus either by histologic studies or by growth in tissue culture remains the only certain diagnostic test.

Early accurate diagnosis has recently become important because of the development of an effective treatment for herpes encephalitis demonstrated that treatment with adenine arabinoside (vidarabine) substantially decreased the mortality rate in biopsy-proven herpes encephalities (73). The effectiveness of this drug was demonstrated to be greatest in patients under 30 years of age and patients whose treatment began before they became comatose. Comatose patients, regardless of age, had a mortality rate of over 50% while patients under 30 years of age who were merely lethargic at the start of treatment had a mortality rate of only 9% (74).

Vidarabine, however, does not prevent the neurologic consequences of herpes and half of the survivors have significant neurologic deficits. The recommended dosage of the drug is 15 mg/kg given over 12 hours at a concentration of 0.7 mg/ml. In a 70-kg man, this results in a 1,500 ml of intravenous infusion merely as a vehicle for the drug. The magnitude of this fluid load in a patient with increased intracranial pressure and an edematous temporal lobe may lead to further increases in intracranial pressure. An equally important factor in the treatment of this disease is the control of increased intracranial pressure associated with frontotemporal edema. Intravenous fluids must be carefully monitored and the judicious use of hyperventilation, steroids, osmotic diuretics, and intracranial pressure monitoring are all important to the treatment program.

Brain biopsy remains strongly recommended prior to beginning treatment with vidarabine (75). The low incidence and mild nature of vidarabine side effects have encouraged the use of this drug without biopsy in suspected herpes encephalitis. At present, it appears most appropriate to treat all herpes encephalitis suspects with vidarabine until the final results of biopsy are obtained. If no histologic or culture-proven herpes infection is discovered after 5 days of treatment, the drug is terminated; if the studies are positive for herpes, treatment is continued for 10 days.

Another drug, Acyclovir, an analogue of guanosine, is currently being tested as an antiherpes agent. A recent Swedish study compared this drug with vidarabine and found a mortality rate of 19% in the Acyclovir group as contrasted with 50% in the vidarabine group (65). It appears likely that Acyclovir may soon be the drug of choice for herpes encephalitis.

Jakob-Creutzfeldt Disease

The importance of Jakob-Creutzfeldt disease in neurosurgical practice is its potential for iatrogenic spread. This rapidly progressive dementing degenerative disease is one of the subacute spongiform encephalopathies, a group which also includes kuru in humans and scrapie in sheep. These diseases are often classed as the "slow virus" diseases, although the nucleic acid and protein structure of a virus has never been demonstrated as the infectious agent. It is most appropriate to refer to these agents as "unconventional agents", since, although they are transmissible, they have never been seen by electron microscopy, produce no immune response in the host, and are resistant to treatments (heat, ultraviolet radiation, nucleases) that usually inactivate viruses.

Transmission of Jakob-Creutzfeldt disease in primates has demonstrated that the number of infectious units in the CNS of a diseased animal is many times greater than the number of units in the original innoculation. Thus the agent not only causes infection, but also replicates (72).

Jakob-Creutzfeldt disease is world wide in distribution, with an incidence of one to two cases per million population. About 10% to 15% of cases are familial. Symptoms usually begin in the fifth or sixth decade. In general they begin with a vague prodrome of fatigue, mild gait abnormalities, and memory deficits. This is followed by a rapidly progressive dementia associated with ataxia, blindness, choreoathetosis, and, most characteristically, myoclonus. Death follows within 8 to 12 months. There are no characteristic changes in the CSF or on CT scan. The EEG may show diffuse slowing and paroxsysmal sharp waves but this is not pathognomonic. Pathologic changes include severe cerebral atrophy, neuronal loss, astrocytosis, and cytoplasmic vacuolization of neurons and astrocytes (status spongiosus). The incubation period in the natural disease appears to be a matter of years rather than months.

The mode of natural transmission of Jakob-Creutzfeldt disease remains unknown. The infectious agent may be transmitted from the cornea, liver, spleen, lung, kidney, and CSF as well as from the brain and spinal cord. In some animal transmission, leukocytes have been involved. The infectivity of human CNS tissue is of paramount importance to neurosurgeons; the disease appears to have been transmitted inadvertently by surgery on several occasions. The usual sterilization methods have no effect on this agent.

Extreme care should be taken during operations on patients with progressive dementia. Biopsy and ventricular shunting procedures should be carried out only after careful consideration. Surgical instruments and depth electrodes used in any procedures on demented patients having no clear etiology should be handled with great respect and specially treated after surgery. Gajdusek *et al.* (25) have shown that autoclaving at 250°F at 15 lb/sq in. of pressure for 1 hour or immersion in 5% sodium hypochlorite (household bleach) will inactivate the agent. There is no clear evidence of medical personnel developing the disease after contact with Jakob-Creutzfeldt patients.

Reye's Syndrome

The development of an acute encephalopathy with fatty degeneration of the viscera, especially the liver, in children during recovery from an acute viral illness was first described in 1963 in Australia (58). It rapidly became evident that this syndrome was world wide in scope and primarily affected children under the age of 18 years. The marked increase in incidence in the United States seen during 1973 to 1974 led to vigorous efforts to discover the etiology and pathogenesis of this disease. Despite these investigations, much essential information remains unknown. The agent of the disease, the etiology of the biochemical abnormalities, and the relations of these changes to the liver dysfunction and to the encephalopathy are not clearly understood. There is still no unifying hypothesis to explain the occurrence and manifestation of Reye's syndrome.

The course of the syndrome is quite predictable. During recovery from a respiratory infection or from chicken pox, a child will develop intractable vomiting. This is quickly followed by delirium, progressing in a few hours to a rapidly decreasing level of consciousness and frequently to coma. Early elevations of SGOT and serum ammonia provide evidence of hepatic dysfunction and the prothrombin time is usually prolonged; serum bilirubin remains normal. CSF examination is unremarkable. As the disease progresses, decerebrate posturing and hyperventilation become prominent. Profound EEG changes may be seen but these generally reflect only a widespread neuronal dysfunction and are not pathognomonic of the disease. Changes in the EEG pattern do, however, reflect the severity of the process and are useful in staging the disease when combined with clinical criteria (44).

In fatal cases, examination reveals a swollen edematous brain and an enlarged liver. Microscopic examination of the brain shows no sign of inflammation or demyelination. Neurons are pyknotic and glial cells are swollen. The liver shows an increase in intracellular fat; these fatty changes are reversible in survivors.

Epidemiologic studies have shown a very strong association between Reye's syndrome and a prior influenza B infection (46). The winter and early spring are times of peak incidence of this syndrome. A small but persistent number of cases follow chicken pox, and other viral infections have also been implicated. The virus may act through a direct or indirect effect on cellular metabolism or may interact with some enhancing factor in the environment. Association of Reye's syndrome with heavy aspirin use had been frequently demonstrated, also suggesting a viral interaction with other factors (66).

The most important factor in the pathogenesis of Reye's syndrome appears to be hyperammonemia. Liver clearance of ammonia is decreased by destruction of the urea cycle enzymes. Arterial ammonia levels may be as high as 1,000 μg/100 mm. The arterial ammonia level is directly related both to the depth of coma and the severity of EEG abnormality as well as the mortality rate (15).

Cerebral edema, probably due to astrocyte swelling, is a major factor in Reye's syndrome. Cerebral edema is almost universal in fatal cases and increased intracranial pressure is common in severely ill children. The high mortality in Reye's syndrome patients is closely associated with increased intracranial pressure. Kindt *et al.* (38) reported a reduction in mortality when (ICP) monitoring and vigorous attempts to decrease raised ICP were added to the standard protocols of supportive treatment. Dramatic reversals from profound coma and decreased mortality rate have been associated with effective ICP control in Reye's syndrome (70). The mortality rate of Reye's syndrome today is one fourth of its level prior to the application of these principles.

Acquired Immune Deficiency Syndrome (AIDS)

Acquired immune deficiency syndrome (AIDS) has spread rapidly in the United States in only 4 years. The number of reported cases rose to over 10,000 by April 1985, and another 10,000 will likely be diagnosed within the next year.

The syndrome is largely confined to homosexual and bisexual males and to intravenous drug abusers of both genders. A significant number of hemophiliacs have also been stricken. The disease appears to be spread almost exclusively via sexual contact, exposure to contaminated needles, and transfusion of blood or blood products. Although homosexuals and intravenous drug abusers still account for nearly 90% of AIDS patients, the prevalance of the disease in female partners of AIDS patients and children born of mothers with AIDS is increasing; the increase in female AIDS cases is paralleled by a more recent incidence of the disease in heterosexual males.

Very early in the investigation of this outbreak it was determined that patients with opportunistic infections and Kaposi's sarcoma had an unexplained deficiency in cell-mediated immune mechanisms, with a selective depletion of T lymphocytes in the T_4 (helper/inducer) subset and hyperactivity of B lymphcytes (51). These deficits particularly impaired the immune response to viral, fungal, and tumor antigens. The importance of this deficiency is reflected in the name of the syndrome, which is now defined as the presence of opportunistic infections and malignant diseases in patients without a known cause for their immune deficiency. Further studies on the high-risk groups have demonstrated a large number of cases of chronic lymphadenopathy, sometimes associated with syndromes suggesting a mild or prodromal form of AIDS, the AIDS-related complex (ARC) (50). Although the ultimate outcome of such patients is unclear, these milder syndromes may represent a "pre-AIDS" state and as many as 20% of such patients may go on to develop full-blown AIDS.

The most likely etiologic agent is a retrovirus first isolated from pre-AIDS or ARC patients and designated as the lymphadenopathy-associated virus (LAV) or human T cell lymphotrophic virus type III (HTLV-III) (5, 26). This virus has a preference for T_4 lymphocytes and produces cytopathic changes and cell death in them. Serologic studies have shown a high incidence of antibodies to LAV/HTLV-III in patients with AIDS and ARC. The incidence in persons with hemophilia A is also high. Seropositivity for HTLV-III is strongly associated with clinical AIDS and the AIDS "prodromes" lending support to the etiologic role of this virus in the disease. An enzyme-linked immunosorbent assay (ELISA) for the antibody is now being used to screen donated blood.

Nearly 40% of patients with fully developed AIDS have neurologic abnormalities (41). In this group of patients nearly one third, or 10% of all AIDS patients, present because of neurologic problems. These complications may be due to CNS involvement and, to a lesser extent, peripheral and cranial neuropathies. The vast majority of intracranial processes are due either to opportunistic infections—viral, fungal or protozoal—or to malignant disease.

Opportunistic infections include subacute encephalitis of presumed viral origin which may be due to cytomegalovirus (CMV) or to direct invasion of HTLV-III. This is the most common viral syndrome, although herpes simplex encephalitis and progressive multifocal leukoencephalopathy (PML) are both infrequently reported. The most common intracranial infection is toxoplasomosis, caused by the intracellular protozoan, *Toxoplasma gondii*. This disease appears more commonly in Haitian AIDS patients than in other groups. Other nonviral infectious agents include the fungi Crypotococcus and Candida and the atypical mycobacterium, *mycobacterium aviam-intracellulare*.

Primary CNS lymphoma, a rare tumor usually seen only in immunosuppressed transplant patients, is found in about 3% of AIDS patients. Systemic lymphoma, with spread to the CNS meninges, is not rare. A few instances of Kaposi's sarcoma metastatic to brain have also been reported.

The neurologic problems in AIDS patients fall into three major categories: a diffuse encephalopathy, often with progressive dementia; an aseptic meningitis of viral or cryptococcal origin; and focal neurologic deficits. Additionally, cerebral infarctions may occur secondary to a nonbacterial thrombotic endocarditis.

Recent studies of AIDS patients with neurologic symptoms found cranial CT abnormalities in a substantial number. Some of these lesions may respond to specific treatment; toxoplasmosis to pyrimethamine and sulfadiazine; cryptococcus to amphotericin B; PML to cytarabine; and lymphoma to radiation therapy. Diagnosis based on CT appearance and blood and CSF serologies is uncertain; however, two or more processes may often be present simultaneously. Definitive diagnosis, therefore, depends on accurate biopsy of the demonstrated lesions and serial CT evaluation of the response to appropriate therapy.

Protection of medical personnel during surgical procedures should include the wearing of gown and gloves when handling blood or tissue, rigorous hand washing, and the meticulous avoidance of scalpel or needle wounds.

FUNGAL INFECTIONS OF THE CENTRAL NERVOUS SYSTEM

Fungi are opportunistic organisms which become pathogenic during special circumstances, including depression of the immune system of the host and prolonged systemic antibiotic therapy. It is uncommon for fungi to invade the CNS. When infection of the CNS does occur, it is usually associated with pulmonary fungal infection and depressed host resistance (79). Involvement of the CNS may be disseminated or focal (Table 7.3).

Disseminated

Meningitis

Fungal meningitis (usually *Cryptococcus neoformans, Coccidioides immitis*, and *Candida albicans*) can be subacute or chronic (55). The clinical signs and symptoms are indistinguishable from tuberculous meningitis or any other chronic meningitis (7). The CSF pleocytosis is lymphocytic, CSF protein is mildly elevated, and CSF glucose is usually reduced. The diagnosis of cryptococcal meningitis is made by culture of the CSF; India ink smears are positive in 50% of cases; capsular antigen of Cryptococcus is detectable in the CSF in about 90% of cases. Coccidioidal infection of the meninges can be determined by a positive complement fixation (CF) test for CSF antibody to the fungus; culture of the CSF is positive in half of the cases. The CT scan is not usually helpful, but it may demonstrate inflammatory changes (48).

TABLE 7.3.
Fungal infection of the CNS

Common organisms	Usual clinical manifestation	Preferred antibiotic
Actinomyces	Abscess	Penicillin
Aspergillus	Meningitis Abscess	Amphotericin B
Candida	Meningitis Encephalitis Brain abscess	Amphotericin B 5-Fluorocytosine
Cryptococcus	Meningitis	Amphotericin B
Histoplasma	Meningitis	Amphotericin B
Nocardia	Meningitis Abscess	Sulfonamides
Mucor	Encephalitis Vasculitis	Amphotericin B

The treatment of fungal meningitis includes amphotericin B, although this drug must be used cautiously. Intravenous therapy alone is generally successful in treating cryptococcal and candidal meningitis (22). The duration of therapy is prolonged, usually lasting 8 to 10 weeks. Therapy may have to be continued for even longer periods if the CSF cultures continue to be positive and the CF titer remains elevated in cases of coccidioidal meningitis, or if the cryptococcal antigen titer in the CSF remains elevated. Recent evidence suggests that 5-fluorocytosine (5-FC), in combination with amphotericin B, is effective in the treatment of cryptococcal meningitis (6).

Coccidioidal meningitis is a more severe infection and requires intrathecal or intracisternal administration of amphotericin B for a successful outcome. Many authors recommend placement of a subcutaneous CSF reservoir for intraventricular administration. However, amphotericin B has significant adverse effects that limit its clinical application.

Encephalitis

Fungal infection of the brain parenchyma is usually associated with meningeal involvement. The process ranges from diffuse inflammation to multiple focal abscesses (16). Mucormycosis exemplifies diffuse fungal encephalitis, occurring most often in patients with diabetes mellitus and compromised immunity. This organism preferentially involves the cerebral vasculature, causing ischemia, thrombosis, and infarction in addition to inflammation. Tissues of the orbit and paranasal sinuses are commonly affected. Treatment includes debridement of infected and devitalized tissue, control of the underlying disease, and systemic amphotericin B. The prognosis is poor despite treatment unless the diagnosis is made early.

Focal

Fungal brain abscess may be single or multiple. The disease is often accompanied by fungal pneumonia. Sometimes a fungal abscess develops after direct contamination of the brain from an adjacent infection. Organisms commonly involved are Actinomyces, Aspergillus, and Nocardia.

An intracranial Actininomyces abscess is usually caused by direct extension of the infection from the ear or mandible. The abscess is often solitary and well encapsulated. Meningitis rarely develops. Treatment consists of drainage and intravenous penicillin for a prolonged period.

Aspergillosis of the CNS is preceded by respiratory involvement. It may develop in various ways, including meningitis, encephalitis, solitary or multiple brain abscesses, and vasculitis. Cerebral mycotic aneurysms may develop. The treatment of Aspergillus abscess is drainage and amphotericin B.

Nocardiosis of the CNS commonly occurs in abscess form, though purulent meningitis may also arise. The abscesses are often multiple and multiloculated. Capsular formation is usually poorly developed. Drainage and systemic sulphonamides are preferred treatment.

ANTIBIOTICS FOR INFECTIONS IN THE CRITICALLY ILL PATIENT

General Considerations

Initiation of proper antimicrobial therapy is essential to minimize the impact of infection. With severe infection and sepsis systemic vascular resistance falls, causing hypotension and end-organ damage. Critically ill patients often have little physiologic reserve. Thus, therapy based on clinical clues must be initiated promptly to minimize organ damage. The need to provide broad spectrum activity usually leads to combination therapy initially, which can be changed to more specific therapy later, based on culture results. In the critically ill patient with neurologic disease, an additional feature of therapy in some situations is the need for CNS penetration (Table 7.4). The list of antimicrobial drugs from which to choose has expanded in recent years, many with important attributes for patients with neurologic disease.

Penicillins

The penicillins can be categorized by their antibacterial spectrum into four classes: (*a*) the natural penicillins, including penicillin G; (*b*) the penicillinase-resistant penicillins such as methicillin, oxacillin, and nafcillin; (*c*) the amino penicillins such as ampicillin; and (*d*) the extended spectrum or antipseudomonal penicillins exemplified by ticarcillin or piperacillin. Members of all four groups remain important therapeutic agents in clinical circumstances encountered in seriously ill neurosurgical patients (52).

The natural penicillins, mainly penicillin G, are commonly used in two settings in the NICU. One is in high doses, up to 500,000 units/kg/day, for the treatment of CNS infections due to susceptible pathogens, while the other is in lower doses for treatment of community-acquired oropharyngeal aspiration pneumonia, pneumococcal, or streptococcal infections. Penicillin G is generally given as the potassium salt and when high doses are used,

TABLE 7.4.
Antibiotic Penetration of CNS

Good penetration with normal meninges	Good penetration with inflamed meninges	Poor or no penetration
Chloramphenicol	Penicillin G	Gentamicin
Sulfonamides	Ampicillin	Tobramycin
Trimethoprim/sulfamethoxazole	Carbenicillin	Amikacin
Rifampin	Nafcillin	Streptomycin
INH	Vancomycin	Amphotericin B
Ethambutol	Tetracycline	Erythromycin
Metronidazole	Moxalactam	Polymixin B
	Cefotaxime	Benzathine penicillin
		Cefazolin

it is important to remember that each million units contains 1.7 mEq of potassium.

Since over 80% of *S. aureus* strains encountered clinically produce penicillinase and thus are not inhibited by penicillin G, the penicillinase-resistant penicillins such as methicillin, nafcillin, and oxacillin are central to the treatment of suspected or proven *S. aureus* infection. The usual dose is from 4 to 12 g/day depending on the severity of infection. These compounds have no activity against Gram-negative bacilli or *Streptococcus faecalis*, but although not as active as penicillin G, do inhibit *Streptococcus pyogenes* and *S. pneumoniae* at achievable concentrations. In some parts of the country, methicillin-resistant *S. aureus* strains are common. These strains appear to be resistant by virtue of altered penicillin-binding proteins. This alteration makes them resistant to all penicillins and cephalosporins.

The major parenteral aminopenicillin is ampicillin. It achieves good CSF levels in the face of inflammation and is most commonly used in neurosurgical settings for treating meningitis, especially that due to *Listeria monocytogenes*. It is also important when combined with gentamicin for the treatment of serious *S. faecalis* infections. For severe infections, 6 to 12 g/day is given intravenously.

The antipseudomonal penicillins play a central role in therapy of infections in ICUs because of the frequency of *P. aeruginosa* in various clinical circumstances. Several new compounds have been developed in this class. Carbenicillin was the first penicillin with activity against Pseudomonas but has been replaced by ticarcillin which is two to four times more active against *P. aeruginosa*. The newly introduced ureidopenicillins, piperacillin, and mezlocillin are active against Pseudomonas and also provide activity for other Gram-negative pathogens such as Klebsiella and Enterobacter not usually inhibited by ticarcillin. Piperacillin is also active in vitro for some strains of *P. aeruginosa* not inhibited by mezlocillin or ticarcillin (24). The expanded spectrum and activity of piperacillin have made it a popular agent for use in ICU settings, especially where resistant strains are prevalent. The usual dosage is 200 to 300 mg/kg/day given intravenously in divided doses every 4 hours, most commonly in combination with an aminoglycoside. Only modest reduction is needed in renal insufficiency with the dose in anuria being 50 mg/kg every 12 hours.

Cephalosporins

There has been an explosion of new compounds in the cephalosporin class (40). The enhanced spectrum and CNS penetration of many of the newer compounds are important features. The first generation compounds, exemplified by cefazolin, remain useful agents as alternatives for the therapy of staphylococcal infection as well as other susceptible pathogens. Unfortunately, therapeutic levels are not achieved in CSF. Among the so-called second generation compounds, cefoxitin remains a very useful agent especially for treatment of suspected or proven *Bacteroides fragilis* infections. Cefuroxime is a relatively new addition to the second generation group of cephalosporins. It improves on the activity of cefazolin for *H. influenzae* and achieves therapeutic levels in the CSF (34). It is useful in treating suppurative upper respiratory infections where mixed infections including *H. influenzae* are anticipated. Usual dosage is 750 mg every 8 hours given intramuscularly or intravenously.

The third generation cephalosporins have provided a major advance in therapy of complicated neurosurgical patients. These compounds, exemplified by cefotaxime, penetrate into CSF to produce therapeutic concentrations allowing treatment of many episodes of Gram-negative meningitis previously requiring intrathecal therapy. Approximately 10% to 15% of serum levels are achieved in CSF with inflammation and this is coupled with enhanced specific activity for many Gram-negative pathogens such as *Escherichia coli*, *Klebsiella pneumoniae*, and *Proteus mirabilis*. The concentrations achieved are not sufficient to be predictably active for staphylococci. Full-dose therapy is recommended when these agents are used to treat post-traumatic or postsurgical meningitis, which in an adult with normal renal function for cefotaxime is 2 g every 4 hours intravenously. These extended spectrum compounds can also be useful for the treatment of nosocomial infections with such pathogens as *Serratia marcescens* and *Enterobacter aerogenes*.

Several additional antimicrobics deserve mention as they are becoming more important in the treatment of patients with neurosurgical disease. The first is an older agent re-emerging in importance, Vancomycin (28). This has happened because of the frequency with which methicillin-resistant *S. aureus* and *S. epidermidis* are being encountered clinically. This agent has not been extensively studied, but does appear to cross into CSF in the face of inflammation. In post-traumatic or postsurgical meningitis, it provides broad activity when combined with a third-generation cephalosporin awaiting specific pathogen identification. Vancomycin is usually given 1 g every 12 hours intravenously with care to be sure that the infusion time is about 1 hour to minimize side effects of flushing with or without hypotension seen with rapid infusion. The drug is eliminated strictly by the kidneys and dosage must be reduced in renal insufficiency.

Another older agent seeing new uses is metronidazole. It provides excellent activity for anaerobic bacteria including *B. fragilis* and penetrates well into the CNS (23). In serious infections, a loading dose of 15 mg/kg given intravenously is preferred with subsequent doses of 7.5 mg/kg given every 6 hours. Metronidazole is eliminated by the liver and in severe liver disease, dosage should be reduced. Neurotoxicity including ataxia has been noted and can be confusing when this agent is used in a regimen for CNS infection, but fortunately neurologic side effects are rare.

REFERENCES

1. Adams, D. H., and Miller, J. D. Herpes simplex encephalitis: Clinical and pathological analysis of herpes simples. Postgrad. Med. J., *49:* 393–397, 1973.
2. Alderson, D., Strong, A., *et al.* Fifteen year review of the mortality of brain abscess. Neurosurgery, *8:* 1–6, 1981.
3. Balch, R. Wound infections complicating neurosurgical procedures. J. Neurosurg., *26:* 41–45, 1967.
4. Baringer, J. R., and Swoveland, P. Recovery of herpes simplex virus from human trigeminal ganglions. N. Engl. J. Med., *288:* 648–650, 1973.
5. Barre-Sinoussi, F., Chermann, J. C., Rey, F., *et al.* Isolation of a T-lymphotropic retrovirus from a patient at risk for acquired immunodeficiency syndrome (AIDS). Science, *220:* 868–871, 1983.
6. Bennett, J. E., Dish, W. E., *et al.* Amphotericin B-fluorocytosine in cryptococcal meningitis. N. Engl. J. Med., *301:* 126–131, 1979.
7. Berger, M. P., and Paz, J. Diagnosis of cryptococcal meningitis. J.A.M.A., *236:* 2517–2518, 1976.
8. Black, P., Graybill, J. R., *et al.* Brain abscess penetration of systemically administered antibiotics. J. Neurosurg., *38:* 705–709, 1973.
9. Britt, R. H., and Enzmann, D. R. Intracranial infections in cardiac transplant recipients. Ann. Neurol., *9:* 107–119, 1981.
10. Burke, L. P., Ho, S. U., *et al.* Multiple brain abscesses. Surg. Neurol., *16:* 452–454, 1981.
11. Caplan, E. S., Hoyt, N. J. Nosocomial sinusitis. *J.A.M.A. 247:* 639–641, 1982.
12. Carey, M. D., Chou, S. N., *et al.* Experience with brain abscesses. J. Neurosurg., *36:* 1–9, 1972.
13. Carton, C. A., and Kilbourne, E. D. Activation of latent herpes simplex by trigeminal sensory root section. N. Engl. J. Med., *246:* 172–176, 1952.
14. Choppin, P. W., and Scheid, A. The role of viral glycoproteins in adsorption, penetration, and pathogenicity of viruses. Rev. Infect. Dis., *2:* 40–61, 1980.
15. Corey, L., Rubin, R. J., and Hattwick M. A. W. Reye's syndrome: Clinical progression and evaluation of therapy. Pediatrics, *60:* 708–714, 1977.
16. Cornell, S. H., and Jakoby, C. G. The varied computed tomographic appearance of intracranial cryptococcosis. Radiology, *143:* 701–707, 1982.
17. DeLouvois, J., Gortval, P., *et al.* Bacteriology of abscesses of the central nervous system; a multicentre prospective study. Br. Med. J., *2:* 981–984, 1977.
18. Donowitz, L. G., Wenzel, R. P., and Hoyt, J. W. High risk of hospital acquired infection in the ICU patient. Crit. Care Med., *10:* 355–357, 1982.
19. Drachman, D. A., and Adams, R. D. Herpes simplex and acute inclusion body encephalitis. Arch. Neurol., *7:* 61–79, 1962.
20. Dunker, R. C. Failure of computed tomographic scanning to demonstrate subdural empyema. J.A.M.A., *246:* 1116–1118, 1981.
21. Dutt, M. K., and Johnston, I. D. A. Computed tomography and EEG in herpes simplex encephalitis. Their value in diagnosis and prognosis. Arch. Neurol., *39:* 99–102, 1982.
22. Everett, B. A., Kusske, J. A., *et al.* Cryptococcal infection of the central nervous system. Surg. Neurol., *9:* 157–163, 1978.
23. Finegold, S. M., Metronidazole. Ann. Intern. Med., *93:* 585–591, 1980.
24. Fu, K. P., and Neu, H. C. Piperacillin, a new penicillin active against many bacteria resistant to other penicillins. Antimicrob. Agents Chemother., *13:* 358–363, 1978.
25. Gajdusek, D. C., Gibbs, C. J., Jr., Asher, D. M., *et al.* Precautions in medical care of, and in handling materials from patients with transmissible virus dementia (Creutzfeldt-Jakob disease). N. Engl. J. Med., *297:* 1253–1258, 1977.
26. Gallo, R. C., Salahuddin, S. Z., Popovic, M., *et al.* Frequent detection and isolation of cytopathic retroviruses (HTLV-III) from patients with AIDS or at risk for AIDS. Science, *224:* 500–502, 1984.
27. George, R., Leibrock, L., *et al.* Long-term analysis of cerebrospinal fluid shunt infections: a 25 year experience. J. Neurosurg., *51:* 804–811, 1979.
28. Geraci, J. E., and Hermans, P. E. Vancomycin. Mayo Clin. Proc., *58:* 88–91, 1983.
29. Gombert, M. E., Landesman, S. H., *et al.* Vancomycin and rifampin therapy for staphylococcal epi-

dermidis meningitis associated with CSF shunts: Report of 3 cases. J. Neurosurg., *55:* 633–636, 1981.
30. Goodman, S. J., and Stern, W. E. Cranial and intracranial bacterial infections. In: *Neurological Surgery*, Ed., 2 pp. 3323–3357, edited by J. Youmans. Philadelphia, 1982.
31. Hand, W. L., and Sanford, J. P. Post traumatic bacterial meningitis. Ann. Intern. Med., *72:* 869–874, 1970.
32. Hardy, T. L., Minor, F., *et al.* Chronic subdural empyema. Surg. Neurol., *16:* 154–156, 1981.
33. Ingham, H. R., and Selkon, J. B. Cerebral abscess. J. Antimicrob. Chemother., *2:* 224–225, 1976.
34. Johanson, O., Cronberg, S., Hoffstedt, B., *et al.* Cefuroxime versus ampicillin and chloramphenicol for the treatment of bacterial meningitis. Lancet, *1:* 295–299, 1982.
35. Johanson, W. G. Prevention of respiratory tract infections. Am. J. Med., *76 (Suppl. 5A):* 69–77, 1984.
36. Johnson, R. T. *Viral Infections of the Nervous System.* Raven, New York, 1982.
37. Kaufman, D. M., Miller, M. H., *et al.* Subdural empyema: Analysis of 17 recent cases and review of the literature. Medicine, *54:* 485–495, 1975.
38. Kindt, G. W., Waldman, J., Kohl, C., Baublis, J. V., and Tucker, R. P. Intracranial pressure in Reye's syndrome monitoring and control. J.A.M.A., *231:* 822–825, 1975.
39. Kunin, C. M. Urinary tract infections. Surg. Clin. North Am., *60:* 223–230, 1980.
40. Landesman, S. H., Corrado, M. L., Shah, P. M., *et al.* Past and current roles for cephalosporin antibiotics in treatment of meningitis. Am. J. Med., *71:* 693–699, 1981.
41. Levy, R. M., Bredesen, D. E., and Rosenblum, M. L. Neurologic manifestations of the acquired immunodeficiency syndrome: Experience at UCSF and review of the literature. J. Neurosurg., *62:* 475–495, 1985.
42. Levy, S. B. Microbial resistance to antibiotics: An evolving and persistent problem. Lancet, *2:* 83–88, 1982.
43. Lindberg, J., Rosenhall, V., *et al.* Long term outcome of *Haemophilus influenzae* meningitis related to antibiotic treatment. Pediatrics, *60:* 1–6, 1977.
44. Lovejoy, F. H., Smith, A. L., Bresnan, M. J., Wood, J. N., Victor, D. I., and Adams, P. C. Clinical staging in Reye's syndrome. Am. J. Dis. Child., *128:* 36–41, 1974.
45. Luken, M. G., III, and Whelan, M. A. Recent diagnostic experience with subdural empyema. J. Neurosurg., *52:* 764–771, 1980.
46. Linneman, C. C., Shea, L., Partin, J. C., Schubert, W. K., and Schiff, G. M. Reye's syndrome: Epidemiologic and viral studies, 1963–1974. Am. J. Epidemiol., *101:* 517–526, 1975.
47. Maki, D. G., Weise, C., and Satafin, H. M. A semiquantitative culture method for identifying intravenous-catheter-related infection. N. Engl. J. Med., *296:* 1305–1309, 1977.
48. McGahan, J. P., Graves, D. S., *et al.* Classic and contemporary imaging of coccidioidomycosis. Am. J. Roentgenol., *136:* 393–404, 1981.
49. McGillicuddy, J. E. Infections of the central nervous system. 2. Viral, including Reye's syndrome. In: *Neurosurgery. The Scientific Basis of Clinical Practice*, edited by A. Crockard, R. Hayward, and J. Hoff, pp. 676. Blackwell, Oxford, 1985.
50. Metroka, L. E., Cunningham-Rundles, S., Pollack, M. S., *et al.* Generalized lymphadenopathy in homosexual men. Ann. Intern. Med., *99:* 585–591, 1983.
51. Mildvan, D., Mathur, U., Enlow, R. W., *et al.* Opportunistic infections and immune deficiency in homosexual men. Ann. Intern. Med., *96:* 700–704, 1982.
52. Neu, H. C. Structure-activity relations of new β-lactam compounds and in vitro activity against common bacteria. Rev. Infect. Dis., 5(Suppl): 319–336, 1983.
53. New, P. F. J., Davis, K. R., *et al.* Computed tomography in cerebral abscess. Radiology, *121:* 641–646, 1976.
54. Nissen, A. J. Intracranial complications of otogenic disease. Am. J. Oto., *2:* 164–167, 1980.
55. Parker, J. C., Cleary, T. J., *et al.* The effects of transient candidemia on the brain. Surg. Neurol., *11:* 44–48, 1979.
56. Pinilla, J. C., Ross, D. F., Martin, T., *et al.* Study of the incidence of intravascular catheter infections and associated septicemia in critically ill patients. Crit. Care Med., *11:* 21–25, 1983.
57. Pons, V., and Hoff, J. Infections of the central nervous system. In: *Current Surgical Therapy of Neurological Disease*, edited by C. Wilson and J. Hoff, pp. 265–275. Churchill-Livingstone, Edinburgh, 1980.
58. Reye, R. D. K., Morgan, G., and Baral, J. Encephalopathy and fatty degeneration of the viscera: A disease entity of childhood. Lancet, *2:* 749, 1963.
59. Rish, B. L. Analysis of brain abscess after penetrating craniocerebral injuries in Vietnam. Neurosurgery, *9:* 535–541, 1981.
60. Rosenblum, M. L., Hoff, J. T., *et al.* Decreased mortality from brain abscess since advent of computerized tomography. J. Neurosurg., *49:* 658–668, 1978.
61. Rotheram, E. B., Jr., and Kessler, L. A. Use of computerized tomography in nonsurgical management of brain abscess. Arch. Neurol., *36:* 25–26, 1979.
62. Rubin, R. H., and Hooper, D. C. Central nervous system infection in the compromised host. Med. Clin. NP, *69:* 281–296, 1985.
63. Samson, D. S., and Clark, K. A current review of brain abscess. Am. J. Med., *121:* 207–219, 1973.
64. Sharif, H. S., and Ibrahim, A. Intracranial epidural abscess. Br. J. Radiol., *55:* 81–84, 1982.
65. Skoldenberg, B., Forsgren, M., Alstig, K., *et al.* Acyclovir versus vidarabine in herpes simplex encephalitis. Lancet, *2:* 707–711, 1984.
66. Starko, K. M., Ray, C. G., Diminquez, L. B., Stromberg, W. L., and Woodall, D. F. Reye's syndrome and salicylate use. Pediatrics, *66:* 859–864, 1980.
67. Stephanov, S., and Joubert, M. J. Large brain abscesses treated by aspiration alone. Surg. Neurol., *17:* 338–340, 1982.
68. Thierry, A., Cortet, P., Michiels, R., Seigneuric, C., Binnert, D., Pelikan, M. C., and Santreaux, J. L.

EEG contributions to early neurosurgical treatment of herpes encephalitis. Neurochirurgie, *24:* 123–128, 1978.

69. Thomas, J. N., and Nel, J. R. Acute spreading osteomyelitis of the skull complicating frontal sinusitis. J. Laryngol., *91:* 55–62, 1977.
70. Venes, J. L., Shaywitz, B. A., and Spencer, D. D. Management of severe cerebral edema in the metabolic encephalopathy of Reye-Johnson syndrome. J. Neurosurg., *48:* 903–915, 1978.
71. Verner, E. F., and Musher, D. M. Spinal epidural abscess. Med. Clin. North Am., *69:* 375–384, 1985.
72. Weiner, L. P., and Fleming, J. O. Viral infections of the nervous system. J. Neurosurg., *61:* 207–224, 1984.
73. Whitley, R. J., Soong, S.-J., Dolin, R., Galasso, G. J., Ch'ien, L. T., Alford, C. A. The Collaborative Study Group: Adenine arabinoside therapy of biopsy-proven herpes simplex encephalitis. N. Engl. J. Med., *297:* 289–294, 1977.
74. Whitley, R. J., Soong, H.-J., Hirsch, M. S., Karchmer, A. W., Dolin, R., Galasso, G., Dunnick, J., Alford, C. A. The NIAID Collaborative Antiviral Study Groups. Herpes simplex encephalitis: Vidarabine therapy and diagnostic problems. N. Engl. J. Med., *304:* 313–318, 1981.
75. Whitley, R. J., Soong, S.-J., Linneman, C. J., Liu, C., Pazin, G., and Alford, C. A. The NIAID Collaborative Antiviral Study Group. Herpes simplex encephalitis: Clinical assessment. *J.A.M.A. 247:* 317–320, 1982.
76. Winn, H. R., Mendes, M., *et al.* Production of experimental brain abscess in the rat. J. Neurosurg., *51:* 685–690, 1979.
77. Yang, S. Y. Brain abscess: A review of 400 cases. J. Neurosurg., *55:* 794–799, 1981.
78. Yoshikawa, T. T., Chow, A. W., *et al.* Role of anaerobic bacteria in subdural empyema: Report of 4 cases and review of 327 cases from the English literature. Am. J. Med., *58:* 99–104, 1975.
79. Young, R. C., Bennett, J. E., *et al.* Fungemia with compromised host resistance: A study of 70 cases. Ann. Intern. Med., *80:* 605–612, 1974.

CHAPTER 8

Convulsive Disorders and Their Management

W. E. DODSON, M.D., and
J. A. FERRENDELLI, M.D.

INTRODUCTION

Seizures are one of the more common neurologic disorders and patients with this problem are encountered frequently in the practice of both medical and surgical neurology. Seizures are manifestations of abnormal neurologic function and are caused by paroxysmal, excessive neuronal discharges. Recognition of seizures and understanding the various etiologies and mechanisms responsible for their expression is essential for their successful diagnosis and treatment. This is true for the patient who has epilepsy, i.e., recurrent seizures over a period of months to years, as well as the individual who suffers only from a single or a few seizures as a result of some acute, transient neurologic illness.

It is the purpose of this chapter to review issues concerning assessment and treatment of seizures occurring in acutely ill neurologic patients. Attention will be focused on situations encountered frequently by neurologic surgeons and particularly in neurosurgical intensive care units. Characteristics, pathophysiologic mechanisms, and etiologies of seizures will be outlined. Approaches to and evaluation of patients with seizures in the intensive care unit will be defined. Finally treatment of various acute seizures will be described in detail. The reader is advised to also refer to other texts and reviews of epilepsy for additional information on the general subject of seizure disorders and their treatment.

Definition of Seizures and Seizure Types

Seizures are classically defined as paroxysmal excessive neuronal discharges that result in abnormal cerebral electrical activity and behavior. Both the abnormal electrical activity, usually measured with EEG, and the abnormal behavioral activity are dependent upon the region of brain involved in the seizure discharge and its duration. At present, seizures are usually described according to the classification of the International League Against Epilepsy, "International Classification of Epileptic Seizures" [Table 8.1 (18, 30)]. In this classification seizures are divided into two major categories: (*a*) partial seizures, which usually begin and are confined to a relatively small region of brain; and (*b*) generalized seizures, which are without local onset and appear to involve the brain bilaterally and symmetrically from the outset. The following are more detailed descriptions of the major varieties of generalized and partial seizures most frequently seen in older children and adults.

Primary or Secondary Generalized Tonic-Clonic Convulsions

These are classical grand mal or major motor seizures. Unconsciousness, violent motor activity, and post-ictal somnolence and confusion are hallmarks of this disorder. Both tonic and clonic phases occur in most individuals, but some patients, especially young children, may exhibit only the clonic or the tonic seizure. "Primary" refers to those seizures lacking identifiable causes. "Secondary generalized convulsions" either begin with a focal clinical or an EEG abnormality or may be followed by focal post-ictal neurologic deficits. Simple or complex partial seizures (see below) may precede secondarily generalized convulsions. Thus primary seizures by definition lack discernible

TABLE 8.1
The International Classification of Epileptic Seizures*

I. Partial
  A. Simple partial seizures
    1. With motor signs
    2. With somatosensory or special sensory symptoms
    3. With autonomic symptoms or signs
    4. With psychic symptoms
  B. Complex partial seizures
    1. Simple partial onset
    2. Impaired consciousness at onset
  C. Partial seizures which secondarily generalize
II. Generalized seizures
  A. Absence seizures
    1. Typical
    2. Atypical
  B. Myoclonic
  C. Clonic
  D. Tonic
  E. Tonic-clonic
  F. Atonic
III. Unclassified epileptic seizures
IV. Status epilepticus

*Commission on Classification and Terminology of the International League Against Epilepsy. Proposal for revised clinical and electroencephalographic classification of epileptic seizures. Epilepsia, *22:* 489–501, 1981.

structural abnormality of brain, whereas secondarily generalized seizures more often are associated with structural abnormalities.

Absence Seizures

These seizures are characterized by brief periods, only seconds long, of unawareness and staring without loss of posture and usually without post-ictal symptoms. Minor movements such as eye blinking or a slight twitching of the arms and face often occur. Infrequently absence seizures are prolonged or frequently repeated. When this occurs there are more vigorous, stereotyped movements of the mouth, face, and sometimes, extremities (automatisms). Atypical absence seizures are characterized by more extensive movement during the seizure than is seen with typical absence. In a severe form these may be associated with head nodding or even sudden loss of postural tone, so called atonic or akinetic seizures known colloquially as drop attacks. These seizure types usually occur in children who have diffusely abnormal EEGs and multiple types of seizures. The combination of atonic seizures, multiple types of seizures, slow spike-wave pattern on EEG, and developmental arrest or regression is known as the Lennox-Gastaut syndrome. Patients with this disorder are prone to developing absence status.

Ictal staring can be caused by either absence seizures or partial complex seizures. Ictal staring caused by partial complex (psychomotor) seizures may be clinically indistinguishable from absence seizures, but usually partial complex seizures last longer than 30 seconds. Patients who have partial complex seizures usually have a history of more typical psychomotor spells with affective, cognitive, or hallucinatory symptoms. Because partial complex seizures usually cause a longer period of unconsciousness than absence seizures, automatisms are more likely to occur here than during absence seizures. But either of these seizure types can cause prolonged confusion and clouded sensorium. In this setting the EEG is particularly helpful in making the right diagnosis.

The EEG is the most certain way to differentiate between absence and partial complex seizures. Absence seizures are usually associated with diffuse spike and wave or poly-spike and wave discharges on the EEG. The 3 Hz spike-wave pattern characteristic of absence seizures associated with petit mal epilepsy is a typical example. Partial complex seizures are usually associated with focal spike activity, most often in the temporal or frontal region, with variable alterations, usually slowing, of background cerebral rhythms while the seizure is occurring.

Partial Seizures

These are classified as either simple or complex depending on whether unconsciousness occurs. Simple partial (focal) seizures are associated with motor, sensory, affective, or other symptoms without loss of consciousness. They may originate in various regions of the cortex and the symptoms or signs usually reflect the site of the localized epileptiform discharge. Complicated affective sensations, distorted perceptions, hallucinations, and other symptoms may be associated with discharges in frontal, cingulate, or temporal cortex. When consciousness is lost in this situation, the seizure type is classified as partial complex. Unconsciousness results when the ictal discharge involves bilateral limbic structures. In partial complex seizures, there may be prior symptoms of a simple partial seizure or unconsciousness may be lost from the outset. Thus simple partial seizures may progress to partial complex seizures and both may spread to cause a generalized tonic-clonic seizure, a so called secondarily generalized convulsion.

Partial seizures are more often symptoms of localized functional and morphologic brain abnormality than generalized seizures. For example, patients with absence seizures of the petit mal type almost never have identifiable structural brain disease. These idiopathic cases, especially where there is a genetic predisposition to epilepsy, are classified as primary epilepsies. Because partial seizures are more likely to be manifestations of focal brain pathology, careful patient evaluation with imaging studies is indicated.

ETIOLOGY OF SEIZURES

Most researchers agree that neurons involved in a seizure discharge exhibit prolonged depolarization which is referred to as a paroxysmal depolarizing shift (PDS). A single brief PDS is accompanied only by a transient cerebral electrical abnormality, usually a single spike on the EEG. A very prolonged PDS or multiple repeated PDSs results in a seizure discharge associated with sustained cerebral electrical abnormalities and clinical seizure activity. Alterations of ionic conductances, particularly calcium, sodium, and potassium contribute to the production of the PDS. Synaptic mechanisms also play a role and excessive excitatory neurotransmitter or diminished inhibitory neurotransmitter influences have both been demonstrated to be involved in the initiation and maintenance of seizure discharges. In summary, it is apparent that several factors contribute to the development of seizures and that no single mechanistic scheme can fully explain the cause of various seizure types or etiologies.

Seizures are symptoms and are not a disease per se. However, many patients with seizure disorders have no discernible cause which can be determined by available diagnostic procedures and their condition is referred to as idiopathic or primary epilepsy. Patients who have an underlying cause for their seizures are said to suffer from symptomatic or secondary epilepsy. Several systemic and neurologic diseases and disorders that cause seizures are discussed below.

Trauma

Head injury is a common cause of seizures. A patient may suffer from one or a few seizures immediately following a head injury. Presumably this is due to the acute mechanical distortion of brain tissue and usually is not predictive of subsequent epilepsy. Seizures that begin weeks to months or even years after a head injury tend to be recurring. The severity of the head injury is directly related to the incidence of post-traumatic seizures. Injuries associated with cerebral contusion, intracranial hemorrhage, skull fracture and/or prolonged unconsciousness are much more likely to lead to seizures than less severe injuries. Brain trauma incident to intracranial surgery can also lead to a seizure disorder and this, too, is probably related to the amount and degree of tissue injury. The incidence of epilepsy following various intracranial surgical procedures has not been adequately investigated and remains uncertain.

The pathophysiologic mechanisms responsible for post-traumatic seizures are not well understood. There is some information indicating that the presence of extravascular blood is a contributing factor to epileptogenesis following CNS trauma. A relatively large hemorrhage usually occurring near the time of head injury mechanically distorts brain tissue and also acts as an irritating focus. This sometimes produces acute seizures which are difficult to control and require surgical removal of the hematoma. Seizures occurring later, usually several days or longer after the injury, seem to result from scarring and secondary gliosis which may be partially a result of oxidized blood products. It is unclear how the gliosis or glial scar following cerebral injury of any type is epileptogenic. A popular idea at present is that these regions of gliosis are not able to maintain the neuronal microenvironment adequately which leads to altered concentrations of extracellular potassium, calcium, and other ions and, in turn, increases neuronal excitability.

Tumors

Most cerebral tumors can cause seizures and those near to or involving cerebral cortex are the most epileptogenic. Tumors are usually associated with recurrent seizures. The seizures produced by tumors appear to be a result of various factors. Ischemia contributes to the cause of seizures in some patients. Mechanical factors, including traction, pressure, and distortion by the tumor or surrounding edema on cerebral cortex are important. Reduction of edema and/or removal of tumor are necessary in the treatment of these patients. In some patients whose tumor is successfully treated, glial scarring produced by either the tumor or its treatment may be a source of continuing seizure activity.

Cerebrovascular Disease

Occlusive cerebral vascular disease and diffuse impairment of cerebral circulation are common causes of seizures. Seizures may occur at the time of the acute ischemic event probably as a result of acute impairment of neuronal and glial metabolism. Embolic infarction seems to be more epileptogenic than thrombotic strokes. Frequent recurrent seizures associated with periodic, lateralized epileptiform discharges on the EEG (often referred to as PLEDS) are most commonly caused by acute cerebral infarction and require intensive antiepileptic drug therapy. Acute hemorrhages and hemorrhagic strokes have the same epileptogenic potential as cerebral trauma and probably cause seizures by the same mechanism described in the section on head injury. Strokes, like trauma, may leave a chemically injured region of brain which can be a source of recurrent seizures. This is one of the most common causes of epilepsy that begins in the elderly.

CNS Infections

Acute meningitis, encephalitis, or brain abscess are frequently associated with seizures. Localized cerebral ischemia as well as direct effects of the inflammation on cerebral structure and metabolism are responsible for the seizures in these diseases. Seizures occurring after the acute inflammatory episode are due to glial scarring.

Metabolic Causes of Seizures

Several systemic diseases and disorders causing metabolic abnormalities can produce seizures. Altered blood cation concentration including hyponatremia and hypernatremia, hypocalcemia, and hypomagnesemia lead to seizures. The many causes of these cation abnormalities will not be repeated here, but it is to be emphasized that seizures resulting from these abnormalities may be resistant to antiepileptic drug therapy and must be treated by restoration of electrolyte balance. Decreased neuronal membrane potential stability and altered ionic conductances are the mechanisms underlying seizures secondary to cation concentration abnormalities.

Hypoglycemia and hypoxia are well known metabolic abnormalities producing seizures. The mechanism(s) by which inadequate glucose or oxygen supply produces seizures in brain has not been ascertained. It seems to be multifactorial and includes impairment of cerebral energy supply with resulting changes in neuronal and glial microenvironment and alterations of synaptic mechanisms, possibly excessive excitatory neurotransmitter action.

Both hepatic and renal failure may be associated with seizures. In both cases accumulation of toxic products which have not been definitely identified are most likely responsible for the seizures. Therefore correction of the metabolic imbalance is the primary, and often the only effective, treatment.

Metabolic disorders are a cause of acute seizures which usually disappear when metabolic balance is achieved. Chronic recurrent seizures are only caused by metabolic abnormalities when the underlying cause has produced cerebral damage or if the metabolic disorder is recurrent.

Drugs and Toxins

Several chemical agents cause seizures by a variety of different mechanisms. Only a few need to be considered with respect to patient care in the neurosurgical intensive care unit, however. Methylxanthines, e.g., theophylline, are directly epileptogenic probably because they block the CNS actions of adenosine which is an inhibitory modulator. Local anesthetics also cause seizures because of their ability to impair sodium conductances in excitable membranes. Local anesthetics, especially lidocaine, are also anticonvulsant at low concentrations. Psychotropic drugs, particularly tricyclic antidepressants, phenothiazines, and some recreational drugs may also produce seizures. The seizures occur most often at toxic concentrations of the drug or in patients who are susceptible to seizures for other reasons. Like metabolic disorders drug-related seizures are not recurrent and require treatment of the underlying cause of the seizures. Drug withdrawal may be associated with seizure activity. All sedative drugs, but particularly barbiturates, alcohol, and hypnotics, can cause seizures when these brain concentrations fall rapidly. Withdrawal of antiepileptic drugs in epileptic patients obviously results in increased seizure frequency and is the most common causes of status epilepticus among patients with epilepsy. This problem is particularly important to remember in any patient who already has a seizure disorder under treatment who then requires surgery of any type. In these patients antiepileptic drugs must be continued in the pre- and postoperative periods.

ASSESSMENT AND TREATMENT OF SEIZURE

In the setting of the neurosurgical intensive care unit one is most concerned with the assessment and treatment of patients with acute seizures, particularly status epilepticus. The most widely accepted definition of status epilepticus is "epileptic seizures that are so frequently repeated or so prolonged as to create a fixed and lasting epileptic condition" (7). Status epilepticus may be convulsive or nonconvulsive. Note that the definition also includes the situations in which seizures are recurrent without recovery of consciousness. Older definitions included a duration of 1 hour or longer. However, because serious neural and systemic metabolic consequences develop earlier, contemporary definitions consider a duration of 30 minutes to be sufficient (78). Therapy should be aggressive if a convulsion continues for 10 minutes or longer.

In most patients status epilepticus stops after the first or second medication (24). If not, it often means that a severe cerebral insult has occurred causing continuing brain irritation. If the etiology is not apparent, the search for the cause should be intensified. But even when the primary cause seems evident, potentially aggravating metabolic or toxic factors must still be excluded. Multiple causes often coexist.

Nonconvulsive status epilepticus, that is continuous, nonconvulsive seizures, result from either continuous absence seizures or from continuous complex partial seizures. Patients in nonconvulsive status have persistently clouded sensoriums and variable amounts of twitching or automatic movement (automatisms). It is not an emergency-like generalized convulsive status. Here it is important to make the right diagnosis in order to select the appropriate antiepileptic drug. Nonconvulsive status may be treated less urgently than convulsive status which is a medical emergency.

Treatment of Convulsive Status Epilepticus

Concurrent with treating status one should seek to determine the cause, making certain that treatable metabolic and infectious causes are treated specifically (Table 8.2). Among patients with prior epilepsy, discontinuation or reduced intake of anticonvulsant medications is a common cause of status epilepticus (1, 69). In the neurosurgical intensive care unit, CNS infections, trauma, hypoxia, drugs and drug withdrawal, and systemic metabolic problems can precipitate status epilepticus (56, 75). Obviously in many instances the status epilepticus is a direct consequence of the patient's reason for being in the intensive care unit (27). On the other hand status epilepticus can cause localized brain edema which might be misinterpreted as tumor or infarction (76).

Status epilepticus is an emergency which requires aggressive therapy and intensive support (Table 8.3). Because oxygenation, blood pressure, and acid-base balance may be disturbed by prolonged convulsions, supportive medical care is just as important as anticonvulsant drug therapy (78, 82). Among all the supportive measures, adequate ventilation ensuring oxygenation and maintaining adequate blood glucose are most important.

The initial steps in therapy are to establish vital signs, protect the airway, give oxygen, draw blood for the laboratory determination of glucose, blood urea nitrogen, electrolytes, and drug levels, and rapidly estimate the blood glucose with a Dextrostix. If the blood glucose cannot be estimated immediately, glucose should be given intravenously as 25% dextrose 1 to 2 ml/per kg in children or 50 ml of 50% glucose in adults, followed by the infusion of intravenous fluid containing 10% dextrose.

When multiple medications are needed to stop the seizures, depression of respiration is expected. Any patient with status epilepticus may need temporary ventilatory assistance.

TABLE 8.2
Etiology of Status Epilepticus*

Drug withdrawal
- Antiepileptic drugs
- Alcohol
- Benzodiazepines
- Short acting barbiturates

Drug therapy and diagnostic agents
- Anticholinergic overdose
  - Antidepressant overdose
    - Maprotoline
- Phenothiazines
  - Fluphenazine
- Antibiotics
  - Penicillin
- Theophylline
- Local anesthetics
- Metrizamide myelography

Trauma

Fluid and electrolyte disturbances
- Water intoxication including SIADH
- Hypocalcemia and hypomagnesemia

Miscellaneous
- ECT (bilateral or unilateral)
- Pyridoxine deficiency or dependency
- Multiple sclerosis
- Eclampsia

Hypoxia

Hypoglycemia

CNS infections
- Meningitis
- Encephalitis
- Brain abscess
- Subdural empyema

Cerebrovascular disease
- Venous thrombosis
- Thromboembolic arterial occlusion

*M. J. Aiminoff and R. P. Simon: Status epilepticus. Causes, clinical features and consequences in 98 patients. Am. J. Med., *69:* 657–666, 1980; A. Pilke, M. Partinene, and J. Kovanen: Status epilepticus and alcohol abuse: An analysis of 82 status epilepticus admissions. Acta Neurol. Scand., *70:* 443–450, 1984.

Some patients with status epilepticus become apneic after only a single drug given in a reasonable dose stops the convulsion. If multiple depressant medications are needed to stop the status epilepticus, mechanical ventilation should be provided before the patient becomes hypoxic.

The sequence of anticonvulsants that are given is to some extent a matter of personal preference. Whatever sequence of drugs is used, it is important that the physician have a plan in mind, use drugs familiar to him, and give them in an adequately large doses (Table 8.4). The primary goal of drug administration is the cessation of seizures, not the production of a particular drug concentration in blood. After the status epilepticus is controlled specific drug levels are helpful in preventing recurrent seizures and regulating long-term therapy. Thus in stubborn or refractory status, it is usually necessary to administer larger doses than certain textbooks recommend. The best drugs to use in very high doses to interrupt refractory status are benzodiazepines and barbiturates. In these situations ventilatory support is usually required.

Our preferred sequence of drugs is a benzodiazepine, either diazepam or lorazepam, followed by phenytoin, phenobarbital, and paraldehyde. Although lidocaine has been advocated by some, we do not recommend it (11, 13). If these fail, anesthetic doses of a barbiturate or diazepam infusion or general anesthesia will stop the convulsions. Note well that in refractory status, seizures may recur as anesthesia is withdrawn if the irritative insult to brain persists. Among the barbiturates, phenobarbital, thiopental, and pentobarbital have been used but the last two are anticonvulsant only at anesthetic doses. Phenobarbital has anticonvulsant action at subanesthetic doses. Also effective are frequently repeated doses or a continuous infusion of diazepam. Inhalation anesthetics such as halothane are effective, too

TABLE 8.3
General Therapy in Treating Status Epilepticus*

Airway-oxygenation

Obtain base line blood samples including drug levels
- Dextrostix estimation of blood glucose

Administer glucose intravenously
- Pediatric dose: 1–2 ml/kg of 25% glucose
- Adult dose: 50 ml of 50% glucose
- Infusion of 10% glucose solution

Consider thiamine, 100 mg IV

Administer antiepileptic drugs (see Table 8.4)

Administer bicarbonate if pH <7.2

Correct fluid and electrolyte disturbances

Consider corticosteroids

EKG and EEG

Specific treatment of etiology

*T. Bleck: Therapy for status epilepticus. Clin. Neuropharmacol., *6:* 255–269, 1983; J. Bruni: Treatment of status epilepticus in adults. Can. Med. Assoc. J., *128:* 531–533, 1983.

TABLE 8.4
Doses of Medications Used in Status Epilepticus

Drug	Route	Pediatric Dose	Adult Dose
Diazepam	IV	0.3 mg/kg (1 mg/yr of age)	10–40 mg
Diazepam	Infusion	0.1–0.3 mg/kg/hr	4–8 mg/hr
Diazepam	PR	0.5 mg/kg	
Lorazepam	IV	1–4 mg	4–8 mg
Clonazepam*	IV	0.25 mg/kg (0.25–2 mg)	1–4 mg
Phenytoin	IV	20 mg/kg	15–20 mg/kg
Phenobarbital	IV	20 mg/kg	15–20 mg/kg
Paraldehyde	IV	0.15 ml/kg diluted	8–10 ml diluted
	PR	0.3 ml/kg	
Pentobarbital	IV	Loading 2.5–4 mg/kg	
	Infusion	0.5 mg/kg/hr	100–500 mg/hr

*Not available in the United States.

(7). At anesthetic doses, some of these agents such as pentobarbital appear to be more likely to reduce cardiac output and produce hypotension than phenobarbital. Despite the complex biopharmaceutical problems associated with continuous intravenous infusions of diazepam, this therapy has gained popularity in the past 5 years. Because of the uncertainty about the dose that is actually delivered to the patient during continuous infusions, we prefer frequent bolus doses of diazepam especially for pediatric patients.

Benzodiazepines

Benzodiazepines have been administered intravenously as both "bolus" and continuous infusions in the treatment of status epilepticus in patients of all ages (3, 5, 24, 34, 35). Diazepam has been used most widely, but other benzodiazepines are equally efficacious in the acute stage, and are longer acting because they are not redistributed out of the brain as is diazepam.

Benzodiazepines are thought to act primarily as γ-aminobutyric acid (GABA) agonists. They increase pre- and postsynaptic inhibition. In the latter case they augment the action of GABA to open the chloride channel, alter membrane conductance, and reduce the probability that the membrane potential will reach the threshold to produce an action potential (59, 98). Benzodiazepines also appear to attenuate the release of excitatory neurotransmitter induced by convulsant drugs and other means, probably by GABA-mediated presynaptic inhibition (59). Presumably the inhibitory actions are initiated at high affinity, stereospecific benzodiazepine receptors. These receptors are closely associated with GABA and barbiturate receptors, all of which are affiliated with the chloride channel which mediates postsynaptic inhibition (67, 89).

Benzodiazepine receptors are dynamically regulated by a variety of factors, including seizure discharges and drug therapy (84). Metrazole-induced seizures increase the number of benzodiazepine receptors in cortex (10). In the rat hippocampus the number of benzodiazepine receptors increases only after a large number of seizures (62). Barbiturates, which also enhance the postsynaptic action of GABA, increase the affinity of the benzodiazepine receptor for benzodiazepines (16, 80). Chronic therapy with benzodiazepines reduces the number of receptors in cultured fetal mouse neurons (77). These actions suggest that benzodiazepines may be more helpful in stopping seizures than in preventing them.

Diazepam therapy begins with intravenous bolus doses injected at rates of 1 mg/m. Giving the dose too rapidly is liable to cause hypotension especially in older patients. The initial dose for children is 1 mg/yr of age up to 10 mg. The initial dose in adults is 10 mg. Even at low doses, transient hypoventilation may be a problem because bolus administration causes very high diazepam levels in blood and brain. For comparison, levels of 100 to 200 ng/ml are anxietolytic whereas peak levels of 5,775 to 10,800 ng/ml result after intravenous (IV) doses of 1 mg/kg in infants (8, 53). When the seizures stop before the entire dose is given, the "bolus" infusion should be discontinued because the additional medication will only act to cause more toxicity.

Despite a considerable notoriety for producing hypoventilation or apnea when given IV in high doses for status, benzodiazepines are relatively safe. Accordingly, high doses can be used when ventilatory support is provided. For example, infants in status epilepticus have received daily doses of 75 to 100 mg; 15 to 25 mg/m^2 have been given to children in acute seizure (3); and newborns have been treated with IV bolus doses of 0.5 to 1 mg/kg (53).

In the setting of status epilepticus, any potent sedative-hypnotic drug that can stop status is capable of causing concomitant hypoventilation. In this situation it appears that the status per se also contributes to this adverse effect. Hypoventilation sometimes follows recommended doses of barbiturates, especially among children who are pharmacologically naive with respect to sedative medication. Benzodiazepines and other sedative hypnotic drugs produce considerably more CNS depression than IV phenytoin which is also effective in treating status.

Diazepam, more than other benzodiazepines, is short-acting as an anticonvulsant. Diazepam enters and exits from the CNS more rapidly than phenobarbital or phenytoin and peak brain concentrations may be obtained within the first minute following a "bolus" dose (73). Because of redistribution into other tissues, brain diazepam concentrations decline rapidly in the first hour after IV infusion. Accordingly, the duration of diazepam's anticonvulsant activity is approximately 20 minutes after an intravenous dose. Therefore a longer-acting drug must be given after diazepam is used to interrupt status, in order to sustain the anticonvulsant effect. Most often phenytoin is given (25).

Because a longer-acting antiepileptic drug must be given to prevent early recurrence of seizures after diazepam is used to stop the status, some physicians recommend the use of phenytoin or phenobarbital as the first drug (24, 28). Before considering other drugs, however, other important points concerning benzodiazepines should be reviewed.

A continuous infusion of diazepam can be considered when status is not controlled by initial bolus doses of antiepileptic drugs or when previously controlled status recurs despite adequate loading doses of longer-acting antiepileptics (5, 7). Before the infusion is started the patient should receive an initial loading dose of 30 to 40 mg. In a majority of patients the initial bolus or loading doses of diazepam stop the convulsion and prolonged infusion is unnecessary. The most widely used infusion rate is 4 to 8 mg/hr for adults (25). In this situation the total daily dose usually reaches 1 to 4 mg/kg (5). The infusion is stopped 3 hours after the last seizure.

When diazepam is given by continuous infusion prolonged sedation is to be expected. Unlike the situation after bolus doses in which sedation is abbreviated by diazepam redistribution out of brain into other tissues, greater amounts of diazepam go into tissue and the levels in blood and brain decline more slowly as the drug is eliminated. The diazepam elimination half-life is in the range of 18 to 24 hours. This should be contrasted with a half-life for redistribution of about 20 minutes.

Placing diazepam into IV solutions creates complex biopharmaceutical problems (5). Diazepam is lipophilic with limited aqueous solubility and it also binds to the infusion apparatus, adhering to plastic tubing and bags. Binding is more extensive to plastic than glass. The adsorption of diazepam to the infusion apparatus causes the dose that is actually delivered to the patient to vary, but it is always less than expected based on the amount of drug put in the IV fluid bottle.

The binding of diazepam to IV infusion paraphernalia is saturable and more of the binding sites become occupied as the infusion progresses over time. Thus the dose that is delivered to the patient usually increases when constant infusion rates are prescribed. Depending on the concentration of diazepam in the infusate, the rate of infusion, the type of IV fluid used, and the time the solution hangs at the bedside, the initial dose may be 29% to 93% less than intended (21, 22, 60, 65).

Diazepam is soluble in D5W, normal saline, Ringer's and lactated Ringer's solutions, if diluted to concentrations of 0.125 mg/ml or less (5). At this concentration potency is maintained for 24 hours (66). When glass IV bottles, plastic tubing, and D5W were used at an infusion rate of 100 ml/hr, with a concentration of 0.1

mg/ml in the original stock infusate, 63% of the drug was recovered initially and 83% was recovered after the apparatus was used for 5 hours.

Because the dose that is actually delivered to the patient can increase as the diazepam infusion is prolonged, it is absolutely essential that the patient's vital signs be monitored frequently as long as the infusion continues. Given the biopharmaceutical problems with diazepam infusions, the intended doses described in reports of IV infusions should be interrupted with caution. It is far better to give frequent small doses than to overdose and impair cardiac output causing hypotension.

The problems of variable dose delivery to the patient that result from diazepam adsorption to the infusion apparatus are circumvented when the dose is injected into the intravenous delivery system as near to the patient as possible. Specifically, the doses used in continuous infusions should be reduced by 25% to 75% if they are to be given by "bolus" injection directly into the patient's indwelling venous catheter or needle. The administration of diazepam is most reliable when frequent small "bolus" doses are given directly into the indwelling catheter or needle.

Despite the potential problems with continuous infusions of diazepam, several reports document that this is an effective way of treating status epilepticus, even among small pediatric patients. For example, infants and newborns in status epilepticus were successfully treated with diazepam given by continuous infusion over several days (3, 33, 53, 91). Continuous diazepam infusions of 1 to 1.5 mg/hr (approximately 0.3 mg/kg/hr) for periods of 6 to 11 days have been used in the treatment of neonatal seizures caused by asphyxia with a good outcome in seven of eight patients (33).

Diazepam is also absorbed rapidly and reliably after rectal administration of diazepam solutions, but not suppositories (47, 48, 63, 64). Rectally administered diazepam is widely used in Europe to interrupt prolonged seizures occurring at home and for the intermittent prophylaxis of febrile seizures in children (32). In fact, rectal absorption is more rapid than that after either oral or intramuscular administration (53). Absorption is slowest after intramuscular administration. After rectal administration, diazepam concentrations are usually maximal in 10 to 60 minutes (2). When diazepam cannot be given intravenously in status, rectal administration is next best.

Other benzodiazepines, particularly clonazepam and lorazepam, appear to be as good or better than diazepam in the IV treatment of status epilepticus because of their more prolonged durations of action (85, 86). Although an intravenous formulation of clonazepam is not marketed in the United States, it is available in other countries (79). Clonazepam in IV doses of 0.25 to 0.75 mg stopped convulsions without serious consequences in 17 children aged 2 weeks to 15 years (19). Recurrent seizures in six children were controlled by repeat dosage, in one patient after IV diazepam had failed. IV lorazepam is as effective as diazepam and like clonazepam should be longer acting (57). In a double-blind comparison of diazepam and lorazepam in adults, 89% were controlled with lorazepam versus 76% with diazepam (54). The incidence (12% to 13%) and severity of side effects were equivalent. The doses of lorazepam that have been used are 4 to 8 mg (43, 55, 96). Lorazepam, like diazepam, can cause apnea and hypotension when given IV in status epilepticus.

In nonconvulsive status, a benzodiazepine such as diazepam may be given intravenously while one observes the EEG for a response. This procedure is not as helpful as it might seem because of the following issues. First, failure of the patient to respond does not indicate that orally administered clonazepam will not work. Second, significant sedation, at least briefly, is a consistent side effect of IV administered diazepam. Third, even when IV diazepam is effective, a longer-acting antiepileptic drug must still be given, just as in convulsive status epilepticus.

Benzodiazepines are the drugs of choice for treating seizures caused by local anesthetics, isoniazide, penicillin, and strychnine and in tetanus (88). Based on animal studies benzodiazepines are the drugs of choice for stopping seizures caused by local anesthetic overdose, including cocaine. Data in humans are insufficient to confirm this theory. Local anesthetics appear to initiate convulsions by first causing spike activity in the amygdala. In animals with bilateral amygdalotomies, local anesthetics do not cause seizures. Benzodiazepines prevent amygdalar spiking caused by local anesthetics.

Phenytoin

Phenytoin is effective in treating status epilepticus (17, 97). Because it is nonsedating, many physicians consider it the first drug to be tried in status epilepticus (55, 61). When nonconvulsive status is caused by complex partial seizures, IV-phenytoin is the drug of choice.

Phenytoin prevents the spread of the epileptic discharge. It antagonizes post-tetanic potentiation and calcium-mediated neurosecretion and neurotransmitter release (98). Phenytoin also inhibits sodium and perhaps calcium conductance in excitable membranes, a property which should limit excessively rapid but not normal rates of neuronal firing (23, 59). Phenytoin has not been found to have any effect on GABA-mediated postsynaptic inhibition and differs in this regard from benzodiazepines and barbiturates. In virtually every experimental model evaluated, phenytoin and carbamazepine have similar actions.

Formulations of phenytoin for IV administration are strongly basic (pH 12) and contain propylene glycol to keep the phenytoin dissolved. This concoction is cardiotoxic, causing cardiac standstill if it is infused too rapidly. Phenytoin is best administered IV while monitoring the EEG and blood pressure. If the heart rate slows meaningfully during the infusion, the infusion rate should be decreased. The recommended infusion rate for adults is 50 mg/min (17). Thus for a generic 70-kg adult given a full-loading dose of 18 mg/kg, approximately 25 minutes is required to infuse the dose. In children the recommended rate is a relatively higher 3 mg/kg/min (28). Elderly patients are more likely to develop hypotension during phenytoin infusion at recommended rates (55). But in any age patient it is necessary to slow or stop the infusion if hypotension or bradycardia occurs.

Because phenytoin precipitates and crystallizes in tissue when given intramuscularly, this route is not recommended. The parenteral solution is sufficiently caustic as to cause skin necrosis if it infiltrates at the IV injection site.

In contrast to benzodiazepines and barbiturates, there is an upper limit to how much phenytoin should be administered if seizures do not stop. No more than 20 mg/kg should be given IV before checking the phenytoin blood level, because excessively high phenytoin levels can cause tonic seizures. Thus if seizures persist after 20 mg/kg of phenytoin has been given, a different antiepileptic drug should be administered. Choreoathetosis is another troublesome though less dangerous consequence of toxic phenytoin levels (44, 51). Choreoathetosis should not be confused with continuing seizure activity, an error that can lead one to inappropriately administer more antiepileptic drugs. If there is a question about the diagnosis, a bedside EEG can settle the issue.

Barbiturates

IV administered phenobarbital is considered by many to be the drug of choice for treating status epilepticus in newborns and small infants. The usual dose is 20 mg/kg, a dose that produces phenobarbital levels in excess of 15 μg/ml in most patients (58). It is also quite effective in older children and adults, but is more sedating than phenytoin. At high doses its potential for causing hypoventilation and apnea, especially among pharmacologically naive patients, should not be forgotten. Furthermore, barbiturates potentiate the depressant effects of benzodiazepines. Both barbiturates and benzodiazepines act to enhance GABA-mediated increases in chloride conductance and postsynaptic inhibition. The combination of barbiturates and benzodiazepine in treating status should be expected to cause hypoventilation or apnea.

In treating status in older children and adults IV doses of 200 to 300 mg are often effective in stopping status but are too low to produce levels in the therapeutic range. Administration rates of 100 mg/min have been reported to be safe and thus phenobarbital can be given fairly quickly, as can diazepam (30). When an initial IV dose of 300 mg is not successful it can be repeated in 20 minutes. In order to achieve a level in the therapeutic range, that is a level of more than 10 μg/ml, the initial loading dose must exceed 10 mg/kg. Thus when the seizures stop after the first IV dose, the remainder of the loading dose can be given more slowly over the next several hours minimizing the chance of respiratory depression.

Among all the antiepileptic drugs considered here, phenobarbital is absorbed most rapidly and reliably after intramuscular injection. In young patients, peak levels are seen in 30 to 120 minutes after intramuscular administration.

Repeated doses of phenobarbital can be used to treat intractable status. Even after high doses suppress respiration, there is a considerable margin for administering more drug before hypotension is produced. In this situation, allowing 20 minutes between doses is adequate for determining that blood pressure has not been affected.

Pentobarbital and thiopental have also been used to treat refractory staus epilepticus (7, 15, 68, 99, 100). There are no controlled studies comparing their efficacy with phenobarbital in this situation. The doses of pentobarbital that have been given are similar to those used to treat intracranial hypertension. In adults pentobarbital infusion rates of 100 to 500 mg/hr have been used. In children loading doses of 2.5 to 4 mg/kg followed by infusion rates of 0.5 mg/kg/hr have been recommended. The EEG may be helpful in determining that electrical seizure activity has been stopped, but it makes no sense to push the dose to the point of electroencephalographic burst suppression or electrocerebral silence if the goal of therapy is to control seizures rather than intracranial hypertension. High doses of pentobarbital are prone to causing hypotension and reduced cardiac output, side effects which may need to be countered by giving dopamine.

Paraldehyde

Rectally or intravenously administered par aldehyde is sometimes effective in treating refractory status epilepticus (13, 20, 36). Paraldehyde is rarely used as the first drug to treat status since the popularity of diazepam and phenytoin have increased.

Paraldehyde is predominantly eliminated by hepatic biotransformation and toxicity is more likely if there is associated liver disease; 20% or less is excreted via the lungs. Paraldehyde can potentiate the metabolic acidosis which usually is present during prolonged convulsions. Pulmonary hemorrhage and noncardiogenic pulmonary edema have been found in some patients who died in status after treatment with paraldehyde. In experimental animals, pulmonary hemorrhage was a consistent finding after rapidly administered, lethally high doses (14). Acidosis is a special problem when the paraldehyde container has been opened or exposed to light causing chemical decomposition to acetaldehyde and acetic acid. Other side effects include hypotension, tachypnea, tachycardia, and fever (9). Bolus doses of 0.3 ml/kg have caused respiratory arrest in children (9, 20).

Whether administered rectally or intravenously, paraldehyde should be diluted first. Intramuscular administration causes sterile abscesses and is not recommended. For IV administration the paraldehyde is diluted to a strength of 10% or less in normal saline. We recommend placing 10 ml of paraldehyde in 500 ml of normal saline producing a 2% solution. The initial dose of up to 0.15 ml/kg or a maximum of 10 ml should be infused slowly, over no less than 20 minutes. At lower dilutions longer infusion times are needed because of volume considerations. The maximal safe dose has not been established.

Rectal administration has been used more in children than adults. The recommended dose is 0.3 ml/kg after the paraldehyde has been diluted 1:10 in oil. Any vegetable oil will do but nonabsorbable mineral oil should be avoided. Recently, it has been recommended that this dose be repeated if the seizures persist for 20 minutes after the first dose (20).

Treatment of Nonconvulsive Status Epilepticus

Nonconvulsive status can result from continuous partial or absence seizures (6, 74). The symptoms include confusional states, aphasia, stupor, and behavioral disturbances misdiagnosed as psychiatric disorders (4, 13, 26, 35, 72, 74, 83). If the issue is in doubt, an EEG should be obtained (31). The EEG may be especially helpful in patients with diffuse brain dysfunction which can also cause automatisms. The correct diagnosis of the seizure type is important because different medications are required. Complex partial status should be treated with a major antiepileptic drug such as phenytoin, carbamazepine, phenobarbital, primidone, or methsuximide. Absence status is best treated with ethosuximide, a benzodiazepine such as clonazepam, acetazolamide, or valproic acid.

In nonconvulsive status, intravenous administration of antiepileptic drugs which might cause apnea generally is not recommended because nonconvulsive status per se is not dangerous to the patient. Oral or rectal loading doses are often used. In this situation the initial dose of the medication is doubled during the time equal to one half-life of the drug. This should produce a therapeutic concentration at the end of that time. With most antiepileptic drugs this rapid initiation of treatment usually causes sedation and varying degrees of inebriation.

The details of administering antiepileptic drugs are found in the section on chronic antiepileptic drug administration (Table 8.4). However, a few points deserve special mention now.

Nonconvulsive status can be treated by any route; however, oral, gavage, or rectal administration is preferred because of safety. Absence status can be treated by ethosuximide (orally or by gavage), acetazolamide (IV, orally, or by gavage), diazepam (rectally or IV), or valproic acid (orally, by gavage, or rectally). Rectally administered valproic acid should be considered for treating absence status when oral administration of the drug is not feasible. Valproic acid, like diazepam, is well absorbed rectally. The usual initial dose is 20 mg/kg of the liquid formulation (81, 92).

Long-Term Management of Epilepsy with Drugs

Although the focus of this chapter is on the treatment of seizures in the intensive care unit, the long-term administration of antiepileptic drugs must also be considered. Patients with prior epilepsy who were previously taking antiepileptic drugs find their way to the neurosurgical ICU. Similarly, patients who first began having seizures in the ICU need to be switched to chronic treatment regimens once the acute convulsions are stopped.

Most antiepileptic drugs are eliminated slowly and 1 to 6 weeks must transpire before drug levels stabilize (Table 8.5). This is true whenever the dose is changed. Thus the patient should always be re-evaluated after enough time has elapsed for a new steady state to be achieved. The situation is further complicated with multiple drug therapy and with phenytoin which has nonlinear, saturable elimination kinetics.

All patients, but especially children and patients taking multiple other drugs, vary greatly in their ability to eliminate antiepileptic drugs which is the major determinant of dosage requirements. Because of this intrinsic variability, no single dose is appropriate for all patients. Patients taking anticonvulsants must be re-evaluated periodically to determine whether their medication is effective and whether there are side effects. Often considerable trial and error is involved before the proper dose is found. When problems occur, either continued seizures or toxicity, drug level measurement is an essential adjunct to adjusting the dose.

The selection of the optimum anticonvulsant drug is made after the patient's seizure type(s) and, when possible, the epileptic syndrome is categorized (40). After the drug is selected, it is important to instruct the patient about epilepsy and its therapy. Anticonvulsant medication must be taken consistently. Patients who are warned about early acute side effects which

TABLE 8.5
Pharmacokinetics of Chronically Administered Antiepileptic Drugs*

Drug	$T_{1/2}$ Range (hr)	Time to Reach Stable Levels (wk)	Dosage Range (mg/kg/day)	Therapeutic Range (μg/ml)
Phenobarbital	30–150	2–3	1–5	10–40
Primidone	6–8	2–3	10–20	8–?†
Carbamazepine	10–30	1	15–25	4–12
Phenytoin	3–60‡	2	4–12	10–20
Methsuximide	18–30	1	10–20	10–20§
Ethosuximide	24–42	1–2	10–70	45–100
Valproic acid	4–15	1/2	10–70	50–100
Clonazepam	16–60	1–2	0.03–0.1	0.02–0.07

*W. E. Dodson: Pharmacology and treatment of epilepsy in children. Clin. Neuropharmacol., *4:* 1-2, 1979.
†Metabolized to phenobarbital.
‡Effective half-life ($T_{1/2}$) varies with level.
§N-desmethyl metabolite.

usually abate as tolerance develops are less likely to unilaterally abandon the medication.

The goal of antiepileptic therapy is to use as few drugs as possible to provide the patient with the optimum life style, balancing the ill effects of seizures against drug toxicity. A majority of patients with epilepsy enjoy complete seizure control with one or two medications. Some patients require several anticonvulsant drugs for seizure control and some cannot be totally controlled with any combination of currently available medications. In the latter circumstances a seizure may be preferable to continuous drug side effects.

As chronic treatment is started, the physician should try to treat the patient with a single drug, so called monotherapy. When an initial medication is ineffective, it should be discontinued. If the initial drug is partially effective, it should be retained while the second is tried. If the second plus the first are effective, one should later attempt to withdraw the first drug, usually a few months after the seizures are controlled.

Barbiturates

Phenobarbital, mephobarbital, and primidone are effective in treating partial seizures, major motor seizures, and febrile seizures but have a high incidence of sedative and behavioral side effects in children. They are very safe and generally inexpensive. When therapy is begun they often cause sedation but patients become tolerant with time. Behavioral side effects are more likely to be enduring and necessitate changing to another drug. Primidone is metabolized to phenobarbital and thus the two should not be given concurrently. Mephobarbital is rapidly metabolized to phenobarbital and does not accumulate to a significant extent; its action and side effects are due to phenobarbital.

Phenytoin

Phenytoin is the most popular for the treatment of partial and major motor seizures in the United States, but is used less than carbamazepine in Europe. Phenytoin dosage is difficult to regulate in some patients because it has saturable, nonlinear elimination kinetics. As the concentration increases, the drug-eliminating mechanisms become progressively saturated and the apparent half-life is prolonged. Thus as the concentration increases, it is necessary to make small increases in dose to avoid extreme increases in concentration and toxicity. This same property makes phenytoin concentrations highly prone to drug interactions.

The neurotoxicity of phenytoin correlates well with the concentration in blood. At levels above 20 mg/liter, most patients have nystagmus; above 30 mg/liter, ataxia; above 40 μg/ml lethargy, choreoathetosis, and seizures occur.

Phenytoin should not be given intramuscularly because absorption is slow and erratic, although eventually complete. In most children twice daily dosage is adequate if the dose is sufficient; in older patients a single daily dose can be taken. Different generic brands of phenytoin are not bioequivalent. Patient should be instructed to choose one brand and stick with it to avoid fluctuating drug levels.

Among all the antiepileptic drugs, phenytoin is the most vulnerable to drug interactions because it is eliminated almost wholly by saturable metabolism in the liver. It is also highly bound (90%) to plasma albumin, a feature that provides another opportunity for drug interactions.

Carbamazepine

Carbamazepine is as effective in treating partial and major motor seizures as phenytoin (94, 95). Carbamazepine has little behavioral and cosmetic toxicity, but causes a usually harmless dose-dependent neutropenia in 10% to 20% of patients. Idiosyncratic aplastic anemia is quite rare (42, 70). The neutropenia is rarely severe enough to require discontinuation, but blood counts and differentials should be checked periodically. If the absolute neutrophile count is 1,200 or less it is necessary to reduce the dose or discontinue the drug. Neurologic side effects include initial sedation to which patients become tolerant, idosyncratic vertigo, and diplopia (90).

Hyponatremia which can be caused by carbamazepine is a potentially serious problem in situations where SIADH occurs and intracranial hypertension is a problem (46, 71). Hyponatremia or water intoxication induced by carbamazepine is rarely symptomatic, occurring only once among 143 patients treated chronically for trigeminal neuralgia (90). Although it occurs in patients of any age, it is more common among elderly patients and is usually mild and asymptomatic (42, 49). Studies of the mechanism of this side effect are inconclusive (37). Early reports suggested that carbamazepine stimulated the release of antidiuretic hormone. More recent studies in patients have found low antidiuretic hormone excretion and normal cyclic AMP among hyponatremic patients (46, 95). No relationship has been found between carbamazepine and antidiuretic hormone levels, a finding which points to a renal mechanism (50).

Carbamazepine induces its own metabolism, a process called autoinduction. Autoinduction takes several weeks to develop maximally. When this occurs, drug concentrations may decline from those which are found after the first 2 or 3 weeks of therapy. This is to be expected and should not be misinterpreted as noncompliance. In some patients it is necessary to increase the dose after autoinduction occurs, that is in the third to sixth week of therapy.

Methsuximide

Methsuximide is chemically related to ethosuximide but has a different spectrum of activity. Methsuximide is effective against major motor seizures and is an important adjunctive drug in the treatment of stubborn partial complex seizures. Its principal side effects are transient sedation when therapy is initiated and inebriation at high concentrations.

Valproic Acid

Valproic acid is most effective in minor motor, absence, and myoclonic seizures but is also a useful adjunct in major motor seizures. Valproic acid is the drug of choice in juvenile myoclonic epilepsy, a rare disorder that causes both generalized tonic-clonic and absence seizures.

Valproic acid has a low incidence of neurotoxicity. Common side effects include transient alopecia, gastrointestinal upset, skin rash, and alterations of appetite. Drug interactions are common. It consistently causes phenobarbital levels to increase and phenytoin levels to decrease. Because valproic acid has a short half-life it must be given in three or more daily doses.

Recently an enteric coated, slow release form of sodium divalproex has become available and is the preferred formulation.

The most serious though rare side effect of valproic acid is hepatic failure (41). This idiosyncratic problem usually occurs in the first 6 months of therapy, most often among young patients who are taking other anticonvulsant drugs. Liver function tests should be obtained before starting valproic acid and periodically during the first months of treatment. Unfortunately, it is not clear which test of liver function is best for the early detection of this side effect. The transaminases are mildly elevated in 15% to 30% of children taking other anticonvulsants and may be only mildly increased in severe valproate-induced hepatotoxicity.

Ethosuximide

Ethosuximide is effective against absence seizures but not staring behavior caused by partial complex seizures. It is ineffective against major motor seizures. Neurologic side effects include hiccups and hallucinations. Systemic toxicity is a moderate problem due to a 10% incidence of rashes. Less often there may be depression, usually transient, of the white blood cell count.

Benzodiazepines

Clonazepam, clorazepate, lorazepam, and diazepam are used in chronic antiepileptic treatment (12). Common indications are infantile spasms and the Lennox-Gastaut syndrome. Less often they are used to treat absence epilepsies like petit mal epilepsy and as adjuncts in stubborn partial seizures.

The principal problem with chronic benzodiazepine administration is the high incidence of sedative and behavioral side effects (93). When given chronically, it is usually necessary to increase the dose slowly, allowing the patient to develop tolerance to the sedative drug actions. Some patients also become tolerant to the anticonvulsant actions. Irritability, disobedience, and reduced attention span are common complaints. In high concentrations clonazepam can cause absence status, also called minor motor stupor. When ineffective, benzodiazepines must be withdrawn slowly over weeks or months because of the high incidence of withdrawal seizures (45).

Acetazolamide

Acetazolamide is a carbonic anhydrase inhibitor which is effective adjunctive therapy in some patients with minor motor seizures. Because it is a sulfonamide, it should be avoided in patients who are allergic to sulfa drugs. The usual dosage is 10 to 20 mg/kg/day. Chronic therapy with this drug causes renal tubular acidosis and osteopenia, rarely with clinically important rickets. Acetazolamide also causes sedation and anorexia in some patients.

REFERENCES

1. Aminoff, M. J., and Simon, R. P. Status epilepticus. Causes, clinical features and consequences in 98 patients. Am. J. Med., *69:* 657–666, 1980.
2. Augrell, S., Berlin, A., Ferngren, H., and Hellstom, B. Plasma levels of diazepam after parenteral and rectal administration in children. Epilepsia, *16:* 277–283, 1975.
3. Bailey, D. W., and Fenichel, G. M. The treatment of prolonged seizure activity with intravenous diazepam. J. Pediatr., *73:* 923–927, 1968.
4. Bateman, D. E., O'Grady, J. C., Willey, C. J., Longley, B. P., and Barwick, D. D. De novo monor status epilepticus of late onset presenting as stupor. Br. Med. J., *287:* 1673–1674, 1983.
5. Bell, H. E., and Bertino, Jr., J. S. Constant diazepam infusion in the treatment of continuous seizure activity. Drug Intell. Clin. Pharmacol., *18:* 965–970, 1984.
6. Berkovic, S. F., and Bladin, P. F. Absence status in adults. Clin. Exp. Neurol., *19:* 198–207, 1983.
7. Bleck, T. Therapy for status epilepticus. Clin. Neuropharmacol., *6:* 255–269, 1983.
8. Booker H. E., and Celesia, G. G. Serum concentrations of diazepam in subjects with epilepsy. Arch. Neurol., *29:* 191–194, 1973.
9. Bostrom, B. Paraldehyde toxicity during treatment of status epilepticus. Am. J. Dis. Child., *136:* 414–415, 1982.
10. Braestrup, C., Schmiechen, R., Neef, G., and Petersen, E. N. Interaction of convulsive ligands with benzodiazepine receptors. Science, *215:* 1241–1243, 1982.
11. Browne, T. R. Paraldehyde, chlormethiazole, and lidocaine for treatment of status epilepticus. In: *Status Epilepticus*, edited by A. V. Delgado-Escueta, C. G. Wasterlain, D. G. Treiman, and R. J. Porter, pp. 509–517. Raven Press, New York, 1983.
12. Browne, T. R., and Penry, J. K. Benzodiazepines in the treatment of epilepsy. Epilepsia, *14:* 277–310, 1973.
13. Bruni, J. Treatment of status epilepticus in adults. Can. Med. Assoc. J., *128:* 531–533, 1983.
14. Burstein, C. L. The hazard of paraldehyde administration. J.A.M.A., *121:* 187–189, 1943.
15. Burton, K., and Holland, J. T. Convulsive status epilepsy: Is there a role for thiopentone-induced narcosis? Clin. Exp. Neurol., *20:* 47–56, 1984.
16. Chiu, T. H., and Rosenberg, H. C. Endogenous modulator of benzodiazepine binding in rat cortex. J. Neuorchem., *36:* 336–338, 1981.
17. Cloyd, J. C., Gumnit, R. J., and McLain, L. W., Jr., Status epilepticus. The role of intravenous phenytoin. J.A.M.A., *244:* 1479–1481, 1980.
18. Commission on Classification and Terminology of the International League Against Epilepsy. Proposal for revised clinical and electroencephalographic classification of epileptic seizures. Epilepsia, *22:* 489–501, 1981.
19. Congdon, P. J., and Forsythe, W. Intravenous clonazepam in the treatment of status epilepticus in children. Epilepsia, *21:* 97–102, 1980.
20. Curless, R. G., Holzman, B. H., and Ramsey, R. E. Paraldehyde therapy in childhood status epilepticus. Arch. Neurol., *40:* 477–480, 1983.
21. Dam, M., and Christiansen, J. Diazepam: Intravenous infusion in the treatment of status epilepticus. Acta Neurol. Scand., *54:* 278–280, 1976.
22. Dasta, J. F., Brier, K., and Schonfield, S. Loss of diazepam to drug delivery systems. Am. J. Hosp. Pharm., *37:* 1176–1178, 1980.
23. DeLorenzo, R. J. Antiepileptic drugs. Phenytoin: Calcium and calmodulin-dependent protein phosphorylation and neurotransmitter release. In: *Antiepileptic Drugs: Mechanisms of Action*, edited by G. H. Glaser, J. K. Penry, and D. M. Woodbury, pp. 399–414. Raven Press, New York, 1980.
24. Delgado-Escueta, A. V., Wasterlain, C., Trieman, D. M., and Porter, R. J. Current concepts in neurology: Management of status epilepticus. N. Engl. J. Med., *306:* 1337–1340, 1982.
25. Delgado-Escueta, A. V., and Enrile-Bacsal, F. Combination therapy for status epilepticus: Intravenous diazepam and phenytoin. In: *Status Epilepticus*, edited by A. V. Delgado-Escueta, C. G. Wasterlain, D. G. Treiman, and R. J. Porter, pp. 477–485. Raven Press, New York, 1983.
26. Dinner, D. A., Lueders, H., Lederman, R., and Gretter, T. E. Aphasic status epilepticus; a case report. Neurology, *31:* 888–891, 1981.
27. Dinsmore, W., Crane, J., and Callender, M. E. Status epilepticus and near hanging. Postgrad. Med. J., *61:* 519–520, 1985.
28. Dodson, W. E. Pharmacology and treatment of epilepsy in children. Clin. Neuropharmacol., *4:* 1–2, 1979.
29. Dodson, W. E. Antiepileptic drug use in newborns and infants. In: *Recent Advances in Epilepsy*, edited by T. A. Pedley and B. S. Meldrum, pp. 231–248. Churchill-Livingstone, New York, 1983.
30. Dreifuss, F. E. Proposal for revised clinical and electroencephalographic classification of epileptic seizures. Epilepsia, *22:* 489, 1981.
31. Engel, J., Jr., Ludwig, B. I., and Fetell, M. Prolonged partial complex status epilepticus EEG and behavioral observations. Neurology, *28:* 863–869, 1978.
32. Franzoni, E., Carboni, C., and Lambertini, A. Rectal diazepam: A clinical and EEG study after a single dose in children. Epilepsia, *24:* 35–41, 1983.
33. Gamstorp, I., and Sedin, G. Neonatal convulsions treated with continuous, intravenous infusion of diazepam. Upsala J. Med. Sci., *87:* 143–14, 1982.
34. Gastaut, H., Naquet, R., Poire, R., and Tassinari, C. A. Treatment of status epilepticus with diazepam (Valium). Epilepsia, *6:* 167–183, 1965.
35. Gastaut, H. Aphasia: The sole manifestation of focal status epilepticus. Neurology, *29:* 1638, 1979.
36. Giacoia, G. P., Gessner, P. K., Zaleska, M. M., and Bouutwell, W. C. Pharmacokinetics of paralde-

hyde disposition in the neonate. J. Pediatr., *104:* 291-296, 1984.
37. Gold, P. W., Robertson, G. L., Ballenger. J. C., Kaye W., Chen J., Rubinow, D. R., Goodwin. F. K., and Post, R. M. Carbamazepine diminishes the sensitivity of the plasma arginine vasopressin response to osmotic stimulation. J. Clin. Edocrinol. Metab., *57:* 952–957, 1983.
38. Goldberg, M. A., and McIntyre, H. B. Barbiturates in the treatment of status epilepticus. In: *Status Epilepticus*, edited by A. V. Delgado-Escueta, C. G. Wasterlain, D. G. Treiman, and R. J. Porter, pp. 499-503. Raven Press, New York, 1983.
39. Geller, H. M., Hoffer, B. J., and Taylor, D. A. Electrophysiological actions of benzodiazepines. Fed. Proc., *39:* 3016–3023, 1980.
40. Gomez, M. R., and Klass. D. W. Epilepsies of infancy and childhood. Ann. Neurol., *13:* 113–124, 1983.
41. Gram, L., and Bentsen, K. D. Hepatic toxicity of antiepileptic drugs: A review. Acta Neurol. Scand. (Suppl.), *97:* 81-90, 1983.
41a. Greenblatt, D. J., Shader, R. I., and Abernathy, D. R. Current status of benzodiazepines (second of two parts). N. Engl. J. Med., *309:* 411–415, 1983.
42. Hart, R. G., and Easton, J. D. Carbamazepine and hematological monitoring. Ann. Neurol., *11:* 309–312, 1981.
43. Homan, R. W., and Walker, J. E. Clinical studies of lorazepam in status epilepticus. In: *Status Epilepticus*, edited by A. V. Delgado-Escueta, C. G. Wasterlain, D. G. Treiman, and R. J. Porter, pp. 493–498. Raven Press, New York, 1983.
44. Howrie, D. L., and Crumrine, P. K. Phenytoin-induced movement disorder associated with intravenous administration for status epilepticus. Clin. Pediatr., *24:* 467–469, 1985.
45. Hyser, C. L., and Drake, M. E. Status epilepticus after baclofen withdrawal. J. Natl. Med. Assoc., *67:* 537-538, 1984.
46. Kalff, R., Houtkooper, M. A., Meyer, J. W., Goedhart, D. M., Augusteijn, R., and Meinardi, H. Carbamazepine and serum sodium levels. Epilepsia, *25:* 390–397, 1984.
47. Kanto, J. Plasma concentrations of diazepam and its metabolites after peroral, intramuscular and rectal administration. Int. J. Clin. Pharmacol., *12:* 427–432, 1975.
48. Kanto, J., Iisalo, E., Kangas, L., and Valvirta, E. A. Comparative study on the clinical effects of rectal diazepam and pentobarbital on small children. Relationship between plasma level and effect. Int. J. Clin. Pharmacol. Therap. Toxicol., *18:* 348–351, 1980.
49. Koivikko, M. J., and Valikangas, S. L. Hyponatremia during carbamazepine therapy in children. Neuropediatrics, *14:* 93–96, 1983.
50. Krause, K. H., Rascher, W., and Berlit, P. Plasma arginine vasopressin concentrations in epileptics under monotherapy. J. Neurol., *230:* 193–196, 1983.
51. Krisshnamoorthy, K. S., Zalneraitis, E. L., Young, R. S. K., and Bernad, P. G. Phenytoin-induced choreoathetosis in infancy: Case reports and a review. Pediatrics, *72:* 831–834, 1983.
52. Kutt, H. Interactions between anticonvulsants and other commonly prescribed drugs. Epilepsia, *25:* S118–S131, 1984.
53. Langslet, A., Meberg, A., Bresden, J. E., and Lunde, P. K. M. Plasma concentrations of diazepam and *n*-desmethyldiazepam in newborn infants after intravenous, intramuscular, rectal and oral administration. Acta Paediatr. Scand., *67:* 699–702, 1978.
54. Leppik, I. E., Derivan, A. T., Homan, R. W., Walker, J., Ramsey, E., and Patrick, B. Double-blind study of lorazepam and diazepam in status epilepticus. J.A.M.A., *249:* 1452–1454, 1983.
55. Leppik, I. E., Patrick, B. K., and Cranford, R. E. Treatment of acute seizures and status epilepticus with intravenous phenytoin. In: *Status Epilepticus*, edited by A. V. Delgado-Escueta, C. G. Wasterlain, D. G. Treiman, and R. J. Porter, pp. 447–451. Raven Press, New York, 1983.
56. Lewkowski, W. Status epilepticus as a complication of fluphenazine treatment. Psychiatr. Pol., *17:* 5–6, 1983.
57. Levy, R. J., and Krall, R. L. Treatment of status epilepticus with lorazepam. Arch. Neurol., *41:* 605–611, 1984.
58. Lockman, L. A., Kreil, R., Zaske, D., Thompson, T., and Virnig, N. Phenobarbital dosage for control of neonatal seizures. Neurology, *29:* 1445–1449, 1979.
59. Macdonald, R. L. Mechanisms of anticonvulsant drug action. In: *Recent Advances in Epilepsy*, edited by T. A. Pedley and B. S. Meldrum, pp. 1–24. Churchill-Livingstone, New York, 1983.
60. MacKichan, J., Duffner, P. K., and Cohen, M. E. Adsorption of diazepam to plastic tubing. N. Engl. J. Med., *301:* 332–333, 1979.
61. Mauguiere, F., Sischer, C., Ferry, S., and Courjon, J. Treatment of parital status epilepticus in adults with diphenylhydantoin (DPH). Rev. Electroencephalogr. Neurophysiol. Clin., *14:* 207–211, 1984.
62. McNamara, J. O., Peper, A. M., and Patrone, V. Repeated seizures induce long-term increase in hippocampal benzodiazepine receptors. Proc. Natl. Acad. Sci. U.S.A., *77:* 3029–3032, 1980.
63. Milligan, N., Shillon, S., Richens, A., and Oxley, J. Absorption of diazepam from the rectum and its effect on interictal spikes in the EEG. Epilepsia, *23:* 323-331, 1982.
64. Milligan, N., Shillon, S., Richens, A., and Oxley, J. Rectal diazepam in the treatment of absence status: A pharmacodynamic study. J. Neurol. Neurosurg. Psychiatry, *44:* 914–917, 1981.
65. Deleted in manuscript.
66. Morris, M. E. Compatibility and stability of diazepam injection following dilution with intravenous fluids. Am. J. Hosp. Pharm., *35:* 669–672, 1979.
67. Olsen, R. W., and Leeb-Lundberg, F. Convulsant and anticonvulsant drug binding sites related to the GABA receptor/ionophore system. In: *Neurotransmitters, Seizures and Epilepsy*, edited by P. L. Morselli *et al.* pp. 151–160. Raven Press, New York, 1983.
68. Partinen, M., Kovanen, J., and Nilsson, E. Status epilepticus treated by barbiturate anaesthesia with

continuous monitoring of cerebral function. Br. Med. J., *282:* 520–521, 1981.
69. Pilke, A., Partinene, M., and Kovanen, J. Status epilepticus and alcohol abuse: An analysis of 82 status epilepticus admissions. Acta Neurol. Scand., *70:* 443–450, 1984.
70. Pisciotta, A. V. Carbamazepine: Hematological toxicity. In: *Antiepileptic Drugs*, edited by D. M. Woodbury, J. K. Penry, and C. E. Pippenger, pp. 553–541. Raven Press, New York, 1982.
71. Rado, J. P., Juhos, E., and Sawinsky, I. Dose-response relations in drug-induced inappropriate secretion of ADH: Effects of clofibrate and carbamazepine. Int. J. Clin. Pharmacol., *12:* 315–319, 1975.
72. Racy, A., Osborn, M. A., Vern, B. A., and Molinari, G. F. Epileptic aphasia: First onset of prolonged monosymptomatic status epilepticus in adults. Arch. Neurol., *37:* 419–422, 1980.
73. Ramsey, R. E., Hammond, E. J., Perchalski, R. J., and Wilder, B. J. Brain uptake of phenytoin, phenobarbital, and diazepam. Arch. Neurol., *36:* 535–539, 1979.
74. Richard, P., and Brenner, R. P. Absence status. Encephale, *6:* 385–392, 1980.
75. Russell, D., Anke, I. M., Nyberg-Hansen, R., Slettnes, O., Sortland, O., and Veger, T. Complex partial status epilepticus following myelography with metrizamide. Ann. Neurol., *8:* 325–327, 1980.
76. Sammaritano, M., Anderamnn, F., Melanson, D., Pappius, H. M., Camfield, P., Aicardi, J., and Sherwin, A. Prolonged focal cerebral edema associated with partial status epilepticus. Epilepsia, *26:* 334–339, 1985.
77. Sher, P. Reduced benzodiazepine receptor binding in cerebral cortical culture chronically exposed to diazepam. Epilepsia, *24:* 313–320, 1983.
79. Simon, R. P. Physiological consequences of status epilepticus. Epilepsia, *26:* S58–S66, 1985.
79. Singh, A., and Le Morvan, P. Treatment of status epilepticus with intravenous clonazepam. Prog. Neuro-Psychopharmacol., *6:* 539–542, 1982.
80. Sklonick, A., Moncada, V., Barker, J. L., and Paul, S. M. Pentobarbital: Dual actions to increase brain benzodiazepine receptor affinity. Science, *211:* 1448–1450, 1981.
81. Snead, O. C., and Miles, M. V. Treatment of status epilepticus in children with rectal sodium valproate. J. Pediatr., *106:* 323–325, 1985.
82. Soderfeldt, B., Blennow, G., Kalimo, H., Olsson, Y., and Seijso, B. K. Influence of systemic factors on experimental epileptic brain injury. Acta Neuropathol., *60:* 81–91, 1983.
83. Somerville, E. R. Tonic status epilepticus presenting as confusional state. Ann. Neurol., *13:* 549–551, 1983.
84. Sonawane, B. R., Yaffe, S. J., and Shapiro, B. H. Changes in mouse brain diazepam receptor binding after phenobarbital administration. Life Sci., *27:* 1335–1338, 1980.
85. Sorel, L., Mechler, L., and Harmant, J. Comparative trial of intravenous lorazepam and clonazepam in status epilepticus. Clin. Ther., *4:* 326–336, 1981.
86. Sorel, L., Mechler, L., and Harmant, J. Etude comparative de l'injection intraveineuse de lorazepam et de clonazepam dans les etats de mal epileptique. Acta Neurol. Belg., *80:* 368–379, 1980.
87. Deleted in manuscript.
88. Stoebner, R. C., Kiser, R. W., Deckerd, J. F., *et al.* Diazepam (Valium) in the treatment of tetanus: A report of five cases. South. Med. J., *63:* 445–447, 1970.
89. Study, R. E., and Barker, J. L. Cellular mechanisms of benzodiazepine action. J.A.M.A., *247:* 2147–2151, 1982.
90. Taylor, J. C., Brauer, S., and Espir, M. L. Long-term treatment of trigeminal neuralgia with carbamazepine. Postgrad. Med. J., *57:* 16–18, 1981.
91. Thong, Y. H., and Abramson, D. C. Continuous infusion of diazepam in infants with severe recurrent convulsions. Med. Ann. D. C., *43:* 63–65, 1974.
92. Thorpy, M. J. Rectal valproate syrup and status epilepticus. Neurology, *30:* 1113–1114, 1980.
93. Trimble, M. R. Anticonvulsant drugs and psychosocial development: Phenobarbitone, sodium valproate, and benzodiazepines. In: *Antiepileptic Drug Therapy in Pediatrics*, edited by P. L. Morselli, C. E. Pippenger, and J. K. Penry, pp. 201–218. Raven Press, New York, 1983.
94. Troupin, A. S. Carbamazepine in epilepsy. Clin. Neuropharmacol., *3:* 15–40, 1978.
95. Troupin, A. S. Carbamazepine reexamined. In: *Recent Advances in Epilepsy*, edited by T. A. Pedley and B. S. Meldrum, pp. 47–56. Churchill-Livingstone, New York, 1983.
96. Walker, J. E., Homan, R. E., Vasko, M. R., Crawford, I. L., Bell, R. D., and Tasker, W. G. Lorazepam in status epilepticus. Ann. Neurol., *6:* 207–213, 1979.
97. Wilder, B. J. Efficacy of phenytoin in treatment of status epilepticus. In: *Status Epilepticus*, edited by A. V. Delgado-Escueta, C. G. Wasterlain, D. G. Treiman, and R. J. Porter, pp. 441–446. Raven Press, New York, 1983.
98. Woodbury, D. M. Experimental models of status epilepticus, and mechanisms of drug action. In: *Status Epilepticus*, edited by A. V. Delgado-Escueta, C. G. Wasterlain, D. G. Treiman, and R. J. Porter, pp. 149–160. Raven Press, New York, 1983.
99. Young, R. S., Ropper, A. H., Hawkes, D., Woods, M., and Yohn, P. Pentobarbital in refractory status epilepticus. Pediatr. Pharmacol., *3:* 63–67, 1983.
100. Young, G. B., Blume, W. T., Bolton, C. F., and Warren, K. G. Anesthetic barbiturates in refractory status epilepticus. J. Neurol. Sci., *7:* 291–292, 1980.

CHAPTER 9

Cerebral Homeostasis and Protection

JOHN D. WARD, M.D., RICHARD J. MOULTON, M.D.,
J. PAUL MUIZELAAR, M.D., Ph.D.,
and ANTHONY MARMAROU, Ph.D.

INTRODUCTION

The concept of cerebral homeostasis and protection would imply that there are certain physiologic mechanisms that must be operative and in balance for the brain to maintain its integrity and to function properly. This concept would further suggest that it is necessary to protect these physiologic mechanisms from disturbance or, if necessary, to restore when disordered.

It is the aim of this chapter to (*a*) describe these physiologic mechanisms by analyzing the parameters of cerebrospinal fluid (CSF) dynamics, cerebral blood flow, intracranial pressure, and brain metabolism; (*b*) to demonstrate how these parameters are altered by certain insults; i.e., trauma, hypoxia, ischemia, etc.; (*c*) to show how these parameters can be monitored; and (*d*) to suggest how the brain can be protected by maintaining these variables in proper balance.

When describing an area that is in a state of flux, there is a temptation to drift into and emphasize these areas that are new, but yet unproven. We will try to avoid this and propose and suggest those principles and techniques that have been proven to be clinically useful. On the other hand, it is useful to indicate concepts that are new and potentially helpful so one can be aware of the current trends and future directions in neurologic intensive care. We will try to indicate these areas clearly so there is no confusion that they are, at this time, speculative in nature. Finally, although the approach and system of care is one which we have found useful, we recognize there are often multiple ways to approach a clinical problem. We will try to elaborate these when possible, giving the benefits and problems encountered with each approach.

CEREBRAL HOMEOSTASIS—PHYSIOLOGY

It is important to have a clear understanding of how the brain functions to maintain cerebral homeostasis. In this section, we will examine the basic physiology of CSF dynamics, cerebral blood flow and metabolism, and intracranial pressure (ICP). Having done this, we will then be in a better position to understand and correct any pathologic alterations in these processes.

CSF Dynamics

CSF Production

It is generally felt that in man about 60% to 70% of CSF is produced by the choroid plexus (153, 202), while the remaining 30% to 40% is from extrachoroidal sites. Ependyma (137) and brain parenchyma (114) are the favored extrachoroidal sites, although it is technically difficult to separate these sites from one another. In man, the CSF formation rate is about 0.35 ml/min, 20 cc/hr or 500 cc/24 hr (33, 96). The removal of this volume of fluid becomes important as will be seen in the discussion of ICP control.

CSF production under normal physiologic conditions initially was felt to be fairly constant (68). However, more recently it has been shown that CSF production may in fact decrease as CSF pressure rises (171, 201). At higher levels of CSF pressure, this may in part be related to a decrease in cerebral perfusion pressure with a decrease in choroid plexus blood flow and a resultant decrease in CSF production (139). Other factors such as hypothermia (173) and serum osmolality (69) can influence CSF production, but at present the clinical relevance of these influences is unknown. Drugs such as furosemide appear to decrease production by its effect on chloride transport, while acetazolamide decreases formation by its action on carbonic anhydrase (33, 107, 154).

CSF Outflow

CSF appears to move by bulk flow from sites of formation to sites of absorption; that is, from lateral ventricle through foramen of Monro to third ventricle to cerebral aqueduct to fourth ventricle to subarachnoid space. In addition to this classical route of CSF flow, others have proposed a bulk flow of CSF through the brain in a "lymph-like" manner (21). This concept has been recently reviewed by Bradbury (14). This concept of bulk flow through the brain of fluid is complex and may play a role in the movement and clearance of cerebral edema fluid under pathologic conditions (100, 148).

CSF Absorption

Under normal circumstances, there is a balance between the rate of CSF formation and the rate of CSF absorption. The rate of absorption is pressure-dependent and increases as CSF pressure increases (33). In addition, resistance to flow seems to diminish at higher than normal physiologic CSF pressures (35). This in turn helps compensate for elevations of ICP by increasing CSF flow and absorption.

The pathway for CSF absorption is felt to be mainly via the arachnoid villi (198, 203). However, there are other sites of absorption such as through the brain, as was mentioned above, as well as through the spinal arachnoid villi (101). This delicate balance between the sites of production and the sites of absorption is often disturbed in the setting of trauma, subarachnoid hemorrhage, and cerebral edema. Often, brain protection consists of taking over the role of absorption until the brain returns to normal and the balance between production and absorption is restored.

Chemical Components of CSF

There is extensive literature on the normal constituents of CSF of which there are many. However, other than for the documentation of infection, the routine use of the identification of CSF constituents to aid in the care of patients has not been used routinely. There are, however, interesting alterations that can occur in the CSF in disease states. The identification of abnormal levels of certain chemicals may have a use in determining the prognosis of patients or the monitoring of certain therapies. We will discuss these when we examine certain disease states of the brain.

Cerebral Blood Flow

The brain demands a constant supply of oxygen, glucose, and other metabolic substrates to carry on its work. This supply must be relatively constant and uninterrupted since the brain has little ability to store important nutrients required for the maintenance of its structural integrity as well as for the expenditure of energy required for its proper function. In practical terms, it is crucial for the brain to have sufficient cerebral blood flow (CBF) to meet its metabolic demands. In normal subjects CBF is usually felt to be around 50 cc/100 g/min (74). Attempts have been made to determine what is adequate flow for the brain. This is obviously a difficult question, the answer to which depends on a wide variety of factors such as age, extent of injury, metabolic demands, as well as others. However, when the level of CBF falls below 18 to 20 cc/100g/min, ischemic damage can occur (75). It should also be remembered that CBF can vary in various regions of the brain and that adequate flow may be measured in some areas, while ischemic flows are occurring elsewhere.

There are at least four variables which have significant effect on CBF. They are (*a*) systemic blood pressure, (*b*) arterial blood gases, (*c*) metabolic demands of the brain, and (*d*) ICP.

If the systemic blood pressure is altered quickly, CBF will change passively with the blood pressure. However, in the normal situation, CBF will quickly return to normal. This ability to restore normal flow in the presence of a changing blood pressure is termed autoregulation. It refers to the change in cerebral vascular resistance that in turn maintains a constant CBF as cerebral perfusion pressure (CPP) changes. CPP is defined as the difference between mean arterial blood pressure (MAP) and ICP; i.e., CPP = MAP − ICP (65, 132). In a normal person, there is usually adequate CBF between MAP of 60 to 150 mm Hg. However, below 60 mm Hg, CBF may passively follow blood pressure changes. This means that at a MAP below 60 mm Hg the cerebral vessels mediating this response are maximally dilated. Above 150 mm Hg, "break through" the vasoconstriction caused by hypertension may occur with passive vasodilatation and disruption of the blood-brain barrier (41). Functionally, signs of cerebral ischemia occur when CBF falls to 50% to 60% of normal (109). Failure to maintain membrane integrity begins to occur when CBF falls and is sustained below 40% of normal (188). It must be remembered that although CPP may indicate adequate CBF under some circumstances, there are situations such as coma where CBF can be quite low while CPP is in an acceptable range, because metabolic demands are diminished; this is called metabolic coupling. When CBF is far above metabolic demands, there is uncoupling.

Arterial blood gases exert a profound effect on CBF. CO_2 is, indirectly, a potent vasoactive substance because it readily crosses the blood-brain barrier and can change extravascular pH instantaneously. CBF will change about 4% per mm Hg change in CO_2 (58). This change is very rapid. With rising PCO_2 there is vasodilation with maximal vasodilatation occurring at a PCO_2 of about 60 mm Hg and the reverse with hypocapnia with maximal vasoconstriction at a PCO_2 of 20 mm Hg. This is the basis for reduction of cerebral blood volume by hyperventilation. The exact cause of this response is not known; however, changes in pH (83, 141, 142) have been implicated as the mediator of the change in cerebral vessel diameter. There may also be extravascular effects of CO_2 on certain areas of the brain which in turn affect the cerebral vasculature (165). The preservation of CO_2 responsiveness is completely independent of that of autoregulation in that it can be present when pressure autoregulation is lost. It is felt that if hypocapnia is prolonged especially at PCO_2 less than 20 mm Hg, that some ischemia occurs with accumulation of lactic acid. This lactic acidosis in turn normalizes CSF pH. This may be the reason CBF tends to return to normal after prolonged hyperventilation (141).

Low PO_2, that is hypoxemia, also causes vasodilatation. When PO_2 falls below 50 mm Hg, considerable vasodilatation can occur (108). However, increasing PaO_2 above normal does not lead to vasoconstriction because the O_2 content of the blood is not increased substantially.

The third significant influence on CBF is metabolism which is a reflection of neuronal activity. This metabolic coupling in simple terms means that under normal circumstances there is a tight coupling between the demands of the cerebral tissue and the blood flowing through the tissue. When the metabolic activity of the tissue increases there is a corresponding increase in CBF such as seen in patients with seizures and other causes of increases of cerebral metabolism (22, 174).

The reverse is also true and this is the basis for the use of barbiturates to decrease cerebral metabolism and hence flow (113). Uncoupling of CBF and demand can occur as with some traumatic coma with a low cerebral metabolic rate of oxygen ($CMRO_2$) and elevated CBF.

In an attempt to understand the relationship between flow and metabolism, the formula of $CMRO_2 = CBF \times AVDO_2$ is useful. In this formula, $CMRO_2$ = the cerebral metabolic rate for oxygen (3.0 to 3.5 ml/100 g/min), CBF = cerebral blood flow, and $AVDO_2$ = the arteriovenous difference for oxygen. CBF is measured by techniques we will describe below and $AVDO_2$ is obtained by measuring the oxygen content in arterial blood and jugular venous blood. What this formula says is that as blood flows through the brain, O_2 is extracted. If there is rapid flow in excess of need, the extraction will be less and $AVDO_2$ low. If the brain's need increases or if flow is low, there will be a greater amount of O_2 extracted with a resultant larger $AVDO_2$. Normal $AVDO_2$ at a PCO_2 of 40n mm Hg is about 6 vol% with a range of roughly 4.0 to 8.5 vol% (78). This normal range requires an upward adjustment as $PaCO_2$ drops since CBF decreases with lower $PaCO_2$.

Thus, in a changing situation where $CMRO_2$ is changing, both CBF and $AVDO_2$ values are necessary to correctly interpret the situation. However, if $CMRO_2$ is fairly constant then by just monitoring the $AVDO_2$ one could determine whether CBF is adequate (130). A discussion of methods has been purposely omitted from this chapter. Briefly, most CBF measurements in the intensive care unit (ICU) are done by using the inhalation method of Obrist (131) and the intravenous modification as proposed by Austin (2). For further discussion as to methods, one is referred to these articles as well as others (87, 189).

Intracranial Pressure

By definition, intracranial pressure (ICP) is that pressure which is obtained when one measures pressure either in the ventricle, subarachnoid, subdural, or epidural space. Ideally, all these pressures should be the same at any given point in time. However, as will be discussed in the section on ICP monitoring, this is not always the case; it probably is more accurate to speak of CSF pressure, subarachnoid pressure, etc. These pressures are under most circumstances similar, so the terminology, ICP, regardless of where it is obtained has generally come into use. We will see that as long as pressures in various locations are equal or close to ventricular pressure, then this is acceptable. If, however, due to certain conditions the pressures measured in the various compartments begin to differ, then it is important to distinguish exactly where ICP is being measured and what pressure it represents. Historically, ICP was first measured in the CSF space by the lumbar route and then in the ventricle (60, 97) therefore, in this discussion we will be referring to CSF pressure in the ventricle when the term ICP is used.

It is important to conceptualize ICP as a pressure that is a result of a constantly changing interplay of several systems. These are (*a*) CSF system; (*b*) brain tissue with its associated intra- and extracellular fluid; and (*c*) cerebral blood volume (CBV) contained in venous, capillary, and arterial vessels (Fig. 9.1). Each of these variables exerts an influence and the end result at equilibrium is what we call ICP. Another important concept to grasp is that of the response of ICP to either an increase in one of the systems or an addition of an extrinsic volume such as a tumor or extra-axial hematoma. This concept was first addressed many years ago and what is known as the modified Monro-Kellie doctrine evolved. This doctrine states

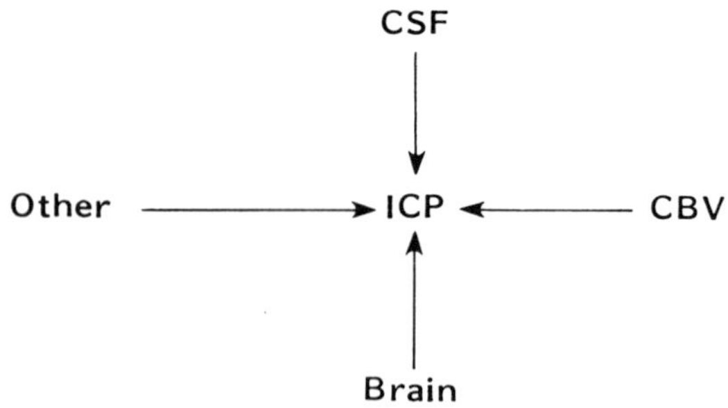

Figure 9.1. Components of intracranial cavity contributing to intracranial pressure (ICP).

that the volume of the craniospinal content is constant and is incompressible (25, 77, 120, 179, 197). Basically, this implies that any volume added to any craniospinal compartment (CSF, blood, brain) must be balanced by an equal loss of volume from another craniospinal compartment or ICP will rise (86). This can be diagrammatically seen in Figure 9.2 where the compartments of blood (arterial and venous), CSF, and brain are represented. Under normal circumstances, these compartments are in equilibrium as a certain resting ICP. As another volume is added the initial response is for the CSF compartment and the venous blood to become smaller because of expression of these fluids out of the intracranial cavity with the resultant effect of no change in ICP. However, eventually at some point in time no further room can be provided; the compensatory mechanisms are exhausted and ICP rises and begins to do so quite rapidly. It can further be seen that subsequent additions of increasingly smaller amounts of volume will cause an increasingly larger elevation of ICP. It will subsequently be shown that, to a large extent, the treatment of elevated ICP relies on the manipulation of these compartments to control ICP and move the patient toward the left part of the curve. It is important to remember also the physiologic concepts described earlier regarding CSF and cerebral blood flow since the various factors discussed earlier all play a role in the development and maintenance of ICP at equilibrium.

As can be seen from Figure 9.2, the initial portion of the curve does not change with the initial addition of an extra volume. That is, due to compensation, the ICP stays the same. However, it is also clear that the intracranial situa-

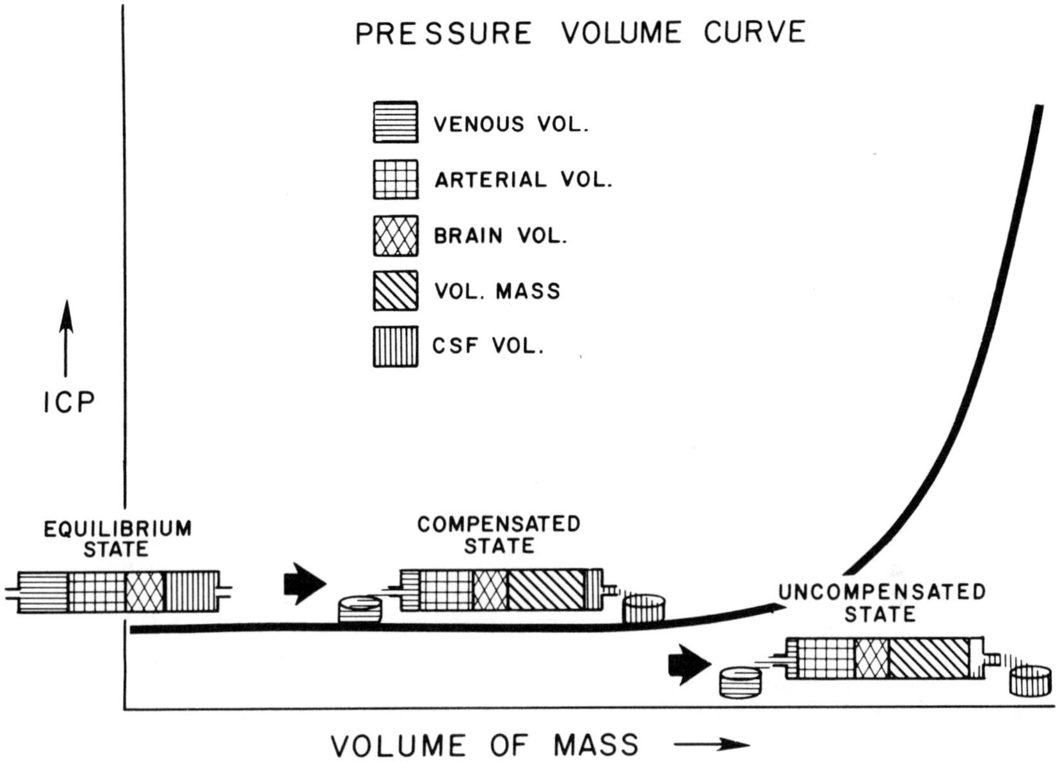

Figure 9.2. Compensation by Intracranial Components to Expanding Mass Lesion. (From J. D. Ward, *et al.*: Intracranial pressure, head injuries, subarachnoid hemorrhage, non-surgical coma and brain tumors. In: *Critical Care, State of the Art*, edited by W. C. Shoemaker and W. L. Thompson, Vol II (R), p. 2, 1981. Reprinted with permission.)

tion is not the same when the brain has all its compensatory mechanisms available compared to the situation when all compensation is exhausted and with further addition of volume, ICP will rapidly rise. Miller was one of the first to address this issue and developed the concept of a volume-pressure response (VPR) and brain elastance. This can be tested by the addition or withdrawal of 1 ml of CSF the associated response was noted. A normal response was a change in ICP of 2 mm Hg or less; a change in ICP of 5 mm Hg or more was considered an abnormal response and indicative of a "tight" brain (119). This change in pressure per change in value $\Delta P/\Delta V$ is termed elastance (94, 116). Compliance decreases as ICP increases. The VPR cannot be predicted and repeated measurements must be performed when there is a change in the resting ICP level. It was noted by Marmarou that if one changes the pressure axis of the curve to a log scale that the resultant curve is a straight line. This led to the development of the concept of the pressure-volume index (PVI) (101). The PVI characterizes the steepness of the pressure-volume curve and is not pressure dependent. In the normal adult, this is about 25 ml, that is 25 cc is required to raise the resting ICP by a factor of 10. It is calculated by the formula:

$$PVI = \frac{\Delta V}{\log_{10} \frac{P_p}{P_o}}$$

where ΔV is the amount injected, P_o is the base line ICP and P_P is the ICP reached after the injection. It can be seen therefore that simply knowing the ICP only gives a glimpse of the actual intracranial situation. The trend now is to not only evaluate the ICP but also try to determine the exact state of the brain in terms of its ability to withstand additional volume and exactly how much additional volume is required to raise ICP to what level. With this knowledge at hand, it can be seen that each patient has their own volume-pressure curve with its own slope and that this curve depends on all of the intracranial contents acting in concert and that the patient's response to additional volume or their volume reserve will be normal if the brain tissue is not swollen, if there is no increase in brain water, if CSF outflow resistance and absorption are normal, if CBF is normal without hyperemia, and if the metabolic demands of the brain are normal. It is therefore evident that any derangement of any or all of these factors can alter ICP and that unless these factors are characterized and measured, it will be difficult to determine (*a*) the exact pathophysiologic process involved, and (*b*) what the best treatment will be. Future directions of ICP measurement will be directed toward a knowledge of the actual state of the brain before it reaches the steep portion of the volume-pressure curve so that the "state" of the brain can be treated rather than just the end result of all of these processes acting; that is, ICP (99).

In addition to the steady elevations of ICP that can occur, there are certain periodic waves that can appear. The most impressive of these is the plateau wave so named because it occurs with a sudden rise of ICP to 50 mm Hg or more, lasts for 5 to 20 minutes and falls back to base line (97). This wave is felt to represent a "tight" brain and the sudden increase in ICP secondary to vasodilatation (152). Today, we often do not see the actual plateau wave since ICP is usually treated once it starts to rise and the wave is aborted. The second type of waves are sharply peaked waves of variable height occurring at frequency of 0.5 to 2/min and often corresponding to changes in respiration. Again, in the acute situation where patients are being ventilated, these waves may not be manifested. Finally, there are waves related to Traube-Hering plots of blood pressure arising 5 to 8 times per minute. There is a current trend to get away from the identification of waves and look more closely at each individual pulse wave and its physiologic meaning. This will be discussed in the next section.

Discussion of ICP would not be complete without some attempt to define what is "normal" ICP. There should be a distinction between what is "normal" ICP and at what level is it appropriate to begin treatment of elevated ICP. In general, 10 mm Hg would be considered a "normal" ICP (97, 117); however, the level at which treatment begins depends on the neurologic condition of the brain, the rapidity with which ICP is rising, the etiology of the ICP elevation, the perfusion of the brain and so forth. This point will be discussed in greater depth later but the message is that, to truly know the level at which increased ICP is dangerous and will influence outcome depends on the clinical condition of the patient as well as a large number of variables. Current practice is to choose a level of 20 to 25 mm Hg in the acute situation. However, this is a "shot-gun" approach and in the future, with more information available, this level will surely be altered.

BRAIN MONITORING

The way one derives more "information" to help answer questions is to monitor the patient. In this section, we will look at ICP monitoring, monitoring of CBF and brain metabolism, the assessment of chemical indicators of brain injury, and electrical monitoring of the brain.

ICP Monitoring

In looking at ICP monitoring, there are several questions that need to be answered. They are (*a*) who needs to be monitored? (*b*) what system should be used? (*c*) how long should the patient be monitored? and (*d*) what are the difficulties encountered with each system?

Which patient should be monitored? ICP monitoring should be used when the risk of not monitoring outweighs the risk of monitoring. In general terms, this means that ICP monitoring should be used in those circumstances where (*a*) the disease process is known to be associated with a significant incidence of intracranial hypertension; (*b*) where this elevation in ICP is felt to be detrimental to brain structure and function; (*c*) where other forms of monitoring are either ineffective or insensitive, i.e., the neurologic examination in a paralyzed head trauma patient; and (*d*) where it is anticipated that therapy aimed at the reduction of elevated ICP will be required. In general, when one or more of these conditions is met, ICP monitoring should be considered. For example, in a comatose patient with a head injury and cerebral contusion on CT not large enough to remove, the risk of elevated ICP is significant and a detectable deterioration in neurologic function might be irreversible. In this situation, ICP monitoring should be used. A patient with a brain tumor with shift who is awake and improving on steroids prior to surgery does not need ICP monitoring. The choice of patients to monitor is dependent on the disease state, the clinical condition of the patient, and the patient's course.

Having decided to utilize ICP monitoring in patient care, the next step is the choice of which type of monitor. Before entering this discussion, an analysis of the advantages and disadvantages of various systems is appropriate. The various methods of ICP monitoring can be divided in several ways. Clinically, it is useful to divide them by their location in the intracranial cavity. That is, they can be intraventricular, subarachnoid, subdural, or epidural. They can be further divided into whether they are fluid coupled or not.

The intraventricular catheter for ICP monitoring, first used by Guillaume and Janny (60), was perfected and shown to be clinically useful by Lundberg (97). It is the current standard against which other methods are compared. Its placement, in experienced hands, is fairly straightforward and its location can be verified by the drainage of fluid and an adequate trace on the oscilloscope. It is usually placed in the frontal horn and is best tunneled from its site of exit from the skull to its point of exit from the scalp. The advantages of the ventricular catheter are (*a*) it can be used therapeutically to drain CSF and control ICP; (*b*) it can be used to determine VPR, PVI, CSF outflow resistance, CSF formation rate and CSF absorption pressure; (*c*) it is accurate. The disadvantages are (*a*) it may be very difficult to insert in patients with cerebral swelling and small ventricles or in patients with significant shift; (*b*) there is a risk of infection; (*c*) there is the risk of hemorrhage.

The major objection to the use of the ventricular catheter is the risk of infection. The risk is dependent first and foremost on length of monitoring ranging from 8% at 5 days to 40% at 12 days (105). It is also dependent on the need for irrigating the system to prevent clogging such as in SAH or intraventricular hemorrhage. A variety of systems can be used, but basically they all consist of a catheter of some type in the ventricle which is fluid coupled to a strain-gauge transducer. There are several manufacturers that sell sets already assembled with attachments for calibration, drainage, and irrigation.

The subarachnoid and subdural devices are considered together since their insertion is similar and their advantages and disadvantages the same. The first subdural-subarachnoid device was the subdural bolt introduced by Vries in 1973 (193). This was simply a hollow-threaded screw that was inserted into the skull through a 1/4″ twist drill hole after the dura had been opened. The screw is inserted until it protrudes just under the dura in the subarachnoid space but not in contact with the brain. It has the advantage of (*a*) being easy to insert; (*b*) has a very low infection rate (151). The disadvantages are (*a*) it can be difficult to insert in very young infants; (*b*) occasionally one can drain CSF but usually not; (*c*) no dynamic ICP testing can be done; and (*d*) there may be a question as to its accuracy under certain conditions. There are studies in which it is concluded that the subarachnoid screw when properly placed reflects intraventricular measurement accurately (98, 184). Other authors feel that the subarachnoid screw may underestimate ICP at higher levels (37, 110). This may well be true in the case where ICP is high and the brain is soft or edematous. This can usually be recognized by a dampening of the waveform. This controversy points out the need to be very familiar with the type of monitoring system one is using.

In addition to the subdural screw, a subdural catheter can also be utilized. This can take the form of a simple No. 5 pediatric tube or one can use a more specialized catheter (205). The principles involved are the same as for the subarachnoid screw.

The third method of monitoring is to use a device in the epidural space. In this method a sensing device is placed in the epidural space usually via a burr hole. Depending on the device, it either sits in the burr hole or is advanced under the edge of the bone. It is important that these devices be coplanar with the dura and that there be no wedging effect. The advantages are (*a*) very easy to insert, and (*b*) virtually no infection. However, the disadvantages are (*a*) they are usually fairly expensive; (*b*) the technology is still evolving to allow for in situ calibration and no drift; (*c*) there can be no drainage; (*d*) there can be no dynamic ICP testing; and (*e*) there still are significant questions as regards accuracy. There have been a number of studies that show that, although these devices parallel intraventricular pressure, epidural devices tend to yield a higher pressure (84, 88, 209).

There is a final group of devices that can be grouped under the term telemetric. These are fully implantable devices which consist of some type of electronic transducer which is telemetered through the intact scalp (156, 208). As yet there are not a sufficient number of studies to determine the accuracy of these devices. There is no question that if they prove accurate and can be rendered sufficiently inexpensive they will fulfill a definite need. There is a constant flow of new, improved devices to measure ICP. However, before adapting a new system one needs to be assured that it is safe, accurate, and easy to insert.

How then is one to decide which device to use to monitor ICP? The best way is to determine the particular needs that the physician and the patient have, balance the advantages and disadvantages, and then make a selection. Figure 9.3 shows a chart which lists the various characteristics of the devices. As can be seen, if the patient is going to require CSF drainage to control ICP and the ventricles are able to be cannulated and dynamic testing is desired, then the ventricular catheter will be selected. If, on the other hand, the ventricles cannot be cannulated or dynamic testing is not required, then some other form of monitoring device should be selected. Another technique is to start with one type, then switch to another if the needs of the patient change. The important thing is that the type of monitoring device be matched to the needs of the patient and that the physician be familiar with the device being used. The proper use of ICP monitoring requires a commitment on the part of both the physician interpreting the information and the nursing staff that is responsible for the daily use of the equipment. It should be remembered that the only thing worse than no information is wrong information. The equipment should be calibrated as often as necessary to ensure accurate readings. In addition, if at any time the waveform from the monitor begins to dampen or if for any reason the physician feels that the device is not functioning properly, then the device should be replaced with a functioning monitor.

Monitoring of CBF and Metabolism

When there is a disproportion between cerebral energy demand and critically required substrate availability in the presence of low CBF, then ischemia can result. Unfortunately, it has been particularly difficult to monitor and ensure adequate CBF to meet metabolic requirements. There are several reasons for this. First, the techniques to adequately and accurately measure CBF require specialized equipment and personnel which are not readily available in

Method	Insertion	Accuracy	Infection	VPR and CSF Drainage
ventricular catheter	problem with small ventricles	excellent	3-5%	yes
subarachnoid screw	little difficulty	good	less	no
epidural transducer	little difficulty	variable	negligible	no

Figure 9.3. Advantages and Disadvantages of Various Techniques of ICP Monitoring. (From J. D. Ward, *et al.*: Intracranial pressure, head injuries, subarachnoid hemorrhage, non-surgical coma and brain tumors. In: *Critical Care, State of the Art*, edited by W. C. Shoemaker and W. L. Thompson, Vol. II(R), p. 6, 1981. Reprinted with permission.)

most hospitals. Secondly, it is often difficult to know and document when ischemia may have occurred. The usual situation is a patient with elevated ICP with a normal blood pressure who is paralyzed. It is difficult to determine when all regions are receiving appropriate blood flow at any given time. Third, the techniques, even if available, are time-consuming and if radioactive methods are used, the number of studies is limited. Finally, the interaction between CBF, ICP neuronal function, and metabolism are complex and only beginning to be understood. However, there is some progress being made in conditions such as head injury (123, 130) and subarachnoid hemorrhage (54, 67). These studies are beginning to be done on a more routine basis and being done earlier in the course of the disease process (124). Recently, in a study by Obrist of a group of head-injured patients, $AVDO_2$ was measured in these patients as well as CBF and $CMRO_2$ (130). They were able to determine that there was good correlation between low $AVDO_2$ and hyperemic blood flows which in a comatose patient represented a CBF of greater than 40 cc/min/100 g. Further, they felt that in those patients who had low CBF, almost all had normal or low $AVDO_2$, which indicated lower rate of metabolism with associated low flows rather than active ischemia. It was also noted by the same group that $CMRO_2$ was stable in many instances with CBF changing frequently with a reciprocal change occurring in $AVDO_2$. If CBF is sufficient for metabolic needs $AVDO_2$ will be in the normal range (PCO_2 40) of 6.3 $\pm$ 1.2. If CBF is elevated above current needs, i.e., hyperemia, $AVDO_2$ will be low and if there is ischemia, that is, flow is insufficient for needs, there will be an increase in $AVDO_2$ usually greater than 8 vol% (PCO_2 40). Whether the monitoring of arterial and jugular oxygen differences will prove to be of value, only time will tell. However, it is a technique that can be done fairly easily with little risk to the patient.

The other aspect of monitoring cerebral metabolism is the serial determination of certain substances in the CSF. This is performed on the premise that either pathologic processes such as acidosis will release chemicals such as lactate into the ventricles which act as a sink or that cells undergoing destruction will release enzymes into the CSF. By determining levels of these substances, it is suggested one can both determine the degree of brain injury and form a prognosis as to outcome (3, 32, 43, 79, 140, 175). While there has been much work done in this area, these markers are not being used on a routine basis as a monitor of neural damage. The measurement of levels of certain substances and correlation of these substances with simultaneous physiologic variables (i.e., CBF, ICP, neurologic function) may result in significant progress in this area.

Electrical Monitoring

Advances in neurologic intensive care have improved the care and survival of seriously ill patients. This has been well documented in the case of severe head injury (5, 118). Many of the more significant advances have been in the monitoring and assessment of cardiac and respiratory status. With the exception of intracranial pressure monitoring, the development of modalities for the continuous measurement of neural status has lagged behind these other areas. One reason is the much greater complexity of the CNS, requiring a proportionately more sophisticated monitoring system. In order to obtain a complete picture of brain function at a given time, it is necessary to know the circulatory, metabolic, mechanical (i.e., ICP), and electrophysiologic status of the brain. This section will concentrate on the current status and possible future directions of electrophysiologic monitoring.

Traditionally, the assessment of neurologic function in the ICU has been carried out by the repetition at a given time interval of an appropriately abbreviated version of the neurologic examination. Most frequently, this takes the form of the Glasgow Coma Score (GCS) (186) with the addition of pupillary reactions, oculocephalic responses, and an assessment of limb strength. Essentially, this comprises an assessment of level of consciousness as well as an examination for evidence of focal functional deficit involving such areas as the brainstem and the motor system pathways. This method of assessment has served clinicians well; however, it does present some serious shortcomings in comatose patients. The first such shortcoming is the intrinsic deficiency of the neurologic examination in the comatose patient. As the patient sinks progressively deeper into coma, the repertoire of patient responses decreases dramatically to a few stereotyped movements to pain. Some additional information can be gleaned from the examination of the brainstem reflexes. Secondly, in even the most straightforward system of patient examination (e.g., the GCS), there is a fairly high degree of interobserver variability (187), and all systems of clinical evaluation introduce a certain degree of subjectivity. The third and most significant shortcoming of the clinical examination is its inability to be used in those patients in whom pharmacologic sedation and/or paralysis are necessary for proper respiratory care or control of ICP. In these patients only the pupillary responses remain to guide the clinician in his assessment of neural function.

Electroencephalography (EEG) and evoked potentials (EP) offer an objective evaluation of patients' neurophysiologic status, both globally and with respect to specific neuroanatomical pathways. There is obvious potential advantage to the use of these techniques as a form of continuous monitoring in the ICU. The following discussion will be limited to the applications of this technology to the clinical monitoring of coma, as this presents the area of greatest potential use for an objective neurophysiologic monitoring system.

Electroencephalography in Coma

A great many studies have been undertaken in the past on patients in coma of different etiologies. The most common finding in coma of all etiologies is slowing of the background frequency (155, 169, 181). The mildest form of this abnormality is slowing of the alpha rhythm and the most severe are burst suppression and electrocerebral silence. Furthermore, changes in the level of consciousness are commonly paralleled by changes in the background frequency, either increasing with improvement, or decreasing with deterioration (62). In post-traumatic coma Dawson *et al.* and Pampiglione have both described a lag in frequency change vis-à-vis change in the clinical status (36, 134). Another feature which has been emphasized by several authors is the reactivity of the EEG to external sensory stimuli, with decreasing reactivity being an indication of increasing depth of coma (155, 169). These findings are not without controversy, however, and Loeb maintains that the depth of coma is related to neither the background frequency of the EEG nor the reactivity to external stimuli (93).

The spontaneous variability of the EEG as a function of the depth of coma has also been stressed. This encompasses a range from monophasic without variability, through diphasic (alternating slow and fast activity) up to normal diurnal variation in the EEG with the presence of normal or near normal sleep activity. These latter patterns have been termed "spindle coma" and have been associated with a good outcome in most series (8, 18, 19, 29, 135). In a large series of post-trauma comatose patients, Bricolo found a fatality rate of 13% in patients with diphasic EEGs with spindles versus 86% mortality in those patients with monophasic EEGs and 100% mortality in those with electrocerebral silence (17). In contrast, Hansotia *et al.* found that in a series of 370 comas of diffuse etiology, the incidence of spindle coma was 5.7%. In these 22 patients there was no relation between the presence of sleep spindles and either depth of coma or outcome. In this same group of 22 patients, the authors were unable to find any relation between reactivity of EEG to external stimuli and prognosis. In all patients except one the background activity consisted of polymorphic slow waves with increase in the background frequency in those patients who improved and decrease in those who worsened clinically (62).

Another EEG subtype of coma is alpha pattern coma. This differs from normal alpha rhythm in that it is diffusely spacially distributed and is not blocked by eye opening or stimulation. This electroencephalographic pattern of coma is most frequently seen in brainstem stroke or diffuse anoxic injury, and is felt by many authors to imply an especially poor prognosis (63, 129, 181, 204). Again, there is some controversy regarding this point, and Sorensen *et al.* have challenged the allegation that there is any special prognostic significance to alpha coma (176).

Thus, in spite of some degree of controversy regarding various EEG patterns and their significance, there is good evidence to believe that serial EEGs in the comatose patient give useful information both as to the depth of coma and changes therein, as well as prognosis.

Another application of EEG monitoring in trauma is the recognition of focal dysfunction.

Several authors have commented on the correspondence of focal EEG findings (usually focal amplitude suppression or focal slowing) and CT, clinical, and autopsy findings (31, 146, 155, 169, 181). Generally, the accuracy of the EEG in identifying focal neural dysfunction is in the range of 50% to 80% in the above series. A potential complicating factor in the recognition of focal change is the fact that in the deeper stages of coma focal change may become lost in the diffuse background abnormality. Previously, much emphasis had been placed on the recognition of EEG patterns associated with specific types of pathologic lesion. Not surprisingly, this proved to be a largely fruitless endeavor (17). In any case this particular concern has been rendered irrelevant by the introduction of the CT scan. With the CT scan available to give more precise anatomic and pathologic information, it would suffice to have EEG monitoring to establish the onset, presence, and degree of neural dysfunction.

The principal disadvantages to the introduction of conventional EEG monitoring to the ICU are the tremendous amounts of data generated by the paper chart recording technique and the necessity of having a trained electroencephalographer present in the ICU for interpretation. In fact, these considerations render the continuous long-term monitoring of the EEG rather impractical. The following section will describe the technical advances in EEG data reduction and simplification of display, and their current application in the ICU setting. Again, the focus will be on the monitoring of traumatic and other forms of coma.

Processed EEG

One of the earliest and simplest forms of data reduction of EEG was the introduction of the Cerebral Function Monitor by Maynard *et al.* (106) in 1969. In this system the EEG is recorded from a single pair of parietal electrodes, on either side of the head. The signal is filtered between 2 and 15 Hz and then undergoes semilogarithmic compression. Finally, it is recorded on a strip chart recorder at very low paper speed (5 cm/hr). The level of the bottom of the trace above base line and the width of the trace indicate the state of cerebral activity. The instrument was designed initially for use with critically ill patients in the ICU. In a study of several types of application of the CFM, including the monitoring of comatose head-injured patients, Sechzer and Ospina found that its greatest utility was in the monitoring of surgical and parasurgical events such as cardiac arrest (164). Schwartz retrospectively studied the utility of the instrument in cardiac surgery and found that it predicted neurologic outcome in 83% of patients (161). In a review of various types of automated EEG processing for intraoperative monitoring, Levy *et al.* concluded that the CFM was best suited for global cerebral insult of large magnitude such as that due to hypoxia or hypotension (90).

A more recent and satisfactory approach to the EEG data reduction problem has been power spectral analysis of the EEG, particularly the Compressed Spectral Array of Bickford (9). The technique involves the fast Fourier transformation of epochs of raw EEG, usually 2 to 4 seconds long, by micro- or minicomputer. The EEG is thereby characterized by power (amplitude squared) and frequency. In the Compressed Spectral Array, power is plotted against frequency and the dimension of time is added by stacking the spectral plots for each epoch one on top of the other. Hidden line suppression may be used to facilitate the display of the data. Other display techniques based on power spectral analysis include density modulation, in which the power at a given frequency is represented by varying densities in gray-scale (49), the spectral edge frequency (155), and topographic mapping of amplitude and frequency data (40). The principal advantages of power spectral analysis are that it offers tremendous data compression without sacrifice of too much information, quantitative information regarding the frequency and amplitude of background activity, and the interpretation of the data does not require specialized training in EEG. The disadvantages of the technique are that transient activity such as spikes are not recognized, and unless one is extremely careful in excluding both physiologic (e.g., eye and cardiac) and electrical artifact from the EEG recording, these will be included in the transformed data and greatly confuse its interpretation (10). Despite these drawbacks, power spectral analysis represents a very promising technology for monitoring the spontaneous activity of the brain. The following paragraphs will describe its use in the monitoring of comatose patients.

By using the compressed spectral array technique, Bricolo has monitored 123 comatose patients (87 with head injury). He described three types of spectrograms: changeable, slow monotonous, and borderline (in which there was an alpha frequency peak which did not change with stimulation). Of those with a changeable spectrogram, 66% survived, whereas 96% of those with a slow monotonous pattern died. Three of five patients with a borderline pattern died. Additionally, he found some correlation between slowing and monotony of the spectrogram over one hemisphere and clinical or radiologic evidence of hemispheric and clinical or radiologic evidence of hemispheric damage on the same side. In six patients with concurrent ICP monitoring, there appeared to be no correlation between ICP and electrical activity (20).

Karnaze et al. monitored the Compressed Spectral Array (CSA) in 24 comatose patients. Based on the presence or absence of spontaneous alteration in the frequency or amplitude of the CSA, the prognostic capability of CSA in patients rendered comatose by head injury or anoxia was equal to that of the Glasgow Coma Score (76). With a classification similar to that of Bricolo, Sironi et al. described a mortality of 13% in those patients with a changeable sleeplike pattern versus 88% mortality in those with slow monotonous records (170). These studies showing a better prognosis with changeable records support those described earlier for conventional EEG.

Steudel described the relationship of quantitative parameters of the EEG power spectrum to prognosis in 50 adult patients with severe brain injuries. He used the relative and absolute powers in the standard EEG frequency bands obtained from the parieto-occipital region. Survival was associated with an increase in the relative and absolute power in the theta and alpha bands during the first week (180). More recently, the persistence or return of a peak in the CSA display between 4 and 13 Hz during the first 10 days of coma has been associated with a good clinical recovery (27).

Again, the above data obtained with power spectral analysis of the EEG reinforce the findings from classical electroencephalography regarding the relationship of changeability, both spontaneous and induced, and background frequency and changes therein to the clinical state of the patient in coma.

Evoked Potentials

From the above it is apparent that the monitoring of the spontaneous EEG is most useful for the deprivation of information concerning the level of consciousness and whether or not this is changing. In addition, information regarding focal hemispheric dysfunction may be inferred from the presence of interhemispheric asymmetries. In contrast, by using evoked potentials, one is able to gain information regarding the functional status of specific neuroanatomical pathways. Hence, the information derived from evoked potentials is complementary to that from EEG rather than redundant.

The most commonly measured evoked responses are the somatosensory potential (SEP), the brainstem auditory evoked potential (BAEP), and the visual evoked potential (VEP). Generation of the evoked responses is similar in all instances. Basically, a peripheral receptor is stimulated (i.e., peripheral or cranial nerve) by using the appropriate stimulus and the electrical response of the cortex and structures along the neuroanatomical pathway intervening between the cortex and the peripheral stimulus site is measured from scalp electrodes. The stimulus is repeated many times and the responses are averaged by computer, thereby removing the random background EEG and leaving the time-locked response. The evoked response in each particular modality has its own form, characterized by several peaks occurring at particular latencies and having a given amplitude. Deviation from normal is identified by changes in latency, number of peaks, peak amplitudes, or a combination of all three. Various grading schema have been evolved which consider some or all of these factors (57, 92, 144). Different EP modalities may be used alone or in combination (i.e., multimodality evoked potentials, MEPs).

Hume and Cant reported on the central conduction time of the SEP (lower brainstem to cortex) in 94 head-injured patients. They found that the persistence of an abnormal conduction time was associated with death and disability. In surviving patients conduction times decreased over the duration of the study. Overall conduction time correlated with outcome in 75% to 84% of patients depending on when the studies were done (73). De la Torre *et al.* found that outcome was correlated with the number of peaks in the SEP (38).

Used alone, visual evoked potentials have been useful in detecting and/or predicting damage to the visual apparatus (optic nerve to occipital cortex) in patients who are unconscious and therefore unable to cooperate with conventional visual examination (46). They have also been found useful in delimiting different stages of coma (195).

The brainstem auditory evoked response is characterized by five waves originating from the cochlear nerve up to the inferior colliculus (56). Hence, the Pl-5 latency measures the conduction time across the brainstem. Additionally, the loss of various components of the BAEP indicates damage at various levels of the brainstem, correlating with loss of pupillary, oculovestibular, and corneal reflexes (55, 163, 191, 192). Complete absence of the response including wave 1 indicates damage to the end organ and therefore one cannot draw any conclusions regarding brainstem function. Loss of all components after wave 1 is an ominous finding, indicating medullary failure and associated with an isoelectric EEG (82, 192). Additionally, BAEPs ave been found to be very resistant to the effects of drugs, including barbiturates (61, 127), thus offering a means of monitoring patients receiving barbiturates for ICP treatment, even when the dosage is sufficient to flatten the EEG (183). The relation of the BAEP to the depth and outcome of coma is less clear-cut, with several authors maintaining that abnormalities are related to neither the depth, duration, nor outcome of coma (55, 61, 92).

A number of authors have reported on the use of a combination of evoked potential responses to study traumatic coma (18, 55, 57, 92, 126, 128, 144, 145). In one study of multimodality evoked potentials, 91% prognostic accuracy was achieved in traumatic coma using a two-category outcome scale (126). In other studies with MEPs, the best correlations between both depth of coma and outcome were achieved by using cortical evoked responses rather than brainstem EPs (92, 144). Serial MEPs may also be used to monitor neural recovery. Newlon *et al.* found that those patients showing a deterioration in evoked responses due to secondary insult had a poor outcome compared with those who showed no such deterioration or those whose evoked responses improved (128).

Toward Real-Time Neurophysiologic Monitoring

There is good evidence to indicate that presently available electrophysiologic techniques can give objective information regarding the status of the central nervous system in severe illness such as coma. To date, these technologies have for the most part been applied intermittently with the principal aim of indicating prognosis. In order to derive maximum benefit from these measurements, they must be used continuously so that the functional state of the brain can be known at all times. As previously discussed, conventional EEG is ill suited to this task. However, power spectral analysis yields almost as much information and is well suited to use in the ICU.

Movement toward real-time continuous neurophysiologic monitoring poses two principal challenges: one involving engineering, and the second involving the scientific and statistical problems inherent in this undertaking. The engineering problem involves the creation of systems for EEG and EP monitoring which are compact, user-friendly, and sufficiently automated so as to reduce the need for constant operator presence, which is both time consuming and extremely costly—so much so that the potential benefits of this technology are at present outweighed by the cost. Nevertheless, particularly in the case of computerized EEG, tremendous technical advances have been made, and real-time stand-alone systems are commercially available for the continuous spectral analysis of the EEG. This brings us to the second problem. The ideal parameters to monitor (e.g., relative or absolute power in the EEG), the frequency of monitoring, the number of channels to monitor to achieve the best balance between cost, convenience, and clinical information, the variability of both EEG and EPs and hence the number of studies and amount of electrophysiologic change required to indicate significant clinical change all remain to be determined.

CEREBRAL HOMEOSTASIS AND TRAUMA

It would be impossible in this chapter to take each acute neurologic problem and show how it alters and impairs cerebral homeostasis. Therefore, only one acute neurologic problem will be examined; that is, head trauma. The principles and relationships examined can be extrapolated to other acute neurologic conditions. There are several reasons for this choice: (*a*) head injury is common; (*b*) there is a large body of knowledge that has been accumulated concerning the affect of mechanical injury on the brain; (*c*) the problems encountered in the care of the head-injured patient demonstrate the entire spectrum of neurologic difficulties; that is, intracranial hypertension, alteration of CBF on ischemia, cerebral edema, metabolic derangement of the brain and so forth, which require all of the current modes of cerebral protection. Furthermore, many of the techniques used in the intensive care of the head-injured patient have already been applied to patients who are demonstrating neurologic deterioration from other causes. We will continue in the same format and examine how trauma to the brain effects (*a*) CSF dynamics, (*b*) CBF and metabolism, and (*c*) intracranial dynamics.

Effects of Trauma on CSF Dynamics

If the injury to the brain is of sufficient severity, CSF information, outflow resistance, and absorption may be affected. If there is alteration of choroid plexus blood flow secondary to shock or cerebral ischemia with or without an associated rise in ICP, CSF formation may decrease (200). If there is indeed clearance by the brain of edema fluid via the ventricular system, then this would simulate an elevated production rate and affect ICP (148, 149). Certain drugs such as furosemide will affect CSF production. In addition, osmolarity will also affect CSF production (69). CSF outflow resistance can be increased in patients with a severe head injury. The presence of blood in the ventricles or shift can impede the flow of CSF. If patients acquire ventriculitis as a complication of monitoring or meningitis associated with a basilar skull fracture, the flow of CSF could also be impeded (34). There is usually a delicate balance between the production and absorption of CSF. If there is significant subarachnoid hemorrhage, absorption can be impaired. It has been shown that there is a 15% incidence of hydrocephalus following a head injury (80), presumably due to blood either in the basal cisterns or in the arachnoid villi interfering with proper absorption.

Since the CSF compartment serves as a compensatory mechanism, any impairment in its absorption capacity may lead to elevation in ICP. Furthermore, if as Reulen postulated (148, 149), CSF pathways may be a route of clearing edema fluid, then impairment of this pathway would aggravate an already difficult situation.

Effect of Trauma on CBF and Metabolism

The effect of head injury on CBF varies with the severity of the injury, the age of the patient and the presence or absence of secondary factors such as shock or elevated ICP, and the time the CBF study is performed. However, if CBF is measured within 6 to 24 hours in general, there seems to be a correlation between the clinical condition of the patient and CBF. That is, the lower the motor score the lower the CBF (124). This is somewhat at variance with other reports, where the range of time after injury, during which patients were studied, was much wider. This does not necessarily mean that the low CBF was the cause of the low motor score. If flow and demand were coupled in these patients, CBF would be low in patients whose brains were damaged to such an extent that metabolic needs were low. There also appears to be a group of patients with normal flow who, when hyperventilated, show values dropping to below acceptable values (18 to 19 cc/min/100 g) with an associated rise in $AVDO_2$ indicating the presence of early ischemia. Therefore, although low flow after head injury is a common response, its correlation with function and metabolism is variable. Decreased CBF is by no means the universal finding in patients with severe head injury. Bruce found a significant number of children with diffuse brain swelling whom he felt represented hyperemia (23). Obrist found a 55% incidence of hyperemia in patients who were comatose and when studied early (130). However, even in these patients, low flows were often obtained either before or after the hyperemic phase.

The other effect of trauma on CBF is that of impairment of autoregulation (91). This is difficult to reliably test since most evaluations are done in a global manner. While loss of autoregulation may be detected, if it is completely absent, regional loss of autoregulation or shunting of blood from one area to another may be difficult to detect (47). Generally, if flows are measured early and are found to be low, then autoregulation is usually impaired. Autoregulation is tested by first obtaining a base line flow, then altering the systemic blood pressure by either raising or lowering it, depending on the clinical situation. As we saw earlier, if autoregulation is intact, the flow should be fairly constant. If however autoregulation is defective, then with a change in systemic blood pressure there should be a corresponding change in CBF. In addition, if the brain is tight, a rise in ICP might also occur. Experimentally, it has also been shown that a generalized loss of autoregulation occurs after head injury, and seems to be related to the severity of injury. Whether or not autoregulation is intact again seems to be a function of how long after injury it is tested since its impairment is probably transient. Whether or not autoregulation is intact has obvious clinical implications. Head-injured patients often have multiple injury and have instability of their vital signs. If CBF is pressure-passive secondary to impaired autoregulation, then any drop in systemic blood pressure puts the patient at risk for ischemic brain damage.

CO_2 reactivity also seems to be affected by trauma (42, 133). In addition, there may be some regional variation in this response. Cerebral metabolism after severe head injury is usually depressed. In fact, there is a very good correlation between $CMRO_2$ and Glasgow Coma Score that is maintained throughout the course of the patient's illness (130). The extent and duration of this impairment again is probably dependent on severity of injury and the presence or absence of other factors such as ischemia and hypoxia.

Intracranial Pressure and Head Injury

Since ICP is a result of the interaction of all the processes discussed so far in this section, many aspects of ICP and trauma have been mentioned. However, in this section increased ICP will be examined from a clinical viewpoint; that is in the setting of a severe head injury how often it is present, can it be controlled, and how often is it the cause of a patient death.

In 1977 the Richmond group examined a series of 160 patients who had severe head injuries and who had ICP monitoring within hours of injury (117). This was expanded to 225 patients in a later report (118). It was found that 70% of all patients with surgical lesions had elevated ICP (greater than 20 mm Hg) and that 30% of these went on to die from or with uncontrolled ICP. If patients had a diffuse injury, that is, with significant neurologic dysfunction but no surgical mass lesion, the incidence of increased ICP was 33% with only 4% of the patients going on to have uncontrolled ICP. If patients had intracerebral contusions that were not operated upon, then the incidence of elevated ICP was 70% with 6% going on to develop uncontrollable ICP. In patients who were operated upon for mass lesion, 50% still had difficulty with ICP elevations over 20 mm Hg, despite adequate surgical therapy. Of 29 children who had ICP monitored, Bruce had 59% incidence of ICP over 20 mm Hg in the first 3 days (23). In summary, ICP is elevated in a significant number of patients from a variety of causes. This ICP elevation is associated with a poorer outcome than if it is not present. Whether the ICP per se is causing the poor outcome or whether it is an effect of a more severe injury is difficult to tell.

In closing this section on the effect of trauma on the brain, it should be stressed that the end result of an injury to the brain is a composite of the primary damage that occurs at the moment of impact and any secondary injury resulting from systemic hypotension, hypoxia, or metabolic disturbances.

Frequently, it is impossible to determine whether a particular low CBF or elevated ICP is due to neural damage or an ischemic insult secondary to shock from a ruptured spleen in a patient whose brain does not autoregulate. It is important therefore in dealing with the head-injured patient to control these secondary insults as vigorously as possible.

CEREBRAL PROTECTION

In the majority of circumstances brain protection is in fact a combination of resuscitation from some sort of insult and then protection from subsequent injury while the brain recovers from this insult. It is the purpose of this section to discuss the utilization of the knowledge and principles, elucidated thus far in this chapter for the treatment of the patient with impending, acute brain failure. First will be a discussion of methods of ICP control, followed by a discussion of preserving an adequate match of CBF and cerebral metabolism and, finally, an examination of other techniques and medications that are useful in brain protection.

ICP Control

In practical terms, three questions need to be answered when confronted with the problem of elevated ICP: (*a*) at what level should ICP be treated? (*b*) how should ICP be treated? and (*c*) what can be changed to correct the ICP elevation?

The first question is difficult to answer since different patients require different levels to be treated to prevent ischemic damage. Within the range of 15 to 40 mm Hg, however, one fact is clear, if the patient starts to deteriorate neurologically, at whatever pressure, treatment should be given: be it at 10, 15, or 20 mm Hg. However, in the majority of circumstances, patients will not acutely change until ICP becomes much higher, usually 40 to 50 mm Hg. The difficulty with waiting until this deterioration occurs is that the resultant damage may not be reversible. Therefore, most clinicians choose an ICP between 20 to 25 mm Hg as a point to commence treatment. There are several reasons for this (*a*) treatment should be started before there is complete exhaustion of compensatory mechanisms, for it is at this point on the volume-pressure curve (Fig. 9.1) that ICP rises precipitously; (*b*) frequently there is a lag period between the time treatment is begun and the time ICP elevation starts to be reversed and, finally, CPP and CBF should be kept well above the threshold at which neuronal damage can occur. As was pointed out, electrical monitoring may help define this treatment threshold with greater clarity.

The treatment of elevated ICP is a two-pronged procedure—there is the treatment itself and, simultaneously, a cause for the ICP elevation is sought. The treatment phase will be dealt with first.

The treatment of elevated ICP is dependent on the manipulation of the compartments mentioned in the first part of the chapter (Fig. 9.2); that is, manipulation of the CSF, blood volume, and brain compartments. The approach and treatment of ICP should be done in a stepwise fashion (Fig. 9.4), trying first one method, then sequentially adding another should the situation demand it. First, the patient if being mechanically ventilated is sedated with narcotics or paralyzed with pancuronium or some comparable agent. The purpose of this is to allow adequate ventilation of the patient and keep the patient from straining against the ventilator. If the patient is not intubated and he is having ICP difficulties, intubation and mechanical ventilation is probably warranted. Next, if ICP elevations persist, the patient is hyperventilated usually to a $PaCO_2$ of around 25 mm Hg. This will in turn cause cerebral vasoconstriction with shrinkage of the blood volume compartment. This effect is usually immediate and if ICP elevation is mild may easily control the situation. Theoretically, the pH of the CSF should adjust to the chronic alkalosis and hyperventilation would become ineffective. However, in practical terms patients can be hyperventilated for many days without losing this response. If ICP continues to rise and if the patient has an intraventricular catheter, then CSF drainage is utilized. It has been estimated that CSF factors may contribute to as much as 30% of the ICP

A. PHYSIOLOGIC CAUSES OF ELEVATED ICP

increased $PaCO_2$ - ABG

decreased serum NA+ - Electrolytes

increased temperature - thermometer

out of phase with respirator - observation

B. STRUCTURAL CAUSES OF ELEVATED ICP

1) hydrocephalus
2) hematoma
3) cerebral edema

→ CT Scan

Figure 9.4. Stepwise Treatment of Elevated ICP. (From J. D. Ward, *et al.*: Intracranial pressure, head injuries, subarachnoid hemorrhage, non-surgical coma and brain tumors. In: *Critical Care, State of the Art*, edited by W. C. Shoemaker and W. L. Thompson, Vol. II(R), p. 8, 1981. Reprinted with permission.)

elevation in certain circumstances such as head injury (101). This is not unreasonable since CSF production can be up to 0.35 cc/min (33). This would amount to about 500 cc/day. If CSF absorption is impaired such as with bleeding from head injury or subarachnoid hemorrhage, the diversion of the fluid can be most helpful. In addition, if in fact the CSF pathway is utilized by the brain as an aid in the resolution of cerebral edema (28, 70), then by draining CSF, control of the ICP should be enhanced. If CSF drainage is used, the patient should be drained against a pressure gradient to prevent the collapse of the ventricles against the catheter. If drainage is insufficient, diuretics are then used. The majority of clinicians use mannitol for ICP reduction. It is easy to use and is not associated with the difficulty of preparation and potential problems of extravasation and hemolysis associated with glycerol (26). However, glycerol if used appropriately, usually in a 10% solution, can be quite effective in ICP control (50, 194).

Mannitol is used as a 20% solution and is infused over a period of 5 to 15 minutes. The dosage varies from 0.25 g/kg up to 1 g/kg depending on the rapidity of the ICP rise. It is desirable to use the smallest amount of mannitol possible to obtain the desired effect (103). During osmotherapy serum osmolality should be kept below 320 mOsm/liter. Often it is difficult to do this in patients who require frequent doses of mannitol. Serum osmolality over 350 mOsm/liter may lead to renal damage (182). The exact mechanism of action of mannitol has been assumed to be due to the drawing out of water from the normal brain where the blood-brain barrier is intact. However, some doubt has been cast on this explanation by the failure to find a decreased water content in brain after the administration of mannitol (185). Recent work has suggested that mannitol changes viscosity which in turn causes vasoconstriction. This in turn causes a decrease in cerebral blood volume with a resultant fall in ICP (125). The mechanism requires that cerebral vessel reactivity be intact. Rebound is explained as an increase in viscosity secondary to dehydration with resultant vasodilatation.

Other diuretics have been used, most notably furosemide (158, 160, 190). In addition, it has been suggested that furosemide and mannitol used in combination have a greater effect than when either is used alone (138, 206). Furosemide in a dose of 20 to 60 mg can be given 30 minutes after mannitol and this may prolong the time required between doses of mannitol allowing the serum osmolality to come toward a more normal range. Furosemide inhibits sodium transport and decreases CSF production (24). However, this is probably not what causes the relatively rapid drop in ICP.

In addition to the above-mentioned drugs lidocaine has also been suggested for the rapid control of elevated ICP (7). In doses of 1.5 mg/kg IV significant drops in ICP were noted. Its effect is thought to be mediated through a vascular mechanism (157). Its duration of action is rather brief. Other intravenous agents have also been proposed such as etomidate, althesin, and midazolam. However, there have been no clinical trials to date to warrant the routine use of these agents.

If the above regimen fails to control intracranial pressure, then the use of barbiturates has been advocated.

Barbiturates have been used in the protection of the brain since 1937 when Horsley described the lowering of cerebrospinal fluid pressure with barbiturates (71). In the early 1970s barbiturates were used in several experimental models to show the beneficial use in experimental stroke in various species (59, 89, 111, 112, 121). More recently, they have been used during bypass surgery (177). The use of barbiturates was applied to other neurologic diseases in humans in which intracranial hypertension played a deleterious role. These include Reye's syndrome (102) and hypoxia (113).

One of the first uses of barbiturates in head-injured patients was reported by Rockoff and associates in a group of 60 patients, some of whom were head injured (150). During the same year Marshall published a report in which both acute and chronic barbiturates were used in head-injured patients (104). It was their feeling that in these patients who were severely injured and had problems with uncontrolled intracranial hypertension that the use of barbiturate coma lowered ICP and improved outcome in patients that would have otherwise died or been vegetative.

Miller cautioned that what was termed uncontrollable intracranial hypertension in the above studies could perhaps have responded to more intensive conventional therapy and that although barbiturate therapy looked promising, the only true way to prove its efficacy was a randomized, controlled trial (115). This was then followed by a number of studies which used high-dose barbiturates in severely head-injured patients (85, 136, 147, 159, 162).

The exact way barbiturates may lower ICP and improve outcome is unknown. There are a number of proposed mechanisms for the usefulness of barbiturates. The first of these suggest a lowering of cerebral metabolism which in turn decreases CBF and results in a fall of ICP (166). Second, it has been proposed that barbiturates block the generation of free radicals and subsequently decrease the amount of brain damage caused by these agents (48). In addition, barbiturates may cause vasoconstriction from direct effects on cerebral vessels. Whether this is totally a result of lowered metabolism or an effect on the vasculature itself is unknown.

Thus, barbiturates are viewed as logical candidates for brain protection due to their ability to reduce metabolism, lower ICP, and suppress the autolytic effects of free radicals.

In Richmond, a controlled study of the use of *prophylactic* barbiturates in severe head injury was undertaken (196). Based on this study the following conclusions can be made: (*a*) the prophylactic use of pentobarbital coma does not appear to improve outcome in their patients; (*b*) the prophylactic use of pentobarbital does not make the control of ICP any easier, nor does it decrease the number of patients who die from uncontrolled intracranial hypertension; (*c*) the use of high-dose pentobarbital is associated with a significant occurrence of arterial hypotension even in patients who have normovolemia and whose arterial and pulmonary capillary wedge pressure and cardiac output are being monitored and in whom IV pressors are used.

What has not been reported is the outcome in patients in whom barbiturates were not given until ICP became a problem. The results of this cooperative study from other institutions are pending.

The use of barbiturates to protect the brain of patients after cardiac arrest has also been evaluated in a clinical trial. The results were reported recently by the brain resuscitation clinical trial group at the sixth ICP meeting held in Glasgow, June 1985. The trial showed no effect in terms of improvement of outcome (15).

In stroke, there as been no adequate randomized clinical trial as to the effectiveness of barbiturates (172), although as was mentioned earlier, there are some experimental data to support its use.

In practical terms, when other modalities for control of ICP have been exhausted, barbiturates may, in some patients, lower ICP. Whether this will improve outcome is debatable.

If barbiturates are to be used careful monitoring of ICP, systemic arterial pressure, cardiac output, pulmonary capillary wedge pressure, and drug levels are required. Usually a bolus (pentobarbital 5 to 10 mg/kg) is given and then an hourly maintenance dose (pentobarbital 3 to 5 mg/kg) is used. It is probably better to use a continuous drip since this may be less likely to affect the patient's blood pressure. The goal is to achieve serum levels of 3.5 to 4.5 mg/100 ml.

The main complication of barbiturates is hypotension which has been shown to occur as high as 50% even when adequate blood volume and cardiac output are maintained (196). Hypotension can be potentially harmful. Thus, the use of high-dose barbiturates may be potentially harmful and their use should be restricted to very controlled circumstances with appropriate brain and systemic monitoring.

The final aspect of elevated ICP control is to determine and correct the cause. When elevated ICP reaches levels that require treatment, it is imperative that the situation be appraised in a systematic way with attention to the basic principles that have been discussed earlier (Fig. 9.4). The first step is to determine whether the elevation is, in fact, real. This is done by a careful assessment of the waveform and a calibration of the equipment. If the value being recorded is accurate, a stepwise assessment of the various causes of elevated ICP is begun. First, physiologic causes are investigated to see if these are responsible for the elevation in pressure. Arterial blood gases are checked to evaluate the control of $PaCO_2$. Serum electrolytes are checked to rule out serum hypo-osmolarity that could cause a shift of water into the brain tissue. Temperature is assessed since increased temperature will increase the need of the brain for O_2 and will increase CBF. The patient's activity is observed to be sure that he is not out of phase with the respirator, causing increased intrathoracic pressure with resultant impaired venous return from the head. One physiologic causes have been excluded, other causes are sought to determine the etiology of the intracranial hypertension. The presence of hydrocephalus, intracranial hematoma, or cerebral edema is usually assessed by means of the CT scan. Obviously, if the rise in ICP is abrupt and high, then treatment must be instituted prior to obtaining the results of all the above tests. However, the treatment can be more effective and precise if the exact cause of the intracranial hypertension is determined.

Maintenance of CBF

With cerebral perfusion pressure and CBF dependent on ICP, many of the techniques for the maintenance of adequate CBF were covered in the section on controlling ICP. However, blood pressure control and rheologic modification and hypothermia can also affect CBF.

As we discussed earlier, when autoregulation is intact, CBF remains the same over a fairly wide range of cerebral perfusion pressures. Acute neurologic insults can impair autoregulation and when this occurs, closer control of blood pressure is required. If blood pressure is allowed to go too high, it can promote blood-brain barrier breakdown (12, 83) with resultant cerebral edema formation (81). Too low a systemic blood pressure can cause or aggravate cerebral ischemia resulting in further neurologic damage. Recently, it has been pointed out that if autoregulation is intact and blood pressure is allowed to drop only a small amount, there is a compensatory cerebral vasodilatation. If the patient is on the steep portion of the volume-pressure curve, this vasodilatation can cause a rise in ICP. This is thought by some to be the generation of plateau waves (152). The most accurate way to determine the appropriate level of blood pressure is to perform CBF measurement along with $AVDO_2$ measurements. This would allow the blood pressure to be manipulated to match CBF to metabolic needs. This has been attempted in a limited number of patients with head injury (122). Since CBF measurements are not readily available, the next best procedure would be to maintain cerebral perfusion pressure in the normal range and follow $AVDO_2$ values to monitor the adequacy of CBF. If $AVDO_2$ values are normal or low, then one would assume flow is at least adequate for metabolic needs.

Lowering viscosity of the blood has been proposed as a means of increasing flow through ischemic parts of the brain (66, 207). This is an active area of investigation at this time in patients with stroke. Assessment of its efficacy awaits appropriate clinical trials.

Hypothermia reduces the cerebral metabolic rate by 7% per degree centigrade and effectively reduces CBF. Hypothermia has been used in the treatment of intracranial hypertension (167). In stroke, however, the results are conflicting. The majority of evidence seems to indicate that its use is limited (72, 178). However, selected patients can be carried through difficult episodes of intractable ICP with hypothermia. The body temperature is lowered to 31°C and maintained at this level until ICP is under control. Then it is slowly allowed to return to normal. Hypothermia can be complicated by either arrhythmias, hyperglycemia, or altered drug metabolism. Fortunately, myocardial irritability is uncommon above 30°C (11).

Medical Therapy for Brain Protection

Steroids have been used for many years in acute neurologic problems. However, the only clinical situations they have consistently been of proven value is in the care of patients with brain tumors (51, 95).

In head injury the situation is less clear. There have been reports of a favorable response to the use of steroids in head injury (44, 52), while others have shown no effect even in large doses (30, 59). More recently, Braakman in a carefully conducted study was unable to demonstrate any difference in outcome (13). Thus, evidence indicates that steroids are ineffective in trauma, useful in patients with edema from brain tumors, and of unproven efficacy in stroke.

Recently, there has been increasing discussion of drugs that affect free radicals in acute neurologic disorders. Basically, a free radical is any substance that has a lone electron in its outer orbit. In this state it has an unusual capacity to initiate chemical chain reactions. These reactions in time are felt to cause tissue damage by a variety of mechanisms which include injury to the ventricles and vascular endothelium (39, 48, 199). A variety of drugs such as barbiturates (48, 53) and mannitol (168) are known to scavenge free radicals.

Currently, free radicals are felt to be a factor in the complex process of cellular damage after certain acute neurologic insults. Treatment which decreases their numbers may, on theoretical grounds, prove helpful. Clinical guidelines are not available at this time.

Calcium channel blockers used with such effectiveness in heart disease have found their way into the treatment of ischemia secondary to vasospasm. Their efficacy is connected with the fact that after ischemia, elevated intracellular calcium can, through a sequence of events, initiate and result in membrane alterations. As a group of drugs the calcium channel blockers are quite varied and provide different effects on different parts of the body (16). Their primary clinical use appears to be in the prevention of vasospasm secondary to subarachnoid hemorrhage. In a recent study nimodipine has been advocated in patients who are neurologically intact to prevent spasm (1). As other drugs are investigated and our knowledge of their action at the cellular level increases, it is likely that these drugs will have a role in patients with cerebral ischemia.

Other drugs such as naloxone (4, 45) have also been advanced as beneficial for cerebral ischemia. This, as well as other new drugs, can only be recommended after appropriate prospective, controlled studies.

CONCLUSION

Obviously to utilize all the above information in the clinical setting is not easy and often is not necessary. In patients with a severe, acute neurologic insult, however, the utilization of current methods and techniques can be lifesaving and more important yield improved outcome of good neurologic quality. As an example of how all these methods of brain protection and resuscitation are used in patient care, the management of a severely head-injured patient is handled at the Medical College of Virginia is presented (6).

When a severely head-injured patient is brought to the neuroscience intensive care unit after appropriate neurosurgical intervention, if indicated, various monitors are inserted. These include an ICP monitor, preferably a ventricular catheter, a radial arterial line, an internal jugular catheter advanced up to the jugular bulb, a central venous line as well as other lines needed for routine intensive care. Base line evaluations of CBF, multimodality evoked potentials and $AVDO_2$ values are obtained. In addition, determinations of PVI, CSF formation, outflow resistance and absorption pressure are performed. Autoregulation is also determined and CSF from the ventricle is sent for lactate determination. If CBF is under 18 cc/min/100 g, then the CBF is repeated at a higher blood pressure to see if CBF can be improved (122). During the patient's course in the ICU, $AVDO_2$, PVI and neurologic examinations are repeated at frequent intervals. ICP, CVP, end tidal CO_2 and systemic blood pressure are monitored continuously. CBF studies are repeated if $AVDO_2$ increases indicating possible ischemia. Evoked potentials are done 12 hours after base line and daily unless there is a change for the worse. If evoked potentials, ICP or PVI begin to show neurologic compromise, a CT is performed to rule out a delayed hematoma. ICP monitoring is continued until ICP is below 20 mm Hg for 24 hours and PVI determinations are above 18 cc. If ICP starts to go over 25 mm HG or if evoked potentials or neurologic examination changes at less than 25 mm Hg, ICP is treated with the methods outlined in this chapter. As patient function and the varied parameters normalize, monitoring is gradually discontinued.

Although this type of intensive care can only be rendered in a few institutions and at present is not the "standard of care," it is evident that this is the direction in which neurologic intensive care is headed. The brain is a complex organ and its protection will, of necessity, involve complex solutions. It will be only through the combination of all the various techniques mentioned as well as those yet to be developed that high quality recovery from severe, acute neurologic injury can be expected.

REFERENCES

1. Allen, G. S., Ahn, H. S., Preziosi, T. J., *et al.* Cerebral arterial spasm. A controlled trial of nimodipine in patients with subarachnoid hemorrhage. N. Engl. J. Med., *308:* 619–624, 1983.
2. Austin, G., Horn, N., Rouke, S., *et al.* Description and early results of an intravenous radioisotope technique for measuring regional cerebral blood flow. Eur. Neurol., *8:* 43–51, 1972.
3. Bakay, R. A. E., and Ward, A. A. Enzymatic changes in serum and cerebrospinal fluid in neurological injury. J. Neurosurg., *58:* 27–37, 1983.

4. Baskin, D. S., and Hosobuchi, Y. Naloxone reversal of ischemic deficit in gerbils by the opiate antagonist naloxone. Science, *25:* 69–71, 1982.

5. Becker, D. P., Miller, J. D., Butterworth, J. F., *et al.* The outcome from severe head injury with early diagnosis and intensive management. J. Neurosurg., *407:* 491-502, 1977.

6. Becker, D. P., Miller, J. D., Young, H. F., Selhorst, J. B., Kishore, P. S. R., Greenberg, R. P., and Rosner, M. J. Diagnosis and treatment of head injury in adults. In: *Neurological Surgery*, edited by J. Youmans, Ed. 2, pp. 1938-2083. W. B. Saunders, Philadelphia, 1982.

7. Bedford, R. F., Persing, J. A., Pobereskin, L., and Butler, A. Lidocaine or thiopental for rapid control of intracranial hypertension? Anes. Analg., *59:* 435–437, 1980.

8. Bergamasco, B., Bergamini, L., Doriguzzi, T., and Fabiani, D. EEG sleep patterns as a prognostic criterion in post-traumatic coma. Electroencephalogr. Clin. Neurophysiol., *24:* 374–377, 1968.

9. Bickford, R. G. Computer analysis of background activity. In: *EEG Informatics. A Didactic Review of Methods and Applications of EEG Data Processing*, edited by A. Remond. Elsevier/North Holland Biomedical Press, Amsterdam, 1977.

10. Bickford, R. G., Brimm, J., Berger, L., and Aung, M. Application of compressed spectral array in clinical EEG. In: *Automation of Clinical Electroencephalography*, edited by P. Kellaway and I. Petersen. Raven Press, New York, 1973.

11. Black, P. R., van Dwanter, S., and Cohn, L. H. Current research review effects of hypothermia on systemic and organ system metabolism and function. J. Surg. Res., *20:* 49–63, 1976.

12. Bleyaert, A. L., Sands, P. A., Safar, P., *et al.* Augmentation of postischemic brain damage by severe intermittent hypertension. Crit. Care Med., *8:*41–47, 1980.

13. Braakman, R., Schouten, H. J. A., Blaauw-van Dishoeck, M., and Minderhoud, J. M. Megadose steroids in severe head injury: Results of a prospective double-blind clinical trial. J. Neurosurg., *58:* 326-330, 1983.

14. Bradbury, M. W. B., and Westrop, R. J. Lymphatics and the drainage of cerebrospinal fluid. In: *Hydrocephalis*, edited by K. Shapiro, A. Marmarou, and H. Portnoy, pp. 69–81. Raven Press, New York, 1984.

15. Brain Resuscitation Clinical Trial Study Group. A randomized clinical trial of barbiturate loading in cardiac arrest survivors. Intracranial Pressure VI, 1986, in press.

16. Brandt, L., Andersson, K-E., Edvinsson, L., and Ljunggren, B. Effects of extracellular calcium and of calcium antagonists on the contractile responses of isolated human pial and messenteric arteries. J. Cereb. Blood Flow Metab., *1:* 339-347, 1981.

17. Bricolo, A. Electroencephalography in neurotraumatology. Clin. Electroencephalogr., *7:* 184–197, 1976.

18. Bricolo, A., Faccioli, F., Turazzi, S., and Pasut, M. L. EEG and evoked potentials in brain stem traumatic lesions. In: *Advances in Neurotraumatology*, edited by R. Villani, I. Papo, and M. Giovanelli. Excerpta Medica, Amsterdam, Oxford, Princeton, 1982.

19. Bricolo, A., Turella, G., Salle, Ore, G., and Terzian, H. A proposal for the electroencephalographic evaluation of acute traumatic coma in neurosurgical practice. Electroencephalogr. Clin. Neurophysiol., *34:* 789, 1973.

20. Bricolo, A., Turazzi, F., Faccioli, F., *et al.* Clinical application of compressed spectral array in long-term EEG monitoring of comatose patients. Electroencephalogr. Clin. Neurophysiol., *45:* 211–225, 1978.

21. Brierley, F. B., and Field, E. J. The connections of the spinal arachnoid space with the lymphatic system. J. Anat., *82:* 153–160, 1948.

22. Brodersen, P., Paulson, O. B., Bolwig, T. G., Bogon, Z. E., Rafaelson, O. J., and Lassen, N. A. Cerebral hyperemia in electrically induced epileptic seizures. Arch. Neurol., *28:* 334–338, 1973.

23. Bruce, D. A., Alavi, A., Bilaniuk, L., Dolinskas, C., Obrist, W., and Uzzell, B. Diffuse cerebral swelling following head injuries in children: The syndrome of malignant brain edema. J. Neurosurg., *54:* 170–178, 1981.

24. Buhrley, L. E., and Reed, D. J. The effect of furosemide on sodium 22 uptake into cerebrospinal fluid and brain. Exp. Brain Res., *14:* 503–510, 1972.

25. Burrows, G. *On Disorders of the Cerebral Circulation and on the Connection Between Affections of the Brain and Diseases of the Heart*, pp. 55–56. Longmans, London, 1846.

26. Cameron, G. P., and Finckh, E. S. The production of an acute hemolytic crisis by the subcutaneous injection of glycerol. J. Pathol. Bacteriol., *71:* 165–172, 1956.

27. Cant, B. R., and Shaw, N. A. Monitoring by compressed spectral array in prolonged coma. Neurology, *34:* 35–39, 1984.

28. Cao, M., Tisheng, H., and Shouzheng, S. Resolution of brain edema in severe brain injury at controlled high and low intracranial pressures. J. Neurosurg., *61:* 707–712, 1984.

29. Chatrian, G. E., White, L. E., and Daly, D. Electroencephalographic patterns resembling those of sleep in certain comatose states after injuries to the head. Electroencephalogr. Clin. Neurophysiol., *15:* 272–280, 1963.

30. Cooper. P. R., Moody, S., Clark, W. L., *et al.* Dexamethasone and severe head injury: A prospective double-blind study. J. Neurosurg., *51:* 307–316, 1979.

31. Courjon, J. Traumatic disorders. In: *Handbook of Electroencephalography and Clinical Neurophysiology*, edited by A. Remono, Vol. 14, Part B. Elsevier, Amsterdam, 1972.

32. Crockard, H. A., and Taylor, A. R. Serial CSF lactate-pyruvate values as a guide to prognosis in head injury coma. Eur. Neurol., *8:* 151–157, 1972.

33. Cutler, R. W. P., Page, L., Galwich, F., *et al.* Formation and absorption of cerebrospinal fluid in man. Brain, *91:* 707–720, 1968.

34. Dacey, R. G. J. R., Scheld, W. M., and Winn, H. R., *et al.* Bacterial meningitis: Selected aspects of cerebrospinal fluid pathophysiology. In: *Neurology*

of Cerebrospinal Fluid, edited by J. J. Wood, pp. 727–738. Plenum Press, New York, 1983.
35. Davson, H., Hollingsworth, G., and Segal, M. B. The mechanism of drainage of the cerebrospinal fluid. Brain, *93:* 665–678, 1970.
36. Dawson, R. E., Webster, J. E., and Gurdjian, E. S. Serial electroencephalography in acute head injuries. J. Neurosurg., *8:* 613–630, 1951.
37. Dearden, M. N., McDowell, G. D., and Gibson, R. M. Assessment of Leeds device for monitoring intracranial pressure. J. Neurosurg., *60:* 123–129, 1984.
38. De La Torre, J. C., Trimble, J. L., and Beard, R. T. Somatosensory evoked potentials for the prognosis of coma in humans. Exp. Neurol., *60:* 304–317, 1978.
39. Demopoulis, H. B., Milvy, P., Kakari, S., and Ransohoff, T. Molecular aspects of membrane structure in cerebral edema. In: *Steroids and Brain Edema*, edited by H. J. Reulen, and Schurmann, pp. 29–39. Springer-Verlag, New York, 1972.
40. Duffy, F. H., Burchfiel, J. S., and Lumbroso, C. T. Brain electrical activity mapping (beam): A method for extending the clinical utility of EEG and evoked potential data. Ann. Neurol., *5:* 309–321, 1979.
41. Ekstrom-Jodal, B., Haggendal, E., Johannson, B., Linder, L. E., and Nilsson, M. J. Acute arterial hypertension and the blood-brain barrier: An experimental study in dogs. In: *Cerebral Circulation and Metabolism*, edited by T. W. Langfitt, L. C. McHenry, Jr., M. Rewich, and H. Wollman. Springer-Verlag, Berlin, 1975.
42. Enevoldsen, E. M., Cold, G., and Jansen, F. T. Autoregulation and CO_2 responses of cerebral blood flow in patients with severe head injury. J. Neurosurg., *48:* 689–203, 1977.
43. Enevoldsen, E. M., and Jensen, F. T. Cerebrospinal fluid lactate and pH in patients with acute severe head injury. Clin. Neurol. Neurosurg., *80:* 213–225, 1977.
44. Faupel, G., Reulen, H. J., Mullen, D., *et al.* Double-blind study on the effects of dexamethasone on severe closed head injury. In: *Dynamics of Brain Edema*, edited by H. M. Passius and W. Feindel, pp. 337–343. Springer-Verlag, New York, 1976.
45. Fallis, R. J., Fisher, M., and Lobo, R. A. A double-blind trial of naloxone in the treatment of acute stroke. Stroke, *15:* 627–629. 1984.
46. Feinsod, M., and Auerbach, E. Electrophysiological examinations of the visual system in the acute phase after head injury. Eur. Neurol., *9:* 56–64, 1973.
47. Fieschi, C., Battistini, N., Bedoschi, A., Baselli, L., and Rossanda, M. Regional cerebral blood flow and intraventricular pressure in acute head injuries. J. Neurol. Neurosurg. Psychiatry, *37:* 1378–1388, 1974.
48. Flamm, E. S., Demopoulos, S. G., Seligman, M. L., and Ransohoff, J. Possible molecular mechanisms of barbiturate-mediated protection in regional cerebral ischemia. Acta Neurol. Scand. (Suppl.), *56:* 150–151, 1977.
49. Fleming, R. A., and Smith, N. T. Density modulation—A technique for the display of three variable data in patient monitoring. Anesthesiology *50:* 543–546, 1979.
50. Frank, M. S. B., Nahata, M. C., and Hilty, M. D. Glycerol: A review of its pharmacology, pharmacokinetics, adverse reactions and clinical use. Pharmacotherapy, *1:* 147–160, 1981.
51. Galicich, J. H., and French, L. Use of dexamethasone in treatment of cerebral edema resulting from brain tumors in brain surgery. Am. Practit., *12:* 169–174, 1961.
52. Gobiet, W., Bock, W. J., Leisegang, J., *et al.* Treatment of acute cerebral edema with high dose dexamethasone. In: *Intracranial Pressure III*, edited by J. W. F. Beks, D. A. Bosch, and M. Brock, pp. 231–235. Springer-Verlag, Berlin, Heidelberg, New York, 1976.
53. Godin, D. V., Mitchell, M. J., and Saunders, B. A. Studies on the interaction of barbiturates with reactive oxygen radicals: Implications regarding barbiturate protection against cerebral ischemia. Can. Anaesth. Soc. J., *29:* 203–210, 1982.
54. Granowska, M., Britton, K. E., Aschar, F., Wright, C. W., Smith, R. R. J., Lee, T. V., and Nimmon, C. C. Global and regional cerebral blood flow: Non-invasive quantitation in patients with subarachnoid hemorrhage. J. Neurosurg., *53:* 153–159, 1980.
55. Greenberg, R. P., Becker, D. P., Miller, J. D., and Mayer, D. J. Evaluation of brain function in severe human head trauma with multimodality evoked potentials. Part 2: Localization of brain dysfunction and correlation with post-traumatic neurological conditions. J. Neurosurg., *47:* 163–177, 1977.
56. Greenberg, R. P., and Ducker, T. B. Evoked potentials in the clinical neurosciences. J. Neurosurg., *56:* 1–18, 1982.
57. Greenberg, R. P., Mayer, D. J., Becker, D. P., and Miller, J. D. Evaluation of brain function in severe human head trauma with multimodality evoked potentials. Part 1: Evoked brain-injury potentials, methods and analysis. J. Neurosurg., *47:* 150–162, 1977.
58. Grubb, R. L., Raichle, M. E., Eichling, J. O., and Ter-Pogossian, M. M. The effects of changes in $PaCO_2$ on cerebral blood volume, blood flow and vascular mean transit time. Stroke, *5:* 630–639, 1974.
59. Gudeman, S. K., Miller, J. D., and Becker, D. P. Failure of high dose steroid therapy to influence intracranial pressure in patients with severe head injury. J. Neurosurg., *51:* 301–306, 1979.
60. Guillaume, J., and Janny, P. Manometric intracranienne continue interet de la methode et premiers resultats. Rev. Neurol. (Paris), *84:* 131–142, 1951.
61. Hall, J. W., and Mackey-Hargadine, J. Auditory evoked responses in severe head injury. Semin. Hearing, *5:* 313–335, 1984.
62. Hansotia, P., Gottschalk, P., Green, P., and Zais, D. Spindle coma: Incidence, clinicopathologic correlates, and prognostic value. Neurology (NY), *31:* 82–87, 1981.
63. Hari, R., Sulkava, R., and Haltia, M. Brain stem auditory evoked responses and alpha pattern coma. Ann. Neurol., *11:* 187–189, 1982.

64. Harner, R., and Naquet, R. Altered states of consciousness, coma, cerebral death. In: *Handbook of Electroencephalography and Clinical Neurophysiology*, edited by A. Remond. Elsevier, Amsterdam, 1975.
65. Harper, A. M. Autoregulation of cerebral blood flow: Influence of arterial blood pressure on the blood flow through the cerebral cortex. J. Neurol. Neurosurg. Psychiatry, *29:* 398–403, 1966.
66. Harrison, M. J. G., Pollack, S., Kendal, B. F., *et al.* Effect of hematocrit on carotid stenosis and cerebral infarction. Lancet, *2:* 114–115, 1981.
67. Heilbrun, M. P., Olesen, J., and Lassen, N. A. Regional cerebral blood flow studies in subarachnoid hemorrhage. J. Neurosurg., *37:*36–44, 1972.
68. Heisey, S. R., Held, D., and Pappenheimer, J. R. Bulk flow and diffusion in the cerebral spinal fluid system of the goat. Am. J. Physiol., *203:* 775–781, 1962.
69. Hochwald, G. M., Wald, G., Demattio, J., *et al.* The effect of serum osmolarity on cerebrospinal fluid volume flow. Life Sci., *15:* 1309–1316, 1974.
70. Hochwald, G. M., Wald, A., and Malhan, C. The sink action of cerebrospinal fluid volume flow. Effect on brain water content. Arch. Neurol., *33:* 334–339, 1976.
71. Horsley, J. G. Intracranial pressure during barbital narcosis. Lancet, *1:* 141–143, 1957.
72. Hossman, K. A. Treatment of experimental cerebral ischemia. J. Cereb. Blood Flow Metab., *2:* 275–297, 1982.
73. Hume, A. L., and Cant, B. R. Central somatosensory conduction after head injury. Ann. Neurol., *10:* 411–419, 1981.
74. Ingvar, D. H., Cronquist, S., Ekberg, R., Risberg, J., and Hoedt-Rasmussenk, K. Normal values of regional cerebral blood flow in man including flow and weight measurements of gray and white matter. Acta Neurol. Scand., *41* (Suppl. 14)*:* 72–78, 1965.
75. Jones, T. H., Morawetz, R. B., Crowell, R. M., *et al.* Threshold of focal cerebral ischemia in awake monkeys. J. Neurosurg., *54:* 773–782, 1981.
76. Karnaze, D. S., Marshall, L. F., and Bickford, R. A. EEG monitoring of clinical coma: The compressed spectral array. Neurology, *32:* 289–292, 1982.
77. Kellie, G. An account of the appearances observed in the dissection of two of three individuals presumed to have perished in the storm of the 3D, and whose bodies were discovered in the vicinity of Leith on the morning of the 4th November 1821 with some reflections on the pathology of the brain. Trans. Med. Chir. Sci. Edinb., *1:* 84–169, 1824.
78. Kety, S. S., and Schmidt, C. F. The nitrous oxide method for the quantitative determination of cerebral blood flow in man: Theory, procedure, and normal values. J. Clin. Invest., *27:* 476–483, 1948.
79. King, L. R., McLaurin, R. L., and Knowles, H. C., Jr. Acid base balance and arterial and CSF lactate levels following human head injury. J. Neurosurg., *40:* 617–625, 1974.
80. Kishore, P. R. S., Lipper, M. H., Miller, J. D., *et al.* Post-traumatic hydrocephalus in patients with severe head injury. Neuroradiology, *16:* 261–265, 1978.
81. Klatzo, I., Wisniewski, H., Steinwall, O., and Streicher, E. Dynamics of cold injury edema. In: *Brain Edema Proceedings of the Symposium*, edited by I. Klatzo, and F. Seddberger. Springer-Verlag, New York, 1967.
82. Klug, N. Brain stem auditory evoked potentials in syndromes of decerebration, the bulbar syndrome, and in central death. J. Neurol., *227:* 219–228, 1982.
83. Kontos, H. A., Raper, A. J., and Patterson, J. L. Analysis of vasoactivity of local pH, Pco_2, and bicarbonate on pial vessels. Stroke, *8:*358–360, 1977.
84. Koster, W. G., and Kuypers, M. H. Epidural measurement of intracranial pressure. In: *Intracranial Pressure IV*, edited by K. Shulman, A. Marmarou, J. D. Miller, *et al.*, pp. 371–376. Springer-Verlag, Berlin, Heidelberg, New York, 1980.
85. Lamas, E., Lobato, R. D., Benitez, J., Munoz, J. L., Cordobes, F., Velasco, L., Rivas, J. J., Prados, J., and Delgado, M. High dose barbiturate therapy for severe post-traumatic intracranial hypertension. In: *Intracranial Hypertension*, edited by S. Ishii, H. Hagai, and M. Brock, pp. 806–808. Springer-Verlag, Berlin, 1983.
86. Langfitt, T. W. Increased intracranial pressure. Clin. Neurosurg., *16:* 436–471, 1971.
87. Langfitt, T. W., and Obrist, W. D. Cerebral blood flow and metabolism after intracranial trauma. Prog. Neurol. Surg., *10:* 14–48, 1981.
88. Levin, A. B. The use of a fiberoptic intracranial pressure monitor in clinical practice. Neurosurgery, *1:* 139–141, 1977.
89. Levy, D. E., and Brierley, J. B. Delayed pentobarbital administration limits ischemia damage in gerbils. Ann. Neurol., *5:* 59–64, 1979.
90. Levy, W. J., Shapiro, H. M., Maruchak, G., and Meathe, E. Automated EEG processing for intraoperative monitoring: A comparison of techniques. Anesthesiology, *53:* 223–236, 1980.
91. Lewelt, W., Jenkins, L. W., and Miller, J. D. Autoregulation of cerebral blood flow after experimental fluid percussion injury of the brain. J. Neurosurg., *53:* 500–511, 1980.
92. Lindsay, K. W., Carlin, J., Kennedy, I., *et al.* Evoked potentials in severe head injury—analysis and relation to outcome. J. Neurol. Neurosurg. Psychiatry, *44:* 796–802, 1981.
93. Loeb, C. Electroencephalographic changes during the state of coma. Electroencephalogr. Clin. Neurophysiol., *10:*, 589–606, 1958.
94. Lofgren, F., Von Essen, C., and Zwetnow, N. N The pressure-volume curve of the cerebrospinal fluid space in dogs. Acta Neurol. Scand. *49:* 557–574, 1973.
95. Long, D. M., Maxwell, R. E., and French, L. D. The effect of glucosteroids upon cold induced brain edema. II. Ultrasound evaluation. J. Neuropathol. Exp. Neurol., *30:* 680–697, 1971.
96. Lorenzo, A. V., Page, L. K., and Watters, G. V. Relationship between cerebrospinal fluid formation, absorption, and pressure in human hydrocephalus. Brain, *93:* 679–692, 1970.

97. Lunberg, N. Continuous recording and control of ventricular fluid pressure in neurosurgical practice. Acta Psychol. Neurol. Scand., *36* (Suppl.): 149, 1960.
98. Magnaes, B. Body position and cerebrospinal fluid pressure. Part I: Clinical studies on the effect of rapid postural changes. J. Neurosurg., *44:* 687–697, 1976.
99. Marmarou, A. Personal communication, 1985.
100. Marmarou, A., Nakamura, T., and Tanaka, K. The kinetics of fluid movement through brain tissue. Semin. Neurol., *4:* 439–444, 1984.
101. Marmarou, A., Shulman, K., and Lamorgese, J. Compartmental analysis of compliance and outflow resistance of the cerebral spinal fluid system. J. Neurosurg., *43:* 523–534, 1976.
102. Marshall, L. F., Shapiro, H. M., Rauscher, A., *et al.* Pentobarbital therapy for intracranial hypertension in metabolic coma. Reye's syndrome. Crit. Care Med., *6:* 1–5, 1978.
103. Marshall, L. F., Smith, R. W., Rauscher, L. H., and Shapiro, H. M. Mannitol dose requirements in brain-injured patients. J. Neurosurg., *48:* 169–172, 1978.
104. Marshall, L. F., Smith, R. W., and Shapiro, H. M. The outcome with aggressive treatment in severe head injury. Part II: Acute and chronic barbiturate administration in the management of head injury. J. Neurosurg., *50:* 26–30, 1979.
105. Mayhall, C. G., Archer, N. H., Lamb, V. A., Spadora, P., Baggett, J. W., Ward. J. D., and Narayan, R. K. Ventriculostomy-related infection: A prospective epidemiologic study. N. Engl. J. Med., *310:* 553–559, 1984.
106. Maynard, D., Prior, P. F., and Scott, D. F. Device for continuous monitoring of cerebral activity in resuscitated patients. Br. Med. J., *4:* 545–546, 1969.
107. McCarthy, K. D., and Reed, D. J. The effect of acetazolamide and furosemide on cerebrospinal fluid protection on choroid plexus carbonic anhydrase activity. J. Pharmacol. Exp. Ther., *189:* 194–201, 1974.
108. McDowall, D. G. Inter-relationship between blood oxygen tensions and cerebral blood flow. In: *Oxygen Measurements in Blood Tissues*, edited by J. P. Payne, and D. W. Hill, pp. 205–214. Churchill-Livingstone, London, 1966.
109. McHenry, L. C., Fazekas, J. F., and Sullivan, J. F. Cerebral hemodynamics of syncope. Am. J. Med. Sci., *241:* 173–178, 1961.
110. Mendelow, D. A., Rowan, J. O., Murry, L., and Kerr, A. E. A clinical comparison of subdural screw pressure measurements with ventricular pressure.
111. Michenfelder, J. D., and Milde, J. H. Failure of prolonged hypocapnia, hypothermia, or hypertension to favorably alter acute stroke in primates. Stroke, *8:* 87–91, 1977.
112. Michenfelder, J. D., Milde, J. H., and Sundt, J. M. Cerebral protection by barbiturate anesthesia. Use after middle cerebral artery occlusion in Jova monkeys. Arch. Neurol., *33:* 345–350, 1976.
113. Michenfelder, J. D., and Theye, A. A. Cerebral protection by thiopental during hypoxia. Anesthesiology, *39:* 510–517, 1973.
114. Milhorat, T. H., Hammock, M. K., Fenstermacher, J. D., *et al.* Cerebrospinal fluid production by the choroid plexis and brain. Science, *173:* 330–332, 1971.
115. Miller, J. D. Barbiturates and raised intracranial pressure. Ann. Neurol., *6:* 189–193, 1979.
116. Miller, J. D. Studies of intracranial pressure and volume in patients with head injury. J. Neurol. Sci., *17:* 217–223, 1973.
117. Miller, J. D., Becker, D. P., Ward, J. D., Sullivan, H. G., Adams, W. E., and Rosner, M. J. Significance of intracranial hypertension in severe head injury. J. Neurosurg., *47:* 503–510, 1977.
118. Miller, J. D., Butterworth, J. F., Gudeman, S. K., Faulkner, J. E., Choi, S. E., Selhorst, J. B., Harbison, J. W., Lutz, H. A., Young, H. F., and Becker, D. P. Further experience in the management of severe head injury. J. Neurosurg., *54:* 289–299, 1981.
119. Miller, J. D., and Garibi, J. Intracranial volume/pressure relationships during continuous monitoring of ventricular fluid pressure. In: *Intracranial Pressure: Experimental and Clinical Aspects*, edited by M. Brock, and H. Dietz, pp. 270–274. Springer-Verlag, Berlin, 1972.
120. Monro, A. *Observations on the Structure and Function of the Nervous System*. Creech and Johnston, Edinburgh, 1783.
121. Moseley, J. L., Laurent, J. P., and Molinari, G. F. Barbiturate attenuation of the clinical course and pathologic lesions in a primate stroke model. Neurology, *25:* 870–874, 1975.
122. Muizelaar, J. P., and Becker, D. P. Induced hypertension for the treatment of cerebral ischemia after subarachnoid hemorrhage: Direct effect on cerebral blood flow. Surg. Neurol., *25:* 317–325, 1986.
123. Muizelaar, J. P., Becker, D. P., Lutz, H. A., and Newlon, P. Cerebral ischemia after severe head injury: Its role in determining clinical status and the possible treatment. In: *Advances in Neurotraumatology*, edited by R. Villani, I. Papo, M. Griovanelli, S. M. Gaini, and G. Tomei, pp. 92–98. Excerpta Medica, Amsterdam, Oxford, Princeton, 1982.
124. Muizelaar, J. P., and Obrist, W. D. Cerebral blood flow and brain metabolism with brain injury. In: *Central Nervous System Trauma Status Report: 1985*, edited by D. P. Becker and J. T. Povlishock, pp. 123–137. NINCDS, NIH, Bethesda, MD, 1985.
125. Muizelaar, J. P., Wei, E. P., Kontos, H. A., and Becker, D. P. Mannitol causes compensatory cerebral vasoconstruction and vasodilation in response to blood viscosity changes. J. Neurosurg., *59:* 822–828, 1983.
126. Narayan, R. J., Greenberg, R. P., Miller, J. D., *et al.* Improved confidence of outcome prediction in severe head injury. A comparative analysis of the clinical examination, multimodality evoked potentials, CT scanning, and intracranial pressure. J. Neurosurg., *54:* 751–762, 1981.

127. Newlon, P. G., Greenberg, R. P., Enas, G. G., and Becker, D. P. Effects of therapeutic pentobarbital coma on multimodality evoked potentials recorded from severely head-injured patients. Neurosurgery, *12:* 613-619, 1983.
128. Newlon, P. G., Greenberg, R. P., Hyatt, M. S., *et al.* The dynamics of neuronal dysfunction and recovery following severe head injury assessed with serial multimodality evoked potentials. J. Neurosurg., *57:* 168-177, 1982.
129. Obeso, J. A., Iragui, M. I., Marti-Masso, J. F., *et al.* Neurophysiological assessment of alpha pattern coma. J. Neurol. Neurosurg. Psychiatry, *43:* 63-67, 1980.
130. Obrist, W., Langfitt, T. W., Jaggi, J. L., Cruz, J., and Gennarelli, T. A. Cerebral blood flow and metabolism in comatose patients with acute head injury. J. Neurosurg., *61:* 241-253, 1984.
131. Obrist, W. D., Thompson, H. K., Wang, H. S., *et al.* Regional cerebral blood flow estimated by ^{133}Xenon inhalation. Stroke, *6:* 245-256, 1975.
132. Olesen, J. Quantitative evaluation of normal and pathological cerebral blood flow regulation to perfusion pressure. Arch. Neurol., *28:* 143-149, 1973.
133. Overgaard, J., and Tweed, W. A. Cerebral circulation after head injury. Part I: Cerebral blood flow and its regulation after closed head injury with emphasis on clinical correlations. J. Neurosurg., *41:* 531-541, 1974.
134. Pampiglione, A. Early neurophysiological assessment after insult to the central nervous system. In: *Outcome of Severe Damage to the Central Nervous System*, CIBA Foundation Symposium 34. Elsevier, Excerpta Medica, North Holland, Amsterdam, 1975.
135. Passouant, P., Cadilhac, J., Delange, M., *et al.* Different electrical stages and cyclic organization of post-traumatic comas: Polygraphic recording of long duration. Electroencephalogr. Clin. Neurophysiol., *18:* 726, 1965.
136. Piatt, J. H., Jr., and Schiff, S. F. High dose barbiturate therapy in neurosurgery and intensive care. Neurosurgery, *15:* 427-444, 1984.
137. Pollay, M., and Curl, F. Secretion of cerebrospinal fluid by the ventricular ependyma of the rabbit. Am. J. Physiol., *213:* 1031-1038, 1967.
138. Pollay, M., Fullenwides, C., Roberts, A., and Stevens, A. Affect of mannitol and furosemide on blood brain osmotic gradient on intracranial pressure. J. Neurosurg., *59:* 945-950, 1983.
139. Pollay, M., Stevens, F. A., and Roberts, P. A. Alteration in choroid plexus blood flow and cerebrospinal fluid formation by increased ventricular pressure. In: *Neurobiology of Cerebrospinal Fluid II*, edited by J. H. Wood, pp. 687-695. Plenum Press, New York, 1983.
140. Rabow, L. Lactate dehydrogenase (LD) hydroxybutyrate dehydrogenase (HBD) and LD-ISO enzymes in brain tissue. Acta Neurochir., *36:* 61-70, 1970.
141. Raichle, M. E., and Plum, F. Hyperventilation and cerebral blood flow. Stroke, *3:* 566-575, 1972.
142. Raichle, M. E., Posner, J. B., and Plum, F. Cerebral blood flow during—after hyperventilation. Arch. Neurol., *23:* 394-403, 1970.
143. Rampil, I. J., Sasse, F. J., Smith, N. T., *et al.* Spectral edge frequency—a new correlate of anesthetic depth. Anesthesiology, *53:* 512, 1980.
144. Rappaport, M., Hall, K., Hopkins, K. H., and Belleza, T. Evoked potentials and head injury. Part I. Rating of evoked potential abnormality. Clin. Electroencephalogr., *12:* 154-166, 1981.
145. Rappaport, M., Hopkins, K. H., Hall, K., and Belleza, T. Evoked potentials and head injury. Part 2: Clinical applications. Clin. Electroencephalogr., *12:* 167-176, 1981.
146. Ravagnati, L., Iaguone, M. M., Sironi, V. A., *et al.* Small cerebral lesions in minor head injuries: CT-EEG correlation. In: *Advances in Neurotraumatology*, edited by R. Villani, I. Papo, M. Giovanelli, *et al.*, pp. 301-303. Excerpta Medica, Amsterdam, Oxford, Princeton, 1982.
147. Rea, G. L., and Rockswold, G. L. Barbiturate therapy in uncontrolled intracranial hypertension. Neurosurgery, *12:* 401-404, 1983.
148. Reulen, H. F., Prioleau, G. R., Tsuyumu, M., *et al.* Clearance of edema fluid into cerebrospinal fluid: Mechanism of resolution for vasogenic brain edema. In: *Brain Edema: Pathology Diagnosis and Therapy. Advances in Neurology*, Vol. 28, pp. 375-381. Raven Press, New York, 1980.
149. Reulen, H. J., Tsuyumu, M., and Prioleau, G. R. Further results concerning the resolution of vasogenic brain edema. In: *Brain Edema: Pathology, Diagnosis and Therapy. Advances in Neurology*, Vol. 28, pp. 375-381. Raven Press, New York, 1980.
150. Rockoff, M. A., Marshall, L. F., and Shapiro, H. M. High dose barbiturate therapy in humans: A clinical review of 60 patients. Ann. Neurol., *6:* 194-199, 1979.
151. Rosner, M. J., and Becker, D. P. ICP monitoring: Complications and their contributory factors. Clin. Neurosurg., *23:* 494-519, 1976.
152. Rosner, M. J., and Becker, D. P. Origin and evolution of plateau waves. J. Neurosurg., *60:* 312-324, 1984.
153. Rougemont, J. D., Ames, A., Nesbitt, F. B., and Hofmann, H. E. Fluid formed by choroid plexus. J. Neurophysiol., *23:* 485-495, 1960.
154. Rubin, R. C., Henderson, E. S., Ommaya, A. K., Walker, M. D., and Rall, D. P. The production of cerebrospinal fluid in man and its modification by acetazolamide. J. Neurosurg., *25:* 430-436, 1966.
155. Rumpel, E., Lorenzi, E., Hackal, J. M., *et al.* The EEG at different stages of acute secondary traumatic midbrain and bulbar brain syndromes. Electroencephalogr. Clin. Neurophysiol., *46:* 487-497, 1979.
156. Rylander, H. G., Taylor, H. L., Wissinger, J. P., and Story, J. L. Chronic measurement of epidural pressure with an induction powered oscillator transducer. J. Neurosurg., *44:* 565-578, 1976.
157. Sakabe, T., Naekawa, T., Ishikawa, T., *et al.* The effects of lidocaine on canine cerebral metabolism

and circulation related to the electroencephalogram. Anesthesiology, *40:* 433–441, 1974.

158. Sampson, D., and Beyer, C. W., Jr. Furosemide in the intraoperative reduction of intracranial pressure in patients with subarachnoid hemorrhage. Neurosurgery, *10:* 167–169, 1982.

159. Saul, T. G., and Ducker, T. B. Effect of intracranial pressure monitoring and aggressive treatment on mortality in severe head injury. J. Neurosurg., *56:* 498–503, 1982.

160. Schettini, A., Stahurski, B., and Young, H. F. Osmotic and osmotic loop diuretics in brain surgery: Effects on plasma and CSF electrolytes and ion excretion. J. Neurosurg., *56:* 679–684, 1982.

161. Schwartz, M. S., Colvin, M. P., Prior, P. F., *et al.* The cerebral function monitor. Its value in predicting the neurologic outcome in patients undergoing cardiopulmonary bypass. Anesthesia, *28:* 611–618, 1973.

162. Schwartz, M. L., Tator, C. H., Rowed, D. W., Reid, S. R., Meguro, K., and Andrew, D. F. The University of Toronto head injury treatment study: A prospective, randomized comparison of pentobarbital and mannitol. Can. J. Neurol. Sci., *11:* 434–440, 1984.

163. Seales, D. M., Rossiter, V. S., and Weinstein, M. E. Brainstem auditory evoked responses in patients comatose as a result of blunt head trauma. J. Trauma, *19:* 347–353, 1979.

164. Sechzer, P. H., and Ospina. J. Cerebral function monitor: Evaluation in anesthesia/critical care. Curr. Therap. Res., *22:* 335–347, 1977.

165. Shalit, M. N., Shimojyo, S., and Reinmuth, J. M. Carbon dioxide and cerebral circulatory control. I. The extravascular effects. Arch. Neurol., *17:* 298–303, 1967.

166. Shapiro, H. M. Anesthesia effects upon cerebral blood flow, cerebral metabolism, and the electroencephalogram. In: *Anesthesia* edited by R. D. Miller, pp. 795–824. Churchill-Livingstone, New York, 1981.

167. Shapiro, H. M., Wyte, R., and Loeser, J. Barbiturate augmented hypothermia for the reduction of persistent intracranial hypertension. J. Neurosurg., *40:* 90–100, 1974.

168. Siesjo, B. K. Cerebral circulation and metabolism. J. Neurosurg., *60:* 883–908, 1984.

169. Silverman, D. Retrospective study of the EEG in coma. Electroencephlogr. Clin. Neurophysiol., *15:* 486–503, 1963.

170. Sironi, V. A., Ravagnati, L., Singoroni, G., *et al.* Diagnostic and prognostic value of EEG compressed spectral analysis in post-traumatic coma. In: *Advances in Neurotraumatology*, edited by R. Villani, I. Papo, M. Giovanelli, *et al.*, pp. 328–330. Excerpta Medica, Amsterdam, Oxford, Princeton, 1982.

171. Sklar, F. H., Reisch, J., Elashvilli, T., Smith, T., and Long, D. M. Effects of pressure on cerebrospinal fluid formation: Nonsteady-state measurements in dogs. Am. J. Physiol., *2394:* 277–284, 1980.

172. Smith, A. L., Hoff, J. T., Nielson, S. L., *et al.* Barbiturate protection in acute cerebral ischemia. Stroke, *5:* 1–7, 1974.

173. Snodgrass, S. R., and Lorenzo, A. V. Temperature and cerebrospinal fluid production rate. Am. J. Physiol., *222:* 1524–1527, 1972.

174. Sokoloff, L. Influence of functional activity on local cerebral glucose utilization. In: *Brain Work: The Coupling of Function, Metabolism and Blood Flow in the Brain*, edited by D. H. Ingvar and N. A. Lasen, pp. 385–398. Academic Press, New York, 1975.

175. Sodd, S. C., Gulati, S. C., Kumar, M., *et al.* Cerebral metabolism following brain injury. II. Lactic acid changes. Acta Neurochir., *53:* 47–51, 1980.

176. Sorensen, K., Thomassen, A., and Wernberg, M. Prognostic significance of alpha frequency EEG rhythm in coma after cardiac arrest. J. Neurol. Neurosurg. Psychiatry, *41:* 840–842, 1978.

177. Spelzler, R. F., Selman, W. R., Roski, R. H., and Bonshelle, C. Cerebral revascularization during barbiturate coma in primates and human. Surg. Neurol., *17:* 111–115, 1982.

178. Steen, P. A., Newberg, L. A., Milde, J. H., and Michenfelder, J. D. Nimodipine improves cerebral blood flow and neurologic recovery after complete cerebral ischemia in the dog. J. Cerebral Blood Flow Metab., *3:* 38–43, 1983.

179. Stern, W. E. Intracranial fluid dynamics: The relationship of intracranial pressure to the Monro Kellie doctrine and the reliability of pressure assessment. J. R. Coll. Surg. Edinb., *9:* 18–36, 1963.

180. Steudel, W. I., and Kruger, J. Using the spectral analysis of the EEG for prognosis of severe brain injuries in the first post-traumatic week. Acta Neurochir., *28:* 40–42, 1979.

181. Stockard, J. J., Bickford, R. A., and Aung, M. H. The electroencephalogram in traumatic brain injury. In: *Handbook of Clinical Neurology*, edited by P. J. Vinken, and G. W. Bruyn, Vol. 23, Injuries of the Brain and Skull, Part I. Elsevier, North Holland, Amsterdam, 1975.

182. Stuart, F. P., Torres, E., Fletcher, D., and Moore, F. D. Effects of repeated and massive mannitol infusion in the dog. Structural and functional changes in kidney and brain. Ann. Surg., *172:* 190–204, 1970.

183. Sutton, L. N., Frewen, T., Marsha, R., *et al.* The effects of deep barbiturate coma on multimodality evoked potentials. J. Neurosurg., *57:* 178–185, 1982.

184. Swann, K. W., and Cosman, E. R. Modification of the Richmond subarachnoid screw for monitoring of intracranial pressure: Improvements in accuracy of placement and mechanical stability. Technical note. J. Neurosurg., *60:* 1102–1103, 1984.

185. Takagi, H., Saitoh, T., Kitahar, T., *et al.* Mechanism of ICP reducing effects of mannitol. In: *Intracranial Pressure V*, edited by S. Ishii, H. Nagai, and M. Brock, pp. 729–731. Springer-Verlag, Berlin, Heidelberg, New York, Tokyo, 1983.

186. Teasdale, G., and Jennett, B. Assessment of coma and impaired consciousness—a practical scale. Lancet *2:* 81–84, 1974.

187. Teasdale, G., Knill-Jones, R., and Van Der Sade, J. Observer variability in assessing impaired con-

sciousness and coma. J. Neurol. Neurosurg. Psychiatry, *41:* 603–610, 1978.

188. Teasdale, G., Rowan, J. O., Turner, J., Grossman, R., and Miller, J. D. Cerebral perfusion failure and cortical electrical activity. Acta Neurol. Scand. *56:* 430–431, 1977.
189. Todd, M. M., Shapiro, H. M., and Obrist, W. D. Cerebral blood flow measurements in critically ill patients. In: *Brain Failure and Resuscitation Clinics in Critical Care Medicine*, Vol. 2, edited by Ake Grenvik, and Peter Safar, pp. 125–154. Churchill-Livingstone, New York, 1981.
190. Tornheim, P. A., McLaurin, R. L., and Sawaya, R. Effect of furosemide on experimental traumatic cerebral edema. Neurosurgery, *4:* 48–52, 1979.
191. Tsubokawa, T., Nishimoto, H., Yamamoto, T., *et al.* Assessment of brainstem damage by the auditory brainstem response in acute severe head injury. J. Neurol. Neurosurg. Psychiatry, *43:* 1005–1011, 1980.
192. Uziel, A., and Benezech, J. Auditory brainstem responses in comatose patients: Relationship with brainstem reflexes and levels of coma. Electroencephalogr. Clin. Neurophysiol., *45:* 515–524, 1978.
193. Vries, J. E., Becker, D. P., and Young, H. F. A subarachnoid for monitoring intracranial pressure. Technical Note. J. Neurosurg., *39:* 416–419, 1973.
194. Wald, S. L., and McLaurin, R. L. Oral glycerol for the treatment of traumatic intracranial hypertension. J. Neurosurg., *56:* 323–331, 1982.
195. Walter, S. T., and Arfel, G. Responses aux stimulations visuelles dan les etats de coma aigu. Et du coma chronique. Electroencephalogr. Clin. Neurophysiol., *32:* 27–41, 1972.
196. Ward, J. D., Becker, D. P., Miller, J. D., Choi, S. C., Marmarou, A., Wood, C., Newlon, P. G., and Kennan, R. Failure of prophylactic barbiturate coma in the treatment of severe head injury. J. Neurosurg., *62:* 383–388, 1985.
197. Weed, L. H. Some limitations of the Monro Kellie hypothesis. Arch. Surg., *18:* 1049–1068, 1929.
198. Weed, L. H. Studies on cerebrospinal fluid. III. The pathways of escape from the subarachnoid spaces with particular references to the arachnoid villi. J. Med. Res., *31:* 51–91, 1914.
199. Wei, E. P., Kontos, H. A., Dietrick, W. D., Povlishock, J. T., and Ellis, E. F. Inhibition by free radical scavengers and by cyclo-oxygenase inhibitors of pial arteriolar abnormalities from concussive brain injury in cats. Circ. Res., *48:* 95–103, 1981.
200. Weiss, M. H., and Werlman, N. Modulation of CSF production by alterations in cerebral perfusion pressure. Arch. Neurol., *35:* 527–529, 1978.
201. Welch, K. Physiology of hydrocephalus. Adv. Neurol., *13:* 247–332, 1975.
202. Welch, K. Secretion of cerebrospinal fluid by choroid plexus of the rabbit. Am. J. Physiol., *205:* 617–624, 1963.
203. Welch, K., and Friedman, V. The cerebrospinal fluid valves. Brain, *83:* 454–469, 1960.
204. Westmoreland, B. F., Klass, D. W., Sharborough, F. W., and Reagan, T. J. Alpha coma. Electroencephalographic, clinical, pathological, and etiologic correlations. Arch. Neurol., *32:* 713–718, 1975.
205. Wilkinson, H. A. The intracranial pressure-monitoring cup catheter. Technical note. Neurosurgery, 1: 139–141, 1977.
206. Wilkinson, H. A., and Rosenfield, S. Furosemide and mannitol in treatment of acute experimental intracranial hypertension. Neurosurgery, *10:* 167–169, 1982.
207. Wood, J. H., Simeone, F. A., Fink, E. A., and Golden, M. A. Hypervolemic hemodilution in experimental focal cerebral ischemia: Elevation of cardiac output, regional cortical blood flow and ICP after intravascular volume expansion with low molecular weight dextran. J. Neurosurg., *59:* 500–509, 1983.
208. Zervas, N. T., Cosman, E. R., and Cossman, B. J. A pressure balanced radiotelemetry system for the measurement of intracranial pressure. A preliminary design report. J. Neurosurg., *47:* 899–911, 1977.
209. Zierski, J. Extradural, ventricular and subdural pressure recording: Comparative clinical study. In: *Intracranial Pressure IV*, edited by K. Shulman, A. Marmarou, J. D. Miller, *et al.*, pp. 371–376. Springer-Verlag, Berlin, Heidelberg, New York, 1980.

CHAPTER 10

The Multiple Trauma Patient in the NICU

LAWRENCE H. PITTS, M.D.,
and DONALD D. TRUNKEY, M.D.

While prehospital and emergency room care and operative management are of extreme importance in the treatment of head-injured patients, no therapy phase is more prolonged or difficult than treatment in the intensive care unit (ICU). These difficulties are compounded in the head-injured victim who, in addition, has injuries to other organ systems. Half of trauma deaths occur from head injury, and 35% to 40% of patients with coma-producing head injury have significant injuries to the face, thorax, abdomen, or extremities. Not surprisingly, mortality rises as the number of injuries increases (Table 10.1). It is in the patient with multiple injuries that intensive care management complexity is greatest. In this chapter, we will discuss ICU organization, systemic pathophysiologic consequences of trauma, and the management of specific injuries to other organ systems commonly seen in patients with severe head injury and multiple trauma.

ICU ORGANIZATION FOR MULTIPLE TRAUMA VICTIMS

As the number of injured organ systems increases, so does the number of physicians involved in the patient's care. It is imperative that there be close co-ordination among the multiple treating specialists, and that the neurosurgeon remain aware of ongoing and proposed treatment to prevent iatrogenic insults to the traumatized brain. The neurosurgeon, by active involvement or by directing therapy, can modify proposed treatments that might jeopardize brain function. The recovery of the brain dictates the quality of survival more than does any other organ system.

The American College of Surgeons has outlined "Optimal Hospital Resources for Care of the Trauma Victim" (19) and specified both hospital resources and organization best suited to the care of trauma patients. Recommended hospital organization includes both a Trauma Service and a Neurosurgical Service, among others. While many hospitals seeking designation as a trauma center will adopt such an organization, most hospitals in the United States have not sought trauma level designation for a variety of reasons but nonetheless continue to treat trauma victims brought to them. Thus, neurosurgeons in various hospitals will face different internal administrative organizations, generally adapted to suit the needs of a given medical care facility and its physicians, and not necessarily the patients.

Trauma management organization in a given hospital will impinge directly on neurosurgical care in an ICU. When patients have only head injury, we believe the neurosurgeon should be the primary treating physician. He should obtain consultation, when appropriate, from other specialists including infectious disease, pulmonary, cardiology, and intensive care specialists and incorporate their treatment suggestions in his overall management. Depending on the quality of support and long-standing arrangements, neurosurgical patients can receive enormous benefit by the involvement of such specialists.

When the patient has multiple injuries, there is a need for a single physician coordinator, a

TABLE 10.1.
Multiple Injuries, Shock, and Death

	Shock %	Death %
Traumatic coma plus 1 other injury	44	48
Traumatic coma plus 2 other injuries	47	66
Traumatic coma plus 3 other injuries	73	66
Traumatic coma plus 4 other injuries	100	78

"captain of the ship." Ideally, this should be a broadly trained surgeon with a thorough understanding of injury physiology. One format, adopted at some trauma centers including our own, is that patients with multiple trauma are admitted to a Trauma Service directed by a general surgeon. This service coordinates overall patient care, freely using consultation and direct management of specific injuries by a variety of surgical or medical specialties such as neurosurgery, orthopaedic surgery, pulmonary medicine, and ICU staffs, among others. After initial resuscitation and care, the Trauma Service becomes the final common pathway for proposed diagnostic studies and treatment of specific organ injuries as well as being responsible for ongoing fluid, nutritional, and ventilatory management. In our institution, the patient is treated for his multiple problems by the appropriate services and eventually transferred, after several days or longer, to that service responsible for the care of the organ system requiring the most active management decisions. Illustrative examples include a patient with splenic rupture and bladder and urethral injuries who initially would be managed by the Trauma Service and then transferred after a few days to the Urology Service until discharged. A patient with head and extremity fractures would be managed initially by the Trauma Service with close co-ordination with Neurosurgical and Orthopaedic Services. The extremity injuries are optimally treated early and the patient transferred to Neurosurgery a few days after this. Because neurotrauma is so common in multiple injury patients and the management of those neural injuries requires close attention by the neurosurgeon, a substantial portion of patients initially admitted to the Trauma Service are eventually transferred to a neurosurgeon for care (approximately 20% in our institution).

The particular system described above obviously requires strong institutional and physician commitments to the care of the trauma victim. Co-ordination and co-operation among a small nucleus of trauma care specialists is essential to this process and appropriate division of responsibility generally is not a problem. The neurosurgeon is a key member of this decision-making and management process because of the frequency of brain and spinal cord trauma. This input is imperative for optimum patient management and prevention of iatrogenic complications.

A substantially different style of trauma patient management involves assigning the patient at the outset to the service responsible for what appears to be the predominant injury. This would typically be the case in smaller hospitals where the volume of trauma might not warrant the formation of a specific Trauma Service, or where a nucleus of physicians specifically interested in trauma care has not been established. In this situation, the neurosurgeon probably will be responsible for patients with severe head injury or spinal cord injury, and he or she will solicit and respond to appropriate consultations from medical or surgical specialties. Since many physicians are uncomfortable in managing patients with neural dysfunction, the neurosurgeon specifically interested in trauma management should be the primary responsible physician in virtually all patients with altered mental status or spine or spinal cord dysfunction. At the same time, he or she accepts substantial responsibility as the primary physician for patients with multiple organ trauma whose hospital course often can be prolonged and complicated. Such a responsibility requires considerable commitment and energy on the part of the treating neurosurgeon and input from appropriate specialists.

Whatever style of trauma patient management is chosen in a given hospital, it is important that the system be defined in advance. This will ensure a smooth and close co-operation by all of the physicians and personnel who jointly are responsible for optimal outcome for the injured patient.

PATHOPHYSIOLOGIC CHANGES AFTER TRAUMA

Many metabolic and physiologic abnormalities in neurosurgical patients are discusssed in several chapters in this volume and will not be reiterated here. With several exceptions to be discussed below, head injury with or without other organ system injury causes metabolic, endocrinologic, hematologic, or infectious problems not dissimilar from other CNS insults. However, because of the profound implications for secondary insult to the traumatized brain caused by ischemia and hypoxia, shock and respiratory dysfunction will be discussed here in relation to the multiple injury victim. Ventilatory disturbances are commonplace in head-injured patients (23, 31). Shock is also seen frequently in these patients (31), and is even more prevalent when multiple injuries are present (35). Shock correlates adversely with outcome after coma-producing craniocerebral trauma (34), and ischemic or hypoxic brain damage has been identified in over half of the patients who died from head injury (15). Finally, animal models of head injury show significant effects of hypoxia (20).Hypotension results in significantly poorer findings on electroencephalographic (EEG) tracings and affects clinical outcome and brain pathologic changes. These facts warrant a further discussion of shock and hypoxia in trauma victims.

Shock

Systemic shock is a failure of tissue perfusion sufficiently great to alter or stop tissue metabolism and to reduce removal of tissue waste products. Significant systemic shock is associated with an inadequate mean arterial pressure (MAP); cerebral shock results from an inadequate cerebral perfusion pressure (CPP) (CPP = MAP minus intracranial pressure).

Traumatic shock can occur with actual or relative hypovolemia. In the face of hemorrhage with normal function of the medulla oblongata and sympathetic nervous system, peripheral vasoconstriction occurs initially diverting blood from organs which tolerate hypotension well, such as skin and muscle, to vital organs such as brain, heart, kidneys, and liver which withstand ischemia poorly. In this early hypovolemic state, blood pressure and pulse may be normal unless the patient assumes an upright position when gravity-induced lower extremity blood pooling precipitates greater hypovolemia with vital sign changes. As systemic shock increases, blood is diverted from abdominal viscera to the critical organs: the brain and heart. In severe shock, even these organs are hypoperfused and begin to fail. Hypovolemia can occur with internal or external hemorrhage or internal "third space" transcapillary fluid loss into injured tissue (crush syndrome), or even into initially normal tissue subject to severe ischemia and disrupted cellular metabolism.

A second type of traumatic shock involves failure of the pump mechanism. Examples include myocardial contusion, pericardial tamponade, systemic air embolism, or tension pneumothorax which prevents adequate venous return. In hypovolemic shock, central venous and left atrial pressures are low and the neck veins are flat. With pump failure, central venous pressures are elevated with resulting engorged neck veins (Fig. 10.1).

Compensatory mechanisms in hypovolemic shock require brainstem and peripheral neural regulation with aortic and carotid baroreceptor afferent input through the vagus nerves, and peripheral and visceral vasoconstriction mediated through the sympathetic nervous system. Thus, with failure of medullary vasoactive centers, widespread arterial and venous dilatation occurs with a relative hypovolemia in this expanded intravascular space. Optimum treatment is to restore volume and accept a slightly reduced MAP. Adequate flow is maintained despite a reduction in peripheral vascular resistance. Only rarely is it necessary to administer vasopressors.

Cerebral shock arises from either or both systemic hypotension from the causes listed above or from intracranial hypertension from intracranial hematomas, brain edema or hyperemia or, uncommonly, hydrocephalus after head injury. Both components of the CPP, i.e. MAP and ICP, require vigorous and simultaneous treatment to limit the magnitude and duration of cerebral ischemia as much as possible.

Maintenance of cellular integrity is an energy-dependent process where energy is supplied generally by aerobic metabolism and

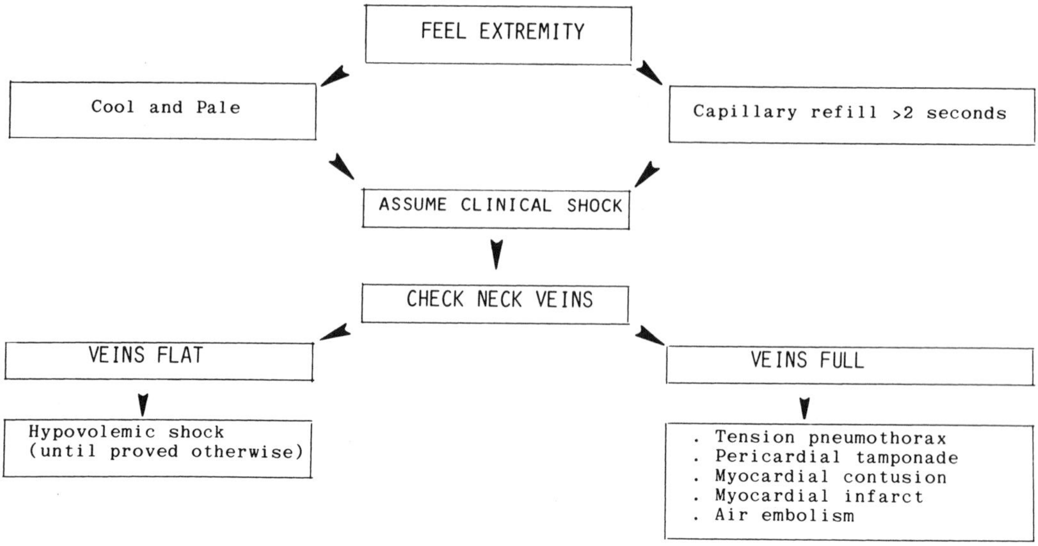

Figure 10.1. Quick assessment of shock.

production of ATP. With ischemic or hypoxic ischemia, high energy phosphate stores are depleted and the cell cannot maintain its usual gradients of high extracellular sodium and intracellular potassium. Intracellular sodium and water increase and extracellular potassium increases. Additionally, calcium ions begin to leak into the cytosol and cannot effectively be sequestered in mitochondria, also an ATP-dependent process. The loss of high energy phosphate compounds such as ATP and phosphocreatine can be extremely rapid with focal cerebral ischemia in experimental animals (Hashimoto and Pitts, unpublished data); the process is probably slower and less dramatic in shock but the cumulative effect probably is similar.

In addition to ATP loss, ischemia also promotes changes in cell membrane phospholipids with increased production of polyunsaturated fatty acids, notably arachidonic acid (7). This compound is readily converted by cyclo-oxygenase to one of several free-radical compounds which can further damage cell membranes. Arachidonic acid also can be metabolized to thromboxane, a potent vasoconstrictor which can further compound focal ischemia.

If cell energy metabolism is sufficiently disordered, mitochondrial and lysosomal membranes also will fail with escape of acid phosphatases and dehydrogenases into the cytosol which further disrupt endoplasmic reticulum and oxidative phosphorylation. Eventually brain electrical function ceases, and in other excitable cells such as cardiac muscle, losses of function impair contractile mechanisms with worsening of systemic shock. If brain or other organ ischemia is severe enough, cells are irretrievably lost and the organism suffers irreparable functional loss or death.

An understanding of some of the microcirculatory changes in shock will aid in understanding later complications sometimes seen in the ICU. Initially with poor tissue perfusion, there is constriction of precapillary arterioles which lowers capillary hydrostatic pressure without altering its oncotic pressure, thus leading to re-entry into vessels of tissue fluids of lower oncotic pressures (capillary refill). This "auto transfusion" can increase intravascular volume sufficiently to compensate shock in some mild cases.

If adequate intravascular volume is not restored, arteriovenous shunts develop which bypass blood around noncritical organs so that circulation to brain and heart can continue. Cells in unperfused tissue must rely on anaerobic metabolism with resulting lactic acidosis and histamine release with further closure of the bypassed microcirculation. Just before cell death, local acidosis and metabolic by-products open the precapillary sphincters, allowing some blood to enter the capillaries. Damaged epithelium initiates the clotting cascade and increased capillary permeability with loss of fluid and protein into the interstitial space. Local changes can be so severe that flow cannot be re-established and there is failure of entire organs such as kidneys or brain in which this failure of recirculation is termed the "no reflow state". If some degree of microcirculation is re-established, a variety of intravascular products and components are swept into the lungs including leukocytes, platelets, lactic acid, and clotting components, thus setting the stage for pulmonary failure.

Stress, such as shock and injury, causes the release of many hormones and initiates inflammatory responses. Catecholamines, both epinephrine and norepinephrine, are released, causing vasoconstriction and decreased perfusion of skin, subcutaneous tissue, kidneys, and arteriolar dilatation with increased flow to skeletal muscle and liver. They increase myocardial blood flow and contractility as well as heart rate and constriction of large veins. The catecholamines promote hemostasis by enhancing both the clotting cascade and platelet aggregation, and stimulate glucose availability by increasing glycolysis, slowing glycogen formation, and increasing gluconeogenesis from amino acids and lactate. Glucocorticoids also promote gluconeogenesis by proteolysis of skeletal muscle into amino acids and their conversion into glucose. Glucocorticoids also stimulate lypolysis with increased free fatty-acid plasma levels.

Systemic shock promotes renin production with conversion to angiotensin II which is both a potent vasoconstrictor and a stimulus for production of the mineralocorticoid aldosterone. This latter compound promotes sodium and water retention by the kidneys in exchange for potassium and hydrogen ion excretion. Antidiuretic hormone (ADH) is released from the posterior hypothalamus in response to shock measured by aortic arch and carotid baroreceptors, with ADH promoting reabsorption of free water from the distal renal tubules in an attempt to support an inadequate circulating volume. Brain endorphins also are increased in some shock states and their effects can be beneficially altered in animal experiments by the administration of the narcotic antagonist, naloxone (18).

There are a host of factors that mediate the inflammatory response following injury. These include kinins, complement, prostanoids, and leukotrienes (arachidonic acid metabolites), endorphins, acute phase proteins, and a myriad of monokines and lymphokines (32). Although these mediators are usually thought of as beneficial following injury, in severe shock these mediators may contribute to the pathophysiology of organ failure. It is beyond the scope of this chapter to detail these events, but uncompensated shock and organ failure may be partly related to an imbalance of these various mediators of inflammation. Treatment modalities directed at one or more of these mediators of inflammation must be viewed with some skepticism at this time since we do not understand all of the various perturbations, and treatment of one mediator may simply imbalance others.

In summary, systemic or cerebral shock results in progressive cellular dysfunction which can lead rapidly to organ failure. In less severe forms, ischemia can compound pre-existing injury. Finally, the body's response to shock can set the stage for delayed organ failure including that of lungs and kidneys whose failure in turn adversely affects primary and secondary brain injuries. These shock states must be recognized and treated early, and treatment continued as long as ischemia is present.

Hypoxia

Many features of pulmonary dysfunction in patients with CNS abnormalities are addressed in a separate chapter in this volume. However, because of the exceedingly important implications of hypoxia for compounding pre-existing traumatic brain injury, some features of pulmonary dysfunction are discussed here as they relate to the head-injury victim.

Head-injury patients manifest hypoxemia in the emergency room with PO_2 below 80 torr in as many as 50% of patients and below 60 torr in nearly one-third. Pulmonary gas exchange often remains compromised in the ICU after emergency room resuscitation and surgery when indicated. A variety of mechanisms have been described to account for these abnormalities.

For all of these reasons, *early and prolonged intubation* usually is used in patients in traumatic coma. Volume ventilators are preferable to pressure-cycled ventilators since the desired goal is a given minute volume which predictably will be delivered by volume ventilators but which can vary considerably with pressure-cycled ventilators in the face of changing lung and chest wall compliance. A variety of ventilator modes with and without positive airway pressure can be selected for optimum ventilation among different patients and pathologies. Positive end-expiratory pressure (PEEP) (1) has been shown in some patients to raise intracranial pressure but this effect generally is unpredictable. However, the improved oxygenation resulting from the use of PEEP may outweigh the effect on ICP which can be addressed by other therapeutic techniques. It is necessary to recognize this effect of PEEP on ICP, to monitor ICP, and to treat it as necessary with or without the application of PEEP. Adequate tidal volume and pulmonary toilet can prevent or dramatically reverse atelectasis with its obligatory arteriovenous shunt which allows blood to traverse the pulmonary circulation without becoming oxygenated and which can result in significant and detrimental hypoxemia.

Intubation and controlled ventilation also will regulate arterial oxygen and carbon dioxide pressures, critical for preventing secondary hypoxic brain damage (21) as well as allowing hyperventilation to produce hypocarbia for ICP reduction. Controlled ventilation and paralysis also virtually eliminate the work of breathing and reduce systemic metabolic demands and lactic acid production by respiratory and skeletal muscle. In short, until patients with severe head injury improve to the point of consistently adequate spontaneous ventilation, intubation and controlled ventilation is an essential part of this management.

In addition to vomiting and aspiration or atelectasis, head-injury victims are subject to bacterial pneumonia, increased extravascular lung water, and occasionally neurogenic pulmonary edema (NPE); they may have some degree of hypoxemia or increased pulmonary shunting with normal chest x-rays (12). Head-injury patients have been described, despite normal chest x-rays, normal arterial CO_2, and normal responsiveness to breathing hypercarbic or hypoxemic gases, who had significant right-to-left shunts (33) that probably were due to areas of low ventilation-perfusion matching (38). One possible explanation is a reduction in functional residual capacity described in some head-injury patients (10). Another possibility is that of increased extravascular lung water described in some head-injury patients (29) which probably precedes NPE.

Actual NPE with copious production of frothy sputum is uncommon in head-injury victims but is a dramatically evident cause of hypoxemia when it occurs. A variety of mechanisms have been proposed including systemic hypertension in response to intracranial hypertension and brainstem ischemia which can cause peripheral vasoconstriction and a shift of blood into the pulmonary vascular bed. The highly compliant pulmonary vascular system can be injured by this sudden increase in volume with subsequent leakage of plasma into the lung parenchyma (41). However, increased lung water can occur in the absence of systemic or pulmonary pressure increases (5, 30). While NPE can cause dramatic hypoxemia, increased lung water can be present in head-injury victims without significant hypoxemia, or with reduced arterial oxygenation that can be corrected easily by an increased fraction of inspired oxygen.

Pneumonia is commonplace in patients with severe head injury. At our institution, bacterial pneumonia occurs in over 80% of comatose patients intubated for longer than 5 days. A variety of mechanisms undoubtedly play a role. Insults such as aspiration may follow decreased gag and cough reflexes or partial upper airway obstruction from relaxed tongue musculature in patients before intubation. Increased lung water in some patients may lead to altered surfactant metabolism or alveolar or macrophage function (24). Comatose patients generally are intubated and suctioned frequently which can lead to iatrogenic pulmonary contamination with eventual development of pneumonia. Nasotracheal tubes reduce sinus drainage on the side of intubation and significantly increase the frequency of maxillary sinusitus, providing a reservoir of infection with relatively easy access to the lungs (37a).

Patients in traumatic coma cannot control their airway such that any vomiting readily leads to aspiration. For varying times after impact there is apnea which may or may not be fatal (26). In surviving patients, however, a period of hypoventilation is common with subsequent atelectasis. In patients with thoracic trauma, pneumo- or hemothorax can compromise ventilation but are readily treated if recognized. Pulmonary contusion also can accompany thoracic trauma and usually resolves with aggressive pulmonary management except in very severe cases when severe bilateral contusion may be incompatible with survival. Abdominal distention from hemorrhage or a paralytic ileus can compromise diaphragmatic excursion, promote atelectasis, and cause aspiration.

It is clear that head-injury patients, particularly those with concomitant thoracic injuries, suffer a variety of pulmonary insults with frequent and easily documented ventilatory abnormalities. The need for preventing systemic hypoxemia with possible resulting secondary brain injury, for control of arterial CO_2 levels for optimum intracranial pressure, for reducing the work of breathing and its metabolic consequences, and for minimizing pulmonary infection, all demand careful attention to and immaculate management of the lungs in the multiple trauma victim.

NON-NEURAL INJURIES IN THE MULTIPLE TRAUMA VICTIM

The following sections will highlight injuries to specific organ systems other than the nervous system, their diagnosis, management, and importance related to neural trauma.

Face and Scalp Injuries

As many as 15% of coma-producing head injuries are associated with severe facial fractures and sometimes with complicated skull and scalp injuries. When an open head injury is complicated by cerebrospinal fluid (CSF) leak, it is important that the dura be repaired at the first surgical procedure if at all possible. This generally requires a more extensive exploration and brain retraction than with hematoma removal alone. The extent of the dural defect often can be identified and repaired with homologous pericranium, temporalis fascia or fascia lata, or by autologous lyophilized cadaver dura. Early CSF leaks through the wound can further be minimized by the use of a lumbar subarachnoid or ventricular catheter attached to a closed drainage system. A ventriculostomy is preferable when there is cerebral swelling since it can be used for ICP monitoring and CSF drainage in the ICU as one method of ICP control.

A variety of facial fractures may be present, the most common being simple zygomatic fractures, orbital blowout fractures, and fractures of the mid-face (LeForte I—transverse fractures of the maxilla; LeForte II—pyramidal fracture of the maxilla extending up to the nasion and laterally to the inferior orbital rim and sometimes the infraorbital rims; LeForte III—craniofacial dysjunction with fractures extending across the orbits and one or both the xygomas with a free-floating section of the mid-face). Zygomatic fractures may produce cosmetic deformities unless repaired. Realignment of the zygoma can be accomplished relatively simply by open or closed techniques from 10 to 14 days after injury as long as the anesthesia required does not have a significant risk for further insult to the traumatized brain. Orbital blowout fractures may require correction to prevent later bothersome diplopia; orbital repair can be delayed for days or weeks after injury.

Mid-facial fractures can extend posteriorly into the ethmoid regions and be accompanied by CSF leak. If surgery is required to minimize cosmetic deformity, we recommend that surgery be done as early as is safe and practical as fracture relocation may enhance spontaneous closure and healing of CSF fistulae. However, in the setting of significant brain injury, careful consideration must be given to the timing of surgery to obtain optimum facial and CSF repair but not to jeopardize the brain with possible insults of hypotension or of anesthesia itself.

Complex scalp injuries including partial avulsions require careful operative management, sometimes including local pedicled scalp rotation flaps or free vascularized cutaneous or myocutaneous grafts requiring microvascular anastomoses (22). If rotation flaps are used, split thickness skin grafts generally are used to cover denuded pericranium or cranial musculature. This may be avoided in vascularized grafts. The nature of the scalp repair generally is not important in the ICU management phase unless there is concomitant CSF leak that may require appropriate CSF draining in the days after surgery. We try to limit external CSF draining by ventriculostomy or lumbar subarachnoid catheters to about 4 days since the risk of infection seems increased thereafter. CSF diversion usually stops CSF leaks entirely during the drainage. If the leak recurs after the drains are removed, a second course of CSF drainage might be considered before attempting definitive repair of the dural fistula.

It must be emphasized that facial injuries, particularly those involving the oropharynx, tongue, or mandible can cause early or delayed airway obstruction which can be fatal. If there is any suggestion of airway compromise, oro- or nasotracheal intubation or tracheostomy should be performed before there is respiratory embarrassment. Delayed soft tissue swelling can produce respiratory compromise in the ICU and requires close observation for early recognition and treatment. Except for impending airway compromise, most facial injuries can be treated semi-electively days or longer after injury.

Neck Injuries

Blunt and penetrating injuries of the neck do occur but are not common, and may or may not require surgical exploration (13). When they are significant, neck injuries can involve either the carotid arteries or occasionally the esophagus, larynx, or trachea. Direct airway injuries are recognized promptly by stridor and respiratory distress. They are best managed by tracheal intubation or tracheostomy and direct surgical exploration either before or after diagnostic studies that include CT scanning.

Cervical arterial injury usually presents with considerable hemorrhage from penetrating wounds and requires emergency surgical exploration and arterial repair. Less frequently, particularly with blunt injuries to the carotid artery, there may be a delayed neurologic progression with hemiparesis and altered levels of consciousness. Traumatic carotid dissections may require acute surgical exploration for repair and hematoma removal. However, others occur in the internal carotid artery distal to the carotid bifurcation in which surgical access is difficult or impossible, in which case an extracranial-intracranial arterial bypass might be appropriate. If the patient does not develop a major hemispheric deficit and does not require specific intervention, even nearly completely occluded carotid arteries may establish normal lumens with time. Arteriovenous malformations occasionally will occur with penetrating neck injuries which lacerate both an arterial branch and a nearby vein. Delayed complications of oral or wound hemorrhage, airway compromise, and sudden neurologic deterioration can represent life-threatening emergencies in the ICU patient and are treated first by securing an airway and second, by hemorrhage control.

Thoracic Injuries

Substantial thoracic trauma occurs in 20% to 25% of patients with coma-producing head injury and in a variety of other trauma victims as well (3). The most common injuries (40%) are fractures of one or more ribs which may produce a flail-chest segment. Almost one-half of patients with a flail segment will require ventilatory support. The remaining patients often require intercostal block or epidural blocks or analgesia. These latter patients must be in the ICU for monitoring. Pulmonary contusion is common and two-thirds can be diagnosed with early chest x-rays. Isolated flail chest has a 16% mortality rate in our institution as does isolated pulmonary contusion. Combined flail chest and pulmonary contusion, however, has a 42% mortality. Early chest films also will show hemothorax or pneumothorax arising from lung parenchymal or bronchial injury. These last two lesions often are present soon after injury but may develop in the ICU, requiring chest tube placement there as the first treatment.

Myocardial contusion can occur with thoracic injuries and present as life-threatening dysrhythmias or cardiac failure. Pericardial tamponade also can present as rapid heart failure with distended neck veins and shock. With tamponade, the cardiac silhouette is enlarged and there can be a dramatic response to pericardiocentesis. In the setting of associated severe head injury, a variety of electrocardiographic (ECG) abnormalities can be seen from ST and T-wave changes to arrhythmias and even Q-waves, most commonly associated with myocardial infarction. Whether these ECG abnormalities arise from CNS injury or from primary myocardial injury, the treatment is the same with management of arrhythmias using lidocaine or procainamide, and treatment of cardiac failure with appropriate cardiac stimulants including digoxin, propranolol and, at times, pressor agents. ECG changes with CNS injury tend to resolve over a few days and myocardial contusion begins to improve within a week although severe myocardial contusion may result in fatal heart failure.

A widened mediastinum seen on chest x-ray is the hallmark for diagnosis of a contained rupture of the thoracic aorta. Optimally this should be ruled out prior to admission to the ICU. Arteriography is still the gold standard for confirmation of this lesion. There is also a significant association between aortic disruption and thoracic spine injuries.

Abdominal Injuries

For the most part, acute life-threatening abdominal injuries will be identified during or shortly after initial emergency room resuscitation of the patient with multiple injuries. Continuing shock or unstable blood pressures should invariably prompt careful abdominal evaluation which, along with chest injuries or pelvic or femoral fractures, can account for substantial internal bleeding. Chest and orthopaedic injuries are readily evaluated by plain x-rays. Hemorrhage from abdominal visceral injuries can be identified reliably with peritoneal lavage, abdominal computed tomography (CT) scanning (40) or, in cases of unexplained shock, emergency laparotomy. In fact, if other major sources of hemorrhage can be excluded, emergency laparotomy is indicated in the multiple trauma victim who is not responding rapidly to volume resuscitation or who has a falling hematocrit. Laparotomy in the patient with severe hypotension can also allow aortic cross-clamping for control of abdominal hemorrhage as well as allowing more rapid restoration of blood pressure to the brain and heart, while allowing identification and direct treatment of the hemorrhage source. Penetrating abdominal wounds thought to have violated the peritoneum almost always warrant exploration. In a few patients with stable vital signs and posterior wounds, observation and conservative management alone may be warranted.

Thus, many multiple trauma victims arrive in the ICU after abdominal exploration and definitive or temporary repair of abdominal injuries. Occasionally, there are patients whose abdominal injuries go unrecognized in the resuscitation phase and first become manifest after arrival in the ICU. The most common clue to these later developing injuries is progressive hypoperfusion which causes peripheral vasoconstriction and cold, clammy extremities, tachycardia, falling urine output, and, finally, falling blood pressure. Progressive anemia documented by serial hematocrits often will occur before other pathophysiologic consequences of shock, and can prompt appropriate abdominal diagnostic investigation such as peritoneal lavage or CT scanning (40).

The major sources of abdominal hemorrhage are the spleen and liver parenchyma, although occasionally with penetrating injuries of the aorta or arterial branches, major hemorrhage or even exsanguination can occur rapidly. With slow bleeding coupled with early resuscitation and continued intravenous fluid administration, circulating volume can be maintained for many hours by which time the patient is in the ICU when severe shock first becomes manifest. A similar volume depletion can occur when initial laparotomy does not stop hemorrhage definitively such as with severe liver injuries that require packing to slow but not entirely stop bleeding, or from retroperitoneal hemorrhage which continues slowly after the initial treatment phases. Again, a falling hematocrit or unstable vital signs signal the need for aggressive diagnostic studies or surgical intervention.

Splenectomy is less commonly carried out today than a decade ago. As trauma surgeons have become aware of postsplenectomy sepsis, attempts have been made to treat splenic parenchymal injuries with a variety of techniques including hemostatic agents, packing and partial splenectomy (6). Indeed, some splenic and liver injuries diagnosed by CT scan are managed expectantly with the caveat that such patients must have careful monitoring and repeated examinations.

Significant hepatic injuries must be treated by some form of local control of hemorrhage. Again a variety of suturing techniques, hemostatic agents and temporary (for several days) packing of the liver may achieve sufficient hemostasis (8). In approximately 5% of patients, partial hepatectomy may be necessary. Injury to the portal vessels requires direct visualization and vascular repair. Injuries to the common bile duct generally are treated with external T-tube drainage of the duct.

Blunt abdominal trauma to the abdomen can rupture hollow organs, including stomach, bowel, and bladder. Free air in the abdomen, seen best on upright or cross-table abdominal x-rays, invariably indicates rupture of part of the gastrointestinal (GI) tract and requires surgical exploration for delineation and repair. Free air also may be seen on CT scans of the abdomen. Ruptured viscera must be repaired or peritonitis and fatal sepsis will ensue.

Blunt and penetrating abdominal trauma can injure the pancreas or gall bladder. The midportion of the pancreas is at greatest jeopardy as it drapes across the upper lumbar spine in the retroperitoneal space. With very severe injuries, total pancreatectomy may be necessary or at times partial pancreatectomy with removal of the distal one-third or two-thirds of the pancreas being necessary. Leakage of pancreatic enzymes into the retroperitoneum or into the peritoneal cavity can cause a severe peritonitis and tissue necrosis with the formation of septic abscesses or pancreatic pseudocysts. This complication of abdominal injury may take several days or longer to develop and can present in the ICU as fever, abdominal pain, peritoneal signs and, in severe cases, as insulin-requiring diabetes mellitus. These abnormalities usually require surgical exploration for cyst or abscess drainage before healing can ensue. Ultrasonography in the ICU can be extremely helpful in delineating cyst or abscess formation.

Occasionally abdominal trauma will cause injury to the gall bladder or common bile duct with jaundice and an elevated direct bilirubinemia. Cholecystograms or cholangiograms may be able to define the extent of injury which usually requires surgical repair.

Slow bleeding into the retroperitoneum (39) might first become manifest in the ICU and can lead to 13% to 20% mortality. If bleeding is arterial in nature, it usually will present in the early postinjury phase but significant venous bleeding may take longer to have an effect on the vital signs. There may be no blood in the peritoneal cavity so that peritoneal dialysis would have negative results. However, CT scanning of the abdomen almost invariably demonstrates the hematoma. In addition, often within 6 to 8 hours of injury, ecchymosis of the flank may appear with retroperitoneal hematomas. In most cases these are not treated surgically but rather by blood and fluid replacement. Four units or more of blood can be sequestered in the retroperitoneum and thus the blood loss can be quite extensive (9). A hematoma that suddenly ruptures into the peritoneal cavity may decompress a hemorrhage site and accelerate intravascular volume depletion with dramatic worsening of vital signs. Although this is uncommon, rapid abdominal distention and blood pressure deterioration with tachycardia would warrant emergency surgical exploration in an attempt to define the source of hemorrhage and control blood loss.

In summary, most major intra-abdominal lesions with rapid blood loss are defined before the patient arrives in the intensive care unit. However, there are significant sources of abdominal organ injury which first become obvious in the ICU and require appropriate management for diagnosis and therapy. Altered vital signs with tachycardia, fluctuating and low blood pressure, decreased urinary output, and falling hematocrit clearly signal potentially life-threatening internal hemorrhage. Abdominal distention by blood or air also requires early recognition and careful evaluation. An abdominal CT scan can delineate a variety of pathologies including focal or generalized hemorrhage and specific organ injury and is the diagnostic procedure of choice in nonemergency situations. Cross-table abdominal films will show intra-abdominal free air and abnormal gas patterns but rarely define specific pathologies. Careful attention must be paid to supporting the patient's blood volume by crystalloid and blood products, and maintenance of adequate blood gases and pH status while a diagnosis is pursued vigorously.

Genitourinary Injuries

Early information regarding the genitourinary (GU) tract is available in most multiple injury victims. Because of the need to assess perfusion status and possible impending shock, an indwelling urethral catheter is inserted to measure urinary output. Assuming that the catheter can be inserted without substantial difficulty (almost always the case in younger and in most older trauma victims), significant urethral injury is unlikely. Although quite nonspecific, hematuria is overwhelmingly the most common signal for GU trauma. Injury to the kidneys, ureters, bladder, or urethra virtually always is accompanied by significant hematuria, discovered on gross inspection or urinalysis after the bladder catheter is inserted. The degree and persistence of blood in the urine and urinary volume mark the need for more detailed GU evaluation.

Trauma victims who have angiography or contrast-enhanced CT studies, particularly those with any degree of hematuria, should have abdominal x-rays or CT scans during dye excretion to evaluate possible renal injury. Abdominal x-rays while the contrast is being excreted usually delineate the calyceal system and provide considerable information regarding the kidney parenchyma and collecting systems. CT scanning offers somewhat more information about the renal parenchyma and can reveal subcapsular, parenchymal, or perirenal hemorrhage. Both x-ray and CT studies can demonstrate renal or urethral displacement and may give information regarding the bladder integrity. If inadequate detail is derived from abdominal x-rays after intravascular contrast studies done for other reasons, a formal intravenous pyelogram may be required. Finally, if there is some questions about bladder injury, a two-view cystogram can be done by using an indwelling urethral catheter for instillation of contrast. The opportunity to obtain these data should not be overlooked during the diagnostic evaluation of multiple trauma victims shortly after initial resuscitation.

If hematuria persists in the ICU and no studies have been done to evaluate GU integrity, an IVP and possibly a cystogram should be considered (17). Barring penetrating GU injuries, the vast majority of injuries can be managed conservatively with excellent resolution and return of normal function. If the patient is allergic to iodine, an abdominal CT scan without contrast may provide adequate information. Renal blood flow and urinary excretion can be evaluated in each kidney with radioisotope studies and essentially can supplant CT studies in patients with iodine allergy. Hematuria which diminishes and ceases within a few days in the face of normal blood urea nitrogen (BUN) and creatinine and in the absence of sepsis can be treated expectantly with little risk of delayed GU dysfunction.

Penetrating GU injuries usually are treated after initial resuscitation, and necessary repairs effected for lacerations of the kidney, ureters, or bladder (36). Even significant renal injuries can be repaired with preserved renal function since the kidney usually can withstand at least an hour of complete ischemia at body temperature, and incomplete ischemia can be tolerated for even longer periods. In a relatively few cases, in order to control severe hemorrhage, a partial nephrectomy may be required.

A more common GU abnormality in the intensive care unit is that of acute tubular necrosis (ATN) following systemic shock (28). Severe ATN can cause renal shutdown with oliguria and an inability to excrete metabolic waste products and potassium. Urine output can fall to unmeasurable levels with a progressive rise in BUN, creatinine, and potassium. The patient's total output falls essentially to insensible losses requiring severe fluid restriction without which the patient can be severely overhydrated with cardiac failure or pulmonary edema. With ATN, the patient's circulating volume generally will be adequate as measured by adequate central venous pressure or left atrial wedge pressures which will exclude a depleted vascular volume as a cause for oliguria. Progressive elevation of BUN and creatinine documented by serial examinations will confirm renal failure. The presence of oliguric ATN severely complicates the management of the neurosurgical patient since fluid restriction and moderate dehydration often is used in a perioperative or postinjury treatment phase. In ATN, hyponatremia is not uncommon and this can enhance cerebral edema formation. Unless the oliguric phase resolves fairly quickly, ATN may require peritoneal or hemodialysis which, with fairly rapid fluid and electrolyte shifts despite careful technique, can further insult the brain. Optimally, oliguric ATN can be converted to nonoliguric ATN with the judicious use of diuretics such as mannitol, taking care to maintain volume and prevent increased ICP.

In less severe forms of ATN, or as oliguric ATN begins to resolve, high urine volumes may be excreted as the renal tubules are unable to concentrate urine. Depending on the urine output, there may or may not be adequate clearance of urea, creatinine, or potassium. Overall fluid balance obviously is much easier to control when the kidneys at least can excrete increased circulating volume. Careful attention to fluid and electrolyte replacement still is imperative and will be dictated by frequent determination of blood electrolytes and the patient's perfusion status. Rarely, severe ATN can cause permanent loss of renal function and, in surviving patients, the need for chronic renal dialysis or transplantation. Far more commonly, ATN resolves completely and normal renal function is restored.

Orthopaedic Injuries

There is an almost endless variety of skeletal abnormalities that can occur in the patient with multiple trauma. While a number of these are easily recognized and treated with excellent results, a delay in diagnosis in some of these injuries is not uncommon and requires particular vigilence in the early treatment and intensive care phase of managing the multiple trauma victim. It seems particularly unfortunate when such a delay compromises the long-range functional outcome of a patient who has satisfactory resolution of his or her other systemic injuries. This worsened outcome can occur with delayed therapy of joint injury fractures, an unrecognized spine instability with delayed injury to the spinal cord, or other unrecognized or undertreated skeletal injuries.

Emergency physicians and trauma teams generally are excellent at recognizing common fractures. Local extremity deformity, swelling, or ecchymosis will focus attention on these fractures which can be confirmed easily by plain radiographs. Fractures or dislocations of small bones of the hands or feet may be more difficult to appreciate by gross examination but some degree of local pain or swelling usually focuses attention on these injuries. Complicated or compound fractures probably will have been treated soon after injury before the patient arrives in the intensive care unit but a few may have to be delayed for later repair in patients who have systemic injuries so severe as to cause unstable vital signs and to make surgery too hazardous. Such extremity fractures will be treated initially by splinting or casting or in some instances by external skeletal fixation and traction such as with femoral or severe tibia-fibular fractures. One complication of extremity fractures which must be carefully assessed in the ICU with or without definitive repair is that of hemorrhage into or edema of the muscles which can swell sufficiently to cause a compartment syndrome with compromise of neural and/or vascular structures. On physical examination, the distal extremity will be cold and have poor capillary refill in the nail beds and a progressive numbness may be noted in those patients in whom sensory function can be tested. Compartment syndromes can rapidly become surgical emergencies requiring appropriate fasciotomies to relieve pressure on the muscles and neurovascular structures before irreversible ischemia has occurred. Compartment syndromes essentially can be eliminated as a significant problem with a high index of suspicion and a low threshold to measure compartment pressures. Occasionally a cast will put pressure focally on an artery or nerve with progressive loss of function over hours or days. This may be difficult to ascertain but must be carefully searched for in the first several days after the patient's arrival in the ICU.

Pelvic fractures are common in patients with multiple injuries resulting from falls or motor vehicle accidents. Such fractures may be minor and of no consequence or may be severe, comminuted, and lead to life-threatening blood losses that require vigorous resuscitation and attempts at hemostasis including arterial embolization or other procedures. CT scanning provides a rapid and accurate evaluation of such injuries (11). When posterior pelvic fractures such as sacroiliac diastasis are present, there may be injury to the nerves of the lumbosacral plexus, most generally from stretch injuries but occasionally from compression by hematomas (43). Many stable pelvic fractures can be treated by bedrest alone and can tolerate some patient movement such as log-rolling. Unstable injuries usually require external skeletal fixation for stabilization and improved control of hemorrhage. Retroperitoneal hemorrhage often exceeds four units as can femoral fractures (9); bone alignment in both cases can dramatically reduce this internal blood loss.

Spine fractures or unstable ligamentous injuries are perhaps the most worrisome of the skeletal injuries accompanying multiple trauma. In awake patients, they generally can be diagnosed by the local pain and at times by the deformity which they cause. In awake patients, nerve root or spinal cord dysfunction would point the way to significant spine involvement.

In confused or unconscious patients, there may be inadequate clinical information to indicate a significant spine injury. This gives rise to the general practice of obtaining at least a lateral cervical spine x-ray in unconscious patients although the actual combination of significant spine injury in coma-producing head injury is only 3–5%. In many situations, there is inadequate radiographic assessment of thoracic or lumbar spine injuries. Delay in diagnosis of these fractures or dislocations periodically gives rise to lawsuits particularly when there may have been increased neural injury. It is wise, particularly in the multiple-injury comatose patient, to obtain not only cervical spine x-rays but anteroposterior and lateral plain radiographs of the thoracic and lumbar spine as well. While not infallible, this approach offers the best opportunity for early recognition and treatment of the potentially unstable spine abnormalities. The management of spine injuries is beyond the scope of this chapter but appropriate recognition clearly is the starting point upon which subsequent therapy is predicated.

Anesthesia and the Multiple Trauma Patient

From the preceding sections, it is clear that a variety of injuries will require return of some multiple trauma victims to the operating room from the ICU in the days or weeks after injury. Unfortunately, many of these trips occur when the patient is far from stable but urgent reoperation nontheless is necessary. Some of these procedures are required to correct life-threatening abnormalities such as continued intrathoracic or intra-abdominal hemorrhage or for abscesses with sepsis uncontrolled by antibiotics. Other urgent procedures may be designed to prevent unacceptable disability which can accrue from untreated compartment syndromes or vascular injury with the threat of destruction of the limbs or other organs including the brain. In these circumstances, the patient must be stabilized to the greatest possible degree and then transported to the operating room for those necessary procedures. Transport now can be accomplished with complete ventilatory support and cardiovascular monitoring, affording the opportunity for continued intensive treatment during transfer to the operating room and thereafter during the surgical procedure. In such instances the benefits, possibly including lifesaving surgical intervention, clearly outweigh these substantial risks. Anesthesia with a variety of inhalational or intravenous agents is administered during continued resuscitation, certainly with greater but unavoidable danger to the patient.

At other times, however, delayed procedures in ICU patients may be necessary but their timing is somewhat more elective. Many facial injuries can be treated 7 to 14 days after injury without compromise of the eventual results. Although they cannot be delayed indefinitely, closure of skin incisions or lacerations often can be delayed for 1 to 2 weeks. A variety of skeletal injuries including definitive operative repair of spine, pelvic, or extremity fractures can be delayed until a patient is metabolically stable and relatively infection-free. Particularly when repair involves the use of implantable protheses, it is important that the patient not be septic at the time of surgery. In some instances, surgery should be done in stable patients in the first week after injury before substantial systemic infections occur. However, once infections are present, surgery often can be delayed until the infection is controlled with a good functional result.

Patients with head injury offer a special challenge regarding delayed surgery. Traumatic intracranial hypertension often persists for 3 to 7 days or longer after injury. Anesthesia with its attendant risks of hypotension and neural stimulation, such as intubation, can provoke additional neural injury. The halogenated hydrocarbon ventilation agents cause vasodilatation and can increase ICP with additional ischemic brain damage. Despite meticulous technique, particularly in patients who are dehydrated or who have compromised circulating volume from other injuries, hypotension can occur with anesthesia, again causing ischemic brain damage. Other unknown mechanisms involving direct cellular metabolism pose a threat to the injured brain undergoing anesthesia.

It is important, therefore, for the neurosurgeon and "captain of the ship" caring for patient to be aware of the additional threats that anesthesia and surgery pose for the neurologically impaired patient. It is imperative that the trauma team be guided by the neurosurgeon, who is more aware than other treating physicians of the patient's cerebral status and the possible risks that anesthesia imposes. This requires that the neurosurgeon be cognizant of plans by other services for treating the patient, and help in weighing the potential benefits and risks from these plans. Whenever possible and whenever unacceptable detriment does not accrue from delay, most procedures should not be done for 5 to 7 days after coma-producing head injury since the brain appears to be least stable during this period of time. After that time, intracranial hypertension usually has resolved, probably indicating improved cerebral blood flow autoregulatory mechanisms and improving neural and glial metabolism. The neurosurgeon will best be able to judge the optimum timing of delayed surgery in patients with neural trauma, and he or she has a substantial responsibility in directing the patient's overall care.

Sepsis

We showed several years ago (2) and more recently (42) that approximately 16% of late trauma deaths are due to sepsis, primarily in the ICU. The most common causes of septic deaths at our institution arise from pulmonary infection. We believe this to be one of the most vexing problems that faces the trauma surgeon in the postinjury period. In contrast to abdominal sepsis or abscesses in extremities, pulmonary sepsis, with the sole exception of empyema, does not lend itself to incision and drainage. Once pulmonary parenchymal sepsis has been established, it is frustrating that we cannot provide drainage and in some instances adequate tissue levels of antibiotics to successfully combat this problem.

The best way currently to treat sepsis is to prevent it. This is difficult, at best, since the problem seems so prevalent. In a study by Schimpff *et al.* (37), it was observed that 48% of patients with severe trauma developed one or more nosocomial infections related to their time in the intensive care unit. We would suggest that there are at least six things that can be done to prevent sepsis in the intensive care unit. The first, and possibly the most important, is to provide adequate pulmonary toilet with relatively aseptic techniques. The intubated and sometimes paralyzed patient is clearly at risk for the build-up of secretions and blood in the airway which can only eventually lead to pulmonary sepsis. One of the major improvements in ICU management over the past 15 years has been the nurse's ability to provide pulmonary toilet in less than optimum conditions with minimum contamination of the upper airway.

A second technique that will minimize infection is to mobilize the patient. This accompanies pulmonary toilet and it allows dependent drainage of the lungs and encourages coughing and avoids stasis. The data from studies in the United States (37) and Europe (4) clearly document the efficacy of early operative reduction of fractures which allows this mobility. In a patient with an injury severity score of 30, which has, according to the American College of Surgeons Trauma Outcome Study, approximately a 28% mortality, a mortality of less than 5% has been achieved in those centers practicing this early reduction. The only contraindications to operative reductions of fractures with the initial anesthetic following injury are hypothermia and hemodynamic instability following the life-saving operations on the head and torso. In these two instances, it is better to take patients to the ICU, warm them, and restore volume before returning to the operating room for fracture fixation. If such mobility cannot be achieved by early fracture fixation, the use of special beds should be strongly considered.

A third mode of preventing infection is to provide adequate nutrition. We start enteral or parenteral nutrition within 48 hours of the injury if it appears that the patient will not be eating on his or her own within 96 hours of the injury.

A fourth way to prevent infection is to have a mandatory policy of removing within 24 hours all lines that were placed in the emergency room. These lines are often placed under adverse and septic conditions and it is imperative that they be replaced under more optimal conditions once the patient has been stabilized in the intensive care unit. Most of our resuscitation lines are cutdowns and once they are removed we have no hesitation in leaving these wounds open to heal by secondary intent or to do delayed primary closure with sterile tapes. Every effort should be made to remove other tubes including Foley catheters, nasogastric tubes, and tube thoracostomy as soon as clinically feasible. It must also be emphasized that the endotracheal tube is a major source of pulmonary sepsis and that every effort should be made to extubate as soon as feasible.

A fifth means of prevention is to avoid prophylactic antibiotics. There is probably no single practice that promotes nosocomial infections as does the injudicious use of antibiotics. There is no evidence of efficacy of prophylactic antibiotics in head injury. The use of antibiotics for chest trauma is controversial with at least two articles in the literature supporting their use (14, 16) and other studies (25, 27) showing that they provide no benefit. Our own personal practice is not to use prophylactic antibiotics unless there is an associated hollow viscus injury such as to the esophagus, or if there has been contamination from an associated abdominal injury. Antibiotics are clearly indicated in patients with hollow viscus injuries in the abdomen, grade 3 compound fractures, untidy soft tissue injuries, and injuries involving joints and tendon sheaths.

A final means of preventing infection is to avoid unnecessary or unproved pharmacologic manipulations of some injuries. A specific example is the use of steroids and diuretics in treating pulmonary contusion which is unsubstantiated by the current literature. It has never made physiologic sense that one can selectively dry out a bruise in the lung. Furthermore, one cannot reduce edema in a pulmonary contusion with steroids without accepting the disadvantage of these agents. Until blinded, randomized, controlled trials show their efficacy, we cannot recommend their use.

SUMMARY

Since severe head injury is so common in multiple trauma victims and plays such an important role in eventual outcome, the neurosurgeon plays an essential role in the early and ongoing care of patients with multiple injuries. He or she is uniquely qualified to assess the level of neural injury and rank its importance in the setting of other system injuries. The care of neural trauma differs somewhat from the care of other injuries, and an overall treatment plan must be developed to integrate all of the necessary therapies designed to restore the patient's health. Although very complex, initial resuscitation and early surgical management of neural and non-neural injuries generally are straightforward and not controversial. Some of the key elements in this early treatment involve physician and facility availability and rapid response to life-threatening injuries. This initial phase usually is over within a few hours of impact, after which time complex management decisions must be made in the intensive care setting. While delayed procedures such as craniotomy for removal of intracerebral hematomas of late onset are sometimes necessary, the neurosurgeon plays a more critical role in nonoperative management of the multiple injury victim in the ICU. One of his most useful functions is to assess the impact of various treatment plans on the nervous system, some of which may have to be altered or delayed until such time as brain or spinal cord function will not be affected adversely by execution of the plan. It is important that the neurosurgeon be aware of the delayed problems that can arise and to have a general plan for their management, either by himself or in collaboration with other trauma specialists.

The preceding remarks should provide a framework for understanding the scope and complexity of some of the multiple organ injuries that can occur and how they are addressed in the intensive care setting. In recognizing these injuries and directing their management, the neurosurgeon provides critical care that cannot be supplied better by other members of the trauma team. Whether "captain of the ship" or a consultant trauma team member, the neurosurgeon must participate actively in intensive care management if the patient is to achieve an optimum outcome after multiple trauma.

REFERENCES

1. Appuzzo, M. L. J., Weiss, M. H., Petersons, V., Small, R. B., Kurze, T., and Heiden, J. S. The effect of positive end expiratory pressure (PEEP) ventilation on intracranial pressure. J. Neurosurg., *46:* 227–231, 1977.
2. Baker, C. C., Oppenheimer, L., and Stephens, B. Epidemiology of trauma deaths. Am. J. Surg., *140:* 144–150, 1980.
3. Besson, A., and Saegesser, F. *Color Atlas of Chest Trauma and Associated Injuries*, Vol. 1, 245 pp. Medical Economics Books, Oradell, NJ, 1983.
4. Border, J. R., Hassett, J. M., and Seibel, R. Blunt multiple trauma (ISS 36), femoral traction and the pulmonary failure—septic state. Ann. Surg., *202:* 283–295, 1985.
5. Bowers, R. E., McKeen, C. R., Park, B. E., and Brigham, K. L. Increased pulmonary vascular permeability follows intracranial hypertension in sheep. Am. Rev. Respir. Dis., *119:* 637–641, 1979.
6. Burtrain, W. L., and Lynn, H. B. Splenorraphy: Changing concepts for the traumatized spleen. Surgery, *86:* 748–760, 1979.
7. Carmona, R. H., Tsao, T. C., and Trunkey, D. D. The role of prostacycline and thromboxane in sepsis and septic shock. Arch. Surg., *119:* 189–192, 1984.
8. Carmona, R. H., Peck, D. Z., and Lim, R. C. The role of packing and planned reoperation in severe hepatic trauma. J. Trauma, *24:* 779–784, 1984.

9. Clarke, R., Fisher, M. R., Topley, E., and Davies, J. W. L. Extent and time of blood-loss after civilian injury. Lancet, *2:* 381–386, 1961.
10. Cooper, K. R., and Boswell, P. A. Reduced functional residual capacity and abnormal oxygenation in patients with severe head injury. Chest, *84:* 29–35, 1983.
11. Dunn, E. L., Berry, P. H., and Connally, J. D. Computed tomography of the pelvis in patients with multiple injuries. J. Trauma, *23:* 378–383, 1983.
12. Frost, E. A. M. The physiopathology of respiration in neurosurgical patients. J. Neurosurg., *50:* 699–714, 1979.
13. Golueke, P. J., Goldstein, A. S., Sclafani, S. J. A., Mitchell, W. G., and Shaftan, G. W. Routine versus selective exploration of penetrating neck injuries: A randomized prospective study. J. Trauma, *24:* 1010–1014, 1984.
14. Goris, R., Gimbrere, J., Van Niekerk, J., Schoots, F., and Booy, L. Early osteosynthesis and prophylactic mechanical ventilation in the multiple trauma patient. J. Trauma, *22:* 895–903, 1982.
15. Graham, D. L., Adams, J. H., and Doyle, D. Ischemic brain damage in fatal non-missile head injuries. J. Neurol. Sci., *39:* 213–234, 1978.
16. Grover, F. L., Richardson, D. J., Fewel, J. G., Arom, K. V., Webb, G. E., and Trinkle, K. J. Prophylactic antibiotics in the treatment of penetrating chest wounds: A prospective double blind study. J. Thorac. Cardiovasc. Surg., *74:* 528–536, 1978.
17. Guice, K., Oldham, K., Eide, B., and Johansen, K. Hematuria after blunt trauma: When is pyelography useful? J. Trauma, *23:* 305–311, 1983.
18. Holaday, J. W., and Faden, A. I. Naloxone reverses the pathophysiology of shock through an antagonism of endorphin system. In: *Neurosecretion and Brain Peptides*, edited by J. B. Martin, S. Reichlin, and K. L. Bick, pp. 421–434. Raven Press, New York, 1981.
19. Hospital and pre-hospital resources for optimal care of the injured patient. Bull. Am. Coll. Surg., *68:* 11–18, 1983.
20. Ishige, N., Pitts, L. H., Hashimoto, T., Nishimura, M., and Bartkowski, H. M. The effect of hypoxia on traumatic brain injury in rats. Part 1: Changes in neurological examination, electroencephalogram and histopathology. Submitted to Neurosurgery.
21. Ishige, N., Pitts, L. H., Pogliani, L., Hashimoto, T., Nishimura, M., Bartkowski, H. M., and James, T. L. The effect of hypoxia on traumatic brain injury in rats. Part 2: Changes in high-energy phosphate metabolism. Submitted to Neurosurgery.
22. Jurkiewicz, M. J., and Hester, T. R. Reconstruction—Head and neck. In: *Clinical Applications for Muscle and Musculocutaneous Flaps*, edited by S. J. Mathes and F. Nahai, pp. 194–217. C. V. Mosby, St. Louis, 1982.
23. Katsurada, K., Yamada, R., and Sugimoto, T. Respiratory insufficiency in patients with severe head injury. Surgery, *73:* 191–199, 1973.
24. LaForce, F. M., Mullane, J. F., Boehme, R. F., Kelly, W. J., and Huber, G. L. The effect of pulmonary edema on antibacterial defenses of the lung. J. Lab. Clin. Med., *82:* 631–648, 1973.
25. LeBlanc, K. A., and Tucker, W. Y. Prophylactic antibiotics and closed tube thoracostomy. Surg. Gynecol. Obstet., *160:* 259–263, 1985.
26. Levine, J. E., Becker, D., and Chun, T. Reversal of incipient brain death from head-injury apnea at the scene of accidents. N. Engl. J. Med., *301:* 109, 1979.
27. LoCurto, J. A., Swan, K. G., Tischeler, C. D., Griffin, C. C., Rocko, J. M., and Blackwood, J. M. Tube thoracostomy in trauma: Antibiotics or not. J. Trauma, in press.
28. Lucas, C. E. Renal consideration in the injured patient. Surg. Clin. North Am., *62:* 133–148, 1982.
29. Mackersie, R. C., Christensen, J. M., Pitts, L. H., and Lewis, F. R. Pulmonary extravascular fluid accumulation following intracranial injury. J. Trauma, *23:* 968–975, 1983.
30. Millen, J. E., and Glauser, F. L. Low levels of concussive brain trauma and pulmonary edema. J. Appl. Physiol., *54:* 666–670, 1983.
31. Miller, J. D., Sweet, R. C., Narayan, R., and Becker, D. P. Early insults to the injured brain. J.A.M.A., *240:* 439–442, 1978.
32. Miller, S. E., Miller, C. L., and Trunkey, D. D. The immune consequences of trauma. Surg. Clin. North Am., *62:* 167–181, 1982.
33. Moss, L. R., Wald, A., and Ransohof, J. Respiratory functions and chemical regulation of ventilation in head injury. Am. Rev. Respir. Dis., *109:* 205–215, 1974.
34. Newfield, P., Pitts, L., Kaktis, J., Hoff, J., and Boggan, J. Influence of shock on survival after head trauma. Neurosurgery, *6:* 596, 1980.
35. Pitts, L. H. Medical complications of head injury. In: *Head Injury*, edited by P. R. Cooper, pp. 327–342. Williams & Wilkins, Baltimore, 1982.
36. Sagalowsky, A. I., McConnell, J. D., and Peters, P. C. Renal trauma requiring surgery: An analysis of 185 cases. J. Trauma, *23:* 128–131, 1983.
37. Schimpff, S. C., Miller, R. M., Polakavetz, S., and Hornick, R. B. Infection in the severely traumatized patient. Ann. Surg., *179:* 352–357, 1974.
37a. Schlobohm, R. Dept. of Anesthesia, San Francisco General Hospital, unpublished data.
38. Schumacker, P. T., Rhodes, G. R., Newell, J. C., Dutton, R. E., Shah, D. M., Scovill, W. A., and Powers, S. R. Ventilation-perfusion imbalance after head trauma. Am. Rev. Respir. Dis., *119:* 33–43, 1979.
39. Selivanov, V., Chi, H. S., Alverdy, J. C., Morris, J. A., and Sheldon, G. F. Mortality in retroperitoneal hematoma. J. Trauma, *24:* 1022–1027, 1984.
40. Sherck, J. P., McCort, J. J., and Oakes, D. D. Computed tomography in thoracoabdominal trauma. J. Trauma, *24:* 1015–1021, 1984.
41. Theodore, J., and Robin E. D. Pathogenesis of neurogenic pulmonary oedema. Lancet, *2:* 749–751, 1975.
42. Trunkey, D. D. Trauma. Sci. Am., *249:* 28–36, 1983.
43. Weis, E. B. Subtle neurological injuries in pelvic fractures. J. Trauma, *24:* 983–985, 1984.

CHAPTER 11

Design and Organization of the Neurosurgical Critical Care Unit

FREMONT P. WIRTH, M.D., PATRICIA VALENZANO, R.N., and DEBRA TILLMAN, R.N.

The development of special care units is not a new concept. Beginning with wards to care for the poor who could not afford medical attention in their homes during the 18th century, this concept has matured with the creation of treatment units for poliomyelitis in the 1950s and subsequently with the creation of burn units (2). During the last 25 years there has been rapid development of the intensive care unit concept to the point that almost all general hospitals have one or more special care units. The creation of neurosurgical intensive care units (NICUs) has been a much more recent phenomenon. Although the number of these units is small, it is increasing. Most neurosurgical intensive care patients are still treated in general or surgical intensive care units.

It is not surprising, therefore, that little has been written about the design and organization of NICUs. In many respects principles of design and organization are those of intensive care units in general. NICUs, however can be designed for the specific needs of patients with nervous system illness. Further benefit is gained from grouping patients with neurologic illness together with nurses trained in and familiar with these diseases. General intensive care unit nurses, while proficient with the cardiovascular and/or respiratory systems, are often uncomfortable caring for patients with disorders of the nervous system.

This chapter is intended to highlight some of these aspects of NICU design and operation. It is important to realize that many NICUs will in fact be neurosurgical and neurologic intensive care units. The principles of design and operation remain the same.

DESIGN

Change is frequently difficult, and the design of an NICU is no exception. Although the design of an NICU may not appear to be a matter of concern for the busy practicing neurosurgeon, input from neurosurgeons is essential for the development of an efficient critical care area. Design cannot be relegated to architects and engineers regardless of their qualifications since the design of an NICU is so highly specialized that even competent hospital designers have had little experience in this area. It is important, therefore, that NICU design be a team effort with input from nursing service, architects, engineers, administrators, and physicians. New technology and sophisticated surgical procedures and management protocols have become much more complex and require more intense observation. Because of the importance of these new capabilities in the intensive care of the neurosurgical patient, the neurosurgeon bears a responsibility for involvement in all phases of NICU design and operation.

Location

Location of the NICU in the hospital reflects many considerations. Congregation of intensive care units in a unified location may be optimum (11). Proximity has many advantages including staffing and ease of patient or staff relocation in circumstances where bed or staff shortages occur in isolated subspecialty units. Unit location adjacent to x-ray facilities, operating room, or laboratory also has obvious advantages including ease of transfer and efficiency in obtaining x-ray and laboratory studies. In a hospital with a busy trauma service, accessibility from the emergency room may be desirable. These considerations are not, however, inviolate. Creation of intensive care areas within the existing hospital may not allow placement of all units together. Furthermore, there are advantages of locating a specialized care unit near that area of the hospital where patients with similar disease processes are treated. Such placement of the unit in a hospital allows development of a unified nursing service under one supervisor for the care of patients with nervous system disease. Continuity of care, staff development, and education may all benefit from this plan and furthermore exchange of staff between acute and less acute care areas can increase awareness of the spectrum of neurologic and neurosurgical disease processes. The authors have had personal experience in two NICUs designed as part of a neurosurgical floor (Barnes Hospital, St. Louis, Missouri; St. Joseph's Hospital, Savannah, Georgia). Both units function well from both staff and patient perspectives.

Size

NICU size must be determined from the case load and complexity of the individual hospital. Optimum unit size has been proposed as six to 12 beds (7). Special care units of less than four beds are not practical to operate and those of more than 12 beds tend to be difficult to administer. Provision should be made for at least one isolation room. The possibility of some less intense observation rooms for care of preoperative subarachnoid hemorrhage patients or observation of seizure patients should also be considered.

Floor Plan

The layout of the NICU and room configuration must to some extent be tailored to the existing structure that is to contain the unit unless a completely new building is to be built. If a new structure is to be designed, a circular or square unit may be most efficient with a central nursing station. Such design allows maximal observation of patients. Alternative designs can, however, be quite functional. If a rectangular or corridor unit is constructed, observation of end rooms can be augmented by closed circuit television. Properly positioned and coupled with monitoring equipment, this can provide intensive care unit rooms where direct vision is not possible. Rooms 1, 2, and 3 (Fig. 11.1) have this monitoring capability and function quite well. TV-monitored rooms are most suitable for patients who do not require the highest acuity levels of NICU care.

There are advantages to both open ward and private room configurations for the NICU. There is a greater flexibility and conservation of space with the open ward design. This, however, frequently results in a noisy, active area where management of patients with diseases such as subarachnoid hemorrhage may be less than optimum. Rooms with solid walls are therefore often preferable, even though they require more square feet of space. Such rooms should open through wide doors or panels, but design must also take into consideration regulations that require that 1 hour fire walls separate patient rooms from corridors (10). In such rooms 150 square feet per room is optimum. With less floor space, the use of ventilators, EEG machines, evoked potential monitoring equipment, cooling blankets, and other devices can make patient care very difficult. Furthermore, it is impossible to resuscitate patients in rooms which are small and filled with equipment.

In the open ward designed intensive care unit, the Joint Commission of Accreditation of Hospitals requires 120 square feet per bed (10). While this may be adequate for the general intensive care unit, it is not sufficient space for the NICU. It is true that less space is necessary in the open ward setting; however, 150 square feet per bed are needed to provide adequate working area. Patient privacy is sacrificed in this situation, and the separation of individual patient's care from one another is difficult. Even with the installation of sinks between each bed, which should be done, such fundamental care practices as hand washing between care of different patients may be neglected. A combination of patient rooms and an open ward (Fig. 11.1) is optimum and offers increased flexibility. Care of the critically ill patient, especially

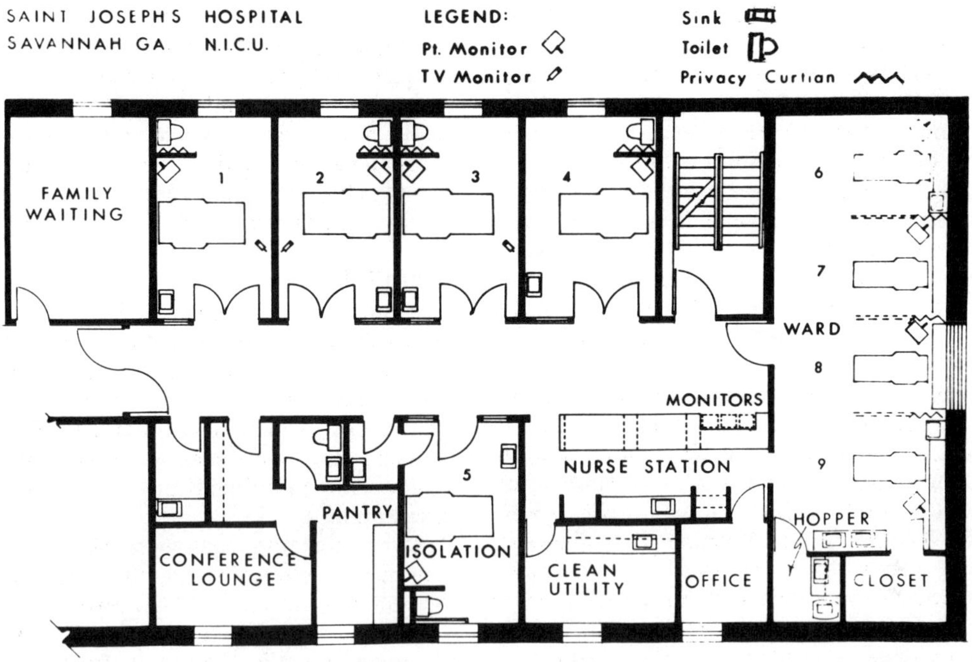

Figure 11.1. Floor plan of a corridor designed unit with large doors on the five patient rooms, each with sinks and toilets behind short privacy walls and a four-bed ward with sinks at bedside. Windows with blinds enhance observation of patients and closed circuit television supplements observation in rooms 1, 2, and 3 which are more remote from the nurse's station. (Neurological Intensive Care Unit, St. Joseph's Hospital, Savannah, Georgia. Reproduced with permission.)

the trauma patient, may be easier in the open ward setting, while management of patients who are post operative or who have subarachnoid hemorrhage or central nervous system infections is clearly enhanced in individual rooms.

Special Features

Windows are an important aspect of NICU design. "ICU psychosis" can result from long stays in highly controlled areas (4). This problem is even greater with central nervous system diseases where the individual is confused by the very nature of his or her illness. Direct visual observation of day and night is also important in maintaining orientation in the NICU patient (8). The inclusion of clocks and large wall calendars in each room, in view of the patient, facilitates orientation of the stressed central nervous system. Even the inclusion of television sets in selected NICU rooms may speed recovery by bringing additional stimuli and information to the NICU patient. Clearly this is not applicable to the ward design where random noise often already exists at greater than optimum levels. In the open ward designed unit, quiet music may modulate some of the noise that results from the other necessary activities of the unit to the benefit of not only the patients but staff.

At least one isolation room should be designed for each NICU. This allows segregation of infected or potentially infectious patients from the remainder of the unit. This room should be designed in close proximity to the nursing station with television monitoring or direct observation through a window (Fig. 11.1, Room 5). Large entry doors through an anteroom with an extra sink enhance isolation of these cases. Appropriately designed ventilation systems with rapid air exchange and separate ventilation ducts, together with a negative pressure vent from the isolation rooms are desirable. In the absence of a suitable isolation room in the NICU, isolation patients should be cared for in a unit with this capability.

Although observation is of primary importance, maintenance of privacy is desirable as well. The use of blinds on windows or curtains across openings is important in this regard, especially for the awake patient. Toilets in the private NICU rooms are desirable. They not only increase patient comfort but speed and simplify nursing care in selected patients. A partial wall is necessary, however, for these facilities to be functional, since patients capable of using toilets will be to some extent conscious of their surroundings and privacy.

Each bed area, whether a room or part of a ward area must have available adequate electrical, suction, and oxygen outlets. Dual oxygen and suction outlets are necessary and three of each are desirable for each bed. Eight to 12 electrical outlets are recommended. NICU patients will often require ventilators, cooling blankets, control units for three to four intravenous lines, and other electrical devices such as electric bed operation and chest tube suction simultaneously. Oxygen may be required for ventilators and for hand ventilation when providing pulmonary care. Suction lines likewise may be required for endotracheal suctioning and nasogastric aspiration simultaneously. A substantial number of the electrical outlets should be connected to emergency power sources, preferably all. These specifications, while more sophisticated than recommended previously, are indicated for the expanded technology presently available (3). Sinks equipped with foot controls, should be placed in each private room and should be located between each bed in the open ward unit.

Common Space

Design of the common space in the NICU is perhaps less the province of the neurosurgeon than the nursing staff. General ICU guidelines recommend that this space be 1 to 1½ times as large as the area assigned to beds (7). This space should be designed to maximize patient visibility and accessibility. Appropriate separate clean and dirty storage areas and adequate charting space are required. A lounge area for the nursing staff is essential for efficient operation and allows space for staff relaxation during breaks. This area should be away from the patient area but in close proximity to the unit in the event of an emergency. A conference room is desirable for both medical conferences and discussions with families. Some degree of isolation of these areas from the activities of the unit is desirable.

The waiting area is also an important part of the unit and should be placed in close proximity to it. At least part of this area, if not all, should be designated as nonsmoking. Furniture should be selected with the realization that families will often spend the night in this area. While this practice may not be desirable it will occur and some provision for this by the inclusion of sofas or reclining chairs results in a benefit to all parties involved.

Monitors

Monitoring equipment of high quality is available from several manufacturers. Selection will be based on many factors including price, design, and interface with existing systems, as well as the availability of service. The latter consideration is especially important as all equipment requires adjustment and repair from time to time.

Basic monitoring equipment should have capabilities of electrocardiographic and respiratory monitoring and at least two, preferably three, channels for pressure monitoring. Not infrequently, particularly in the trauma patient, monitoring of intracranial, arterial, and venous pressure will be desired simultaneously as well as in certain other selected cases. Computer programming capability for cardiac output measurements is also desirable, particularly in any unit where trauma patients are monitored. Interface between monitoring systems and central hospital data management systems should also be considered. This is an expanding field and promises immediate access to laboratory and other data which may be particularly applicable in the NICU patient. The possible application of such systems to the automated control of medications, respirators, and other aspects of NICU care should also be considered as such capability is rapidly developing.

Electroencephalography monitoring equipment with computer averaging ability may also be desirable depending upon the types of diseases treated. Monitoring of evoked potentials in the NICU is an expanding technique; however, portable equipment brought to the NICU may be more practical for this type of assessment. The ability to trend and record data is also desirable, especially where intracranial pressure monitoring is undertaken. Ideally computer storage and retrieval of many parameters of patient data should be possible. If this data can then be printed for inclusion in the chart, nursing care may be made much more efficient and accuracy enhanced.

STAFFING

Every critical care area should have a medical director whose responsibility it should be to oversee the administrative and educational needs of the unit (3). This individual should have special interest and competence in nervous system critical care and should serve as a liaison between medical staff, nursing service, and administration. The director or his designee must be readily available to the unit and during periods of high utilization may need to assist in assigning priorities to patients for admission and discharge. Although the presence of the unit director or his designee in the unit at all times might be desirable, this is not mandatory or practical. Consultants in anesthesia, intensive care, pulmonary, and cardiac medicine should also be readily available to the unit, but it is not appropriate to expect these specialists to assume the overall direction or supervision of a designated neurosurgical critical care unit. Their assistance, however, in the management of patients can be invaluable. The NICU should have admission and discharge criteria. Admission should be restricted to patients with diseases of the nervous system requiring intensive care. Admission privileges should be restricted to physicians with special training and competence in the evaluation and care of the nervous system. Such restriction of admission privileges is necessary in any critical care area if a high standard of care is to be maintained.

It is important for NICU policy and procedures to be reviewed periodically. The NICU should be a part of the intensive care unit committee structure and this will assure this supervision (6). Detailed standing orders should exist for the treatment of emergencies and these should be reviewed periodically by the intensive care unit committee (3). Standing orders are also appropriate for management of endotracheal and tracheostomy tubes, intravenous, intra-arterial, and urinary diversion catheters and intracranial pressure monitoring devices.

Nursing

A critical factor in the NICU is the nursing staff. The quality of patient care will depend to a large extent on the ability, training, and dedication of nursing personnel. The specific nursing structure will be dictated by the organization of the individual hospital. Our experience and that of others, however, indicates that organization of the NICU and neurology and neurosurgery nursing units under one supervisor has advantages. Staff communication, development, and education are all enhanced by such a structure. Close physical proximity of the NICU and the nursing units for neurosurgery and neurology can facilitate this organizational concept. The addition of a clinical specialist in neurosurgery and neurology assigned to these units can also enhance education and care.

The ratio of nurses to patients may vary slightly depending upon the acuity levels of individual patients in the NICU. The basic requirement, however, is a minimum of one critical care nurse for every two NICU patients (3). We have found that for a nine-bed NICU one head nurse, five registered nurses, one nurse technician, one unit secretary, and one male nursing assistant are needed for the 7:00 AM to 3:00 PM shift. For the 3:00 PM to 11:00 PM shift five staff nurses, one nurse technician, one unit secretary, and one male nursing assistant are needed. For the 11:00 PM to 7:00 AM shift four staff nurses, one nurse technician, and one male nursing assistant are sufficient. It is essential that ancillary nursing personnel be available to assist in the care of NICU patients, but because of the complex technology and frequent medication doses required, registered nurses with critical care training must undertake most of the patient care.

The subspecialty of neuroscience nursing is well recognized and has been defined (9). All nurses in the NICU should have critical care training and certification. Training modules in various NICU disciplines, cardiology, neurology-neurosurgery, and others, should be arranged by the individual hospital to assist in certification of the nursing staff (5). For these modules to be meaningful educational experiences, the input of physicians interested in and competent in nervous system critical care is required. This can be time well spent in the long-term, especially for the physician in the community hospital, where resident physicians may not be available to assist in critical care patient assessment. In this situation, trained, competent critical care nurses are capable of quite reliable patient assessment. Many short courses are also available at regional and national meetings to assist in certification and re-certification. The hospital should insist on the proper certification of its NICU nurses and should assist them in obtaining the necessary specialty training. Moreover, continuing education and re-certification of nurses in the NICU is to be encouraged. Six hours of re-certification is required at present by the Joint Commission of Accreditation of Hospitals and another 30 hours of continuing education is required at our institution annually for re-certification of critical care nurses (1).

REFERENCES

1. Accreditation Manual for Hospitals/1984 Joint Commission on Accreditation of Hospitals, 99 pp. Joint Commission on Accreditation of Hospitals, Chicago, 1984.
2. Bendixen, H. H., and Kinney, J. M. History of intensive care. In: *Manual of Surgical Intensive Care*, edited by J. M. Kinney, H. H. Bendixen, and S. R. Powers. W. B. Saunders, Philadelphia, 1977.
3. Grenvik, A., and Safar, P. Staffing patterns and equipment. In: *Manual of Surgical Intensive Care*, edited by J. M. Kenny, H. H. Bendixen, and S. R. Powers. W. B. Saunders, Philadelphia, 1977.
4. Hansell, H. N. The behavioral aspects of noise on man: The patient with intensive care unit psychosis. Heart Lung, *13:* 59–65, 1984.
5. Kahn, J. N. Trends in the educational process for the critical care nurse. Crit. Care and Med., *3:* 123, 1975.
6. Kenny, J. M., and Bendixen, H. H. Administrative and operating procedures. In: *Manual of Surgical Intensive Care*, edited by J. M. Kenny, H. H. Bendixen, and S. R. Powers. W. B. Saunders, Philadelphia, 1977.
7. Kenny, J. M., and Walter, C. W. The design of an intensive care unit. In: *Manual of Surgical Intensive Care*, edited by J. M. Kenny, H. H. Bendixen, and S. R. Powers. W. B. Saunders, Philadelphia, 1977.
8. Roberts, S. L. Behavioral concepts and the critically ill patient, Chap. XIV, 291–309 pp. Prentis Hall, Inc., Englewood Cliffs, NJ, 1976.
9. Standards of Neurological and Neurosurgical Nursing Practice, American Nurses Association, Kansas City, MO, 1977.
10. U. S. Department of Health, Education and Welfare: Minimum Requirements of Construction and Equipment for Hospital and Medical Facilities, Chapt. 7, U. S. Government Printing Office, Washington, DC, 1979.
11. Weil, M. H., and Shubin, H. Centralized hospital care for the critically ill. In: *Clinical Anesthesia*, edited by P. Safar. F. A. Davis, Philadelphia, 1974.

Index

Page numbers in italics denote figures; those followed by "t" denote tables.

C

I